$$\frac{lower\ CSI}{CHL.\ SAT.\ F.\ INDEX} =$$

Also by Sonja L. and William E. Connor
THE NEW AMERICAN DIET

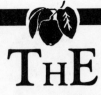

THE

NEW AMERICAN
DIET SYSTEM

Sonja L. Connor, M.S., R.D.,
and
William E. Connor, M.D.

SIMON & SCHUSTER

New York • London • Toronto • Sydney • Tokyo • Singapore

Simon & Schuster
Simon & Schuster Building
Rockefeller Center
1230 Avenue of the Americas
New York, New York 10020

Designed by Carla Weise, Levavi & Levavi
Manufactured in the United States of America

1   3   5   7   9   10   8   6   4   2

Library of Congress Cataloging in Publication Data

Connor, Sonja L.
The new American diet system / Sonja L. Connor and William E.
Connor.
p.   cm.
Includes index.
1. Low-cholesterol diet.   2. Low-cholesterol diet—Recipes.
3. Food—Cholesterol content.   I. Connor, William E., date.
II. Title.
RM237.75.C65   1991
613.2'8—dc20   90-20518
                                                                 CIP

ISBN 0-671-68705-0

To the scientists who have worked towards a "single number" since the early sixties and to our patients and the children and adults of the Family Heart Study in the Hollywood district of Portland, Oregon, who inspired us to develop the Cholesterol–Saturated Fat Index.

ACKNOWLEDGMENTS

Soon after it was recognized that dietary factors had a powerful influence on the blood cholesterol level, there was an intense wish among scientists to provide a numerical expression for those factors. This is important because what we eat inevitably affects our blood cholesterol level over a lifetime. And the blood cholesterol level determines the extent to which coronary arteries become plugged with the fatty plaques of atherosclerosis and cause heart disease.

An important clue related to the effect diet has on the blood cholesterol level came from the University of Texas at Dallas where scientists Joseph Goldstein and Michael Brown discovered the principal way that cholesterol is removed from the blood via a specific mechanism in the liver cells. This mechanism is the LDL receptor. Next, other scientists at the same institution, Dietschy and Spady, showed in animals how cholesterol and saturated fat in the diet operate to raise the blood cholesterol level, again through the LDL receptor in the liver. Foods containing cholesterol and saturated fat were found to cause the receptor to be less active in its ability to remove cholesterol from the blood.

Keys, Anderson, and Grande came up with the first mathematical expression in 1962 to relate change in diet with change in the blood cholesterol level. This was amplified by Hegsted and his associates from the Harvard School of Public Health and ultimately resulted in the Cholesterol Index of Foods by Donald Zilversmit of Cornell. There the matter rested until a chance conversation on the beach at Asilomar, California (at the Deuel Conference on Lipids) between Don Zilversmit and one of us (Sonja Connor) led to a further clarification of the issue. From that conversation came the realization that we needed to use the equations derived from metabolic feeding studies *not* to predict change in blood cholesterol levels, but to help determine a proper weighting for the cholesterol and saturated fat content of foods that would allow them to be combined into a single number. This led to the Cholesterol–Saturated Fat Index of Foods that ranks foods with respect to both their cholesterol and saturated fat contents, thus allowing for more meaningful comparisons of foods than had hereto been available.

We acknowledge the important contributions of these and other scientists whose work paved the way for the development of the single number concept, the Cholesterol –Saturated Fat Index (CSI).

Special appreciation goes to David Rorvik, a writer with a style we like very much, and to Joyce Gustafson, a dietitian who is a keen critic and a good cook. They contributed greatly to the preparation of this book.

These concepts would never have come to fruition without the several decades of past research support, again gratefully acknowledged, from the National Heart, Lung and Blood Institute and the Clinical Research Centers of the Division of Research Resources of the National Institutes of Health, and the American Heart Association (Oregon Affiliate), and for the financial support of these institutions by U.S. taxpayers and generous supporters of medical research.

Finally, we wish to make it clear that we do not *own* the Cholesterol–Saturated Fat Index (CSI). Our wish is for it to be used as widely and in as many ways as people find helpful. If you have ideas about using the CSI, please feel free to develop those ideas.

CONTENTS

PART

I

The CSI: What It Is and Why We Need It

CHAPTER

1

The CSI:
The "Magic Number" That
Can Help Save Your Life

THERE'S MORE TO IT THAN JUST CHOLESTEROL

By now, a majority of Americans know that too much dietary cholesterol, a type of fat found only in foods of animal origin, can seriously endanger health. "Cholesterol consciousness" has swept the land. This is both good and bad: good because cholesterol, in excess, is harmful; bad because, by focusing entirely on cholesterol, many people are overlooking an equally dangerous dietary component—*saturated fat.*

Many assume that cholesterol and saturated fat are the *same* thing. They are *not*. Many of the food products that are now being advertised as "reduced cholesterol" or "cholesterol-free" often contain significant quantities of the saturated fats that, every bit as much as cholesterol, contribute to increased blood cholesterol levels that lead to coronary heart disease and strokes.

Reliance on such products can produce a false sense of security. In addition, focusing on cholesterol to the exclusion of other dietary hazards, especially saturated fats, tempts people to try quick cholesterol "self-cures," such as megadoses of the vitamin niacin, which, in themselves, can imperil health.

This whole issue is very confusing because some foods that are low in cholesterol are high in saturated fat, such as tropical vegetable oils. (We'll differentiate among the different types of fat in Chapter 4 of Part II. For now, you need only be aware that saturated fats are those that are

13

generally solid at room temperature, such as shortenings, chocolate, palm oil, and coconut oil.) The opposite is also true: Some foods that are high in cholesterol are low in saturated fats—for instance, shellfish. In order to make wise, healthful food choices, we need to get a handle on *both* of these nutrients.

To better understand why this is so critical, consider the shellfish we just mentioned (lobster, shrimp, crab). Because the cholesterol content of shellfish, ounce for ounce, is one and a half to two times higher than that of poultry and red meats, people have been led to believe that they would be better off eating steak than lobster. This is not a sound belief. True, some shellfish have a cholesterol content as much as *twice* that of poultry and red meat, *but*—and this is the vital "but" that is frequently overlooked—the amount of saturated fat in shellfish is so very much lower than that of steak that it turns out to be a far healthier choice than the typically purchased cuts of red meats. Conversely, some of those "cholesterol-free" products that are being so heavily touted these days are actually laden with saturated vegetable fats (such as palm or coconut oil), so that some of them are actually worse than similar products *with* cholesterol.

If you are beginning to wring your hands in despair over the seeming complexity of all this, take heart. We have devised a unique—perhaps even revolutionary—*Cholesterol-Saturated Fat Index* (CSI) that instantly ranks foods by their total "atherogenic potential," that is, by their ability to raise the total and LDL cholesterol level in the blood and create the kind of atherosclerotic conditions that contribute to heart attacks and strokes.

Atherosclerosis—sometimes called "hardening of the arteries"—is that process in which deposits of cholesterol, fat, and calcium build up inside artery walls, narrowing and hardening them, diminishing and sometimes entirely obstructing the flow of blood to the heart and brain when a blood clot forms. Dietary fat can also affect blood clot formation, as we will discuss later in Chapter 4 of Part II.

It's no wonder some of our patients and friends call the CSI "the magic number." When you know the CSI of different foods, you can immediately rate them and compare them one with another. *The higher the CSI of any given food, the greater the risk to health. The lower the CSI, the better that food is for your arteries and your health in general.* In a *single* score, the CSI succinctly sums up the risks and benefits of each food choice, taking into account and scientifically weighing the relative influences of *both* cholesterol *and* saturated fat.

WHAT THE CSI IS AND WHAT IT CAN DO FOR YOU

The CSI is one of the most important developments of our thirty years of research in nutrition and heart disease. It was developed, in part, through an ambitious five-year dietary study of 233 randomly selected American families. That study, funded by the National Institutes of

Health, contributed significantly to the refinement of our nutritional recommendations, which are summarized in our previous book, *The New American Diet* (Simon and Schuster, 1986; Fireside, 1988). It was in that book that we first introduced the CSI concept to the lay public, and, though we described it only briefly there, it proved to be one of the most popular features of that book. Our "official"—that is, scientific—introduction of the CSI appeared in the form of a paper published in the medical journal *The Lancet* (1986). A considerably expanded exposition of the CSI has more recently been published in *The Journal of the American Dietetic Association* (1989).

The CSI is a modification of a mathematical construct called a "regression equation" that has been computed from metabolic feeding studies designed to lower the blood cholesterol level. The final formulation permits us to weight the cholesterol and saturated fat in food properly and to calculate, with a high degree of confidence, the potential for any given food to raise the blood cholesterol level and promote processes that contribute to heart disease and stroke. Though derived from complex studies, the final equation (based on earlier equations of researchers Keys, Hegsted, and Zilversmit) is quite simple: CSI = 1.01 × grams of saturated fat + 0.05 × milligrams of cholesterol. But you needn't bother with that equation because we've done all the computations for you—for most foods and many mixed dishes, including even franchised fast foods!

Before we proceed to show you how exciting and helpful the CSI can be in a number of contexts, you need to understand a little more about the underlying significance of and the need for this new rating and food-evaluation system. We have already mentioned the dangers of relying upon decreasing dietary cholesterol alone to prevent heart disease. The surgeon general, in 1988, found that up to *100 million* Americans remain at high risk of developing heart disease, many at relatively early ages. That risk will *remain* high until Americans realize there's more to the prevention challenge than just decreasing dietary cholesterol.

The latest and best research is making it quite evident that the real key to prevention is not so much to lower total blood cholesterol levels but, rather, to lower blood levels of *low-density lipoprotein (LDL)* cholesterol, the real culprit in coronary heart disease. Cholesterol and LDL are removed from the blood by specific receptors in the cells of the liver. The LDL receptor, discovered in the 1980s by Nobel Prize winners Brown and Goldstein, is like a pocket into which the LDL molecule in the blood fits and is thereby removed.

There are many factors that can affect the number and activity of the LDL receptors. Genetic factors are very important. Also important are dietary factors—the very factors that are the subject of this book: dietary cholesterol and saturated fat. Both of these nutrients in the diet will *decrease* the number of LDL receptors and thus *elevate* the blood cholesterol level and the LDL concentration.

With the CSI to guide you, you can easily reduce your intakes of dietary cholesterol and saturated fat. You don't need to understand the medical research, all you have to do is follow the dietary guidelines in this book. You will find that the lowest CSI foods are fruits, vegetables, grains, and beans. When you choose these foods, as you surely will, to lower your CSI intake, you will automatically increase your intake of "soluble" fiber—that very popular cholesterol-lowering nutrient also found in oat bran.

Nutrition researchers have long called for a system such as the CSI (see, for example, *New England Journal of Medicine*, 1985), noting that until a unified score—a single number—could be devised to evaluate the blood cholesterol–elevating and heart disease–promoting potential of foods, there would be no real hope of making the large-scale dietary changes required to prevent the disease that is still the scourge of the entire Western world and the number one killer of Americans. Without that single number, it was argued, neither doctor nor layperson would be able to cope with the complexities of diet, and our eating— and disease—patterns would remain largely unchanged.

We believe that the CSI finally provides the new and long-awaited "magic number." In this book you will learn how to use it to rank and compare hundreds of different foods. You can use it to evaluate the relative risks and benefits of single foods, mixed dishes, individual meals, an entire day of meals, a week, a month, or even a lifetime of meals. We'll give you goals and guidelines to further amplify the usefulness of the CSI.

You will find specific CSI chapters related to meats, chicken, and fish; dairy products and eggs; fats, oils, margarines, salad dressings, and nuts; fruits, vegetables, grains, and beans; snacks, appetizers, and beverages; breakfasts; lunches; dinners; and desserts. In each of these chapters, you'll find visual aids in addition to the detailed CSI listings for the various foods, to better help you understand and utilize the CSIs and the CSI goals for each food category. Each chapter will guide you toward the best CSI choices. CSIs are especially helpful in sorting out the best choices for various meats, cheeses, fats, dairy products, desserts, and snacks. Even some vegetable fats, including chocolate, palm oil, coconut oil, and all highly hydrogenated vegetable fats are free of cholesterol but high in saturated fats. Egg yolks have a lot of cholesterol but not so much saturated fat. Meats and cheeses vary widely in their relative fat and cholesterol content, as do many snacks and desserts. In every case, the CSI provides a quick, easy, accurate way of comparing these foods and making the best choices to meet a variety of dietary goals you can choose from. Information is also provided that enables you to compare the CSIs of traditional recipes with those of altered versions of the same recipes, versions that deliver far lower—and thus healthier—CSIs without sacrificing taste or texture. The lower-CSI recipes can be found in Part III of this book.

Table 1 provides some CSI examples to give you a "taste" of how helpful our magic number can be. In each category the CSIs are for identical quantities of each food or dish. Since the CSI is determined from the amounts of cholesterol and saturated fat in a food, a bigger serving size will have a higher CSI and a smaller serving size a lower CSI. Remember, the higher the number, the greater the potential to raise your blood cholesterol level. Italicized

TABLE 1
THE CHOLESTEROL–SATURATED FAT INDEX (CSI) OF SELECTED FOODS

	CSI		CSI
White fish, 3 ounces	3	*Party Carrot Cake,* 3" × 3¼"	3
Chicken (light meat, no skin), 3 ounces	4	Carrot cake (typical), 3" × 3¼"	14
Shrimp (⅔ cup), 3 ounces	9		
Pot roast (blade, chuck, arm), 3 ounces	15	*Brownies,* 2½" × 2½"	1
		Brownies (typical, frosted), 3" × 3"	20
Cottage cheese (low-fat 1%), ½ cup	<1		
Cottage cheese (regular 4%), ½ cup	4	*Very Skinny Burger,* 1	5
		Quarter pounder, 1	13
Dorman's Light cheese, 1 ounce	<1		
Kraft Light Naturals, 1 ounce	4	*Acapulco Enchilada,* one 6"	3
Cheddar or Monterey Jack, 1 ounce	8	Chicken enchilada, one 6"	7
Milk (skim), 1 cup	<1	Spaghetti with *Beef-Mushroom Spaghetti*	1
Milk (1% fat), 1 cup	2	*Sauce,* 1½ cups	
Milk (2% fat), 1 cup	4	Spaghetti with meat sauce, 1½ cups	6
Milk (whole), 1 cup	7		
		Green pepper-mushroom-onion pizza	9
Typical frozen yogurt, 1 cup	6	(thin crust), ¼ of 14"	
Typical gourmet ice cream, 1 cup	30	Combination pizza (thin crust), ¼ of 14"	20
Mock Sour Cream, ½ cup	2	*Skinny "French Fries,"* 1 cup	<1
Sour cream (20% fat), ½ cup	18	French fries, 1 cup	5
Imitation sour cream, ½ cup	20		
		Potato Salad, 1 cup	1
Dill Dip, ¼ cup	1	Potato salad (typical), 1 cup	10
Sour cream dip, ¼ cup	8		
		Homemade Cream Soup Mix,	<1
Spanish Omelet, ⅙ recipe	tr.	equivalent of 1 can	
Omelet (plain), 2 eggs	27	Cream of mushroom (condensed,	6
		undiluted), 1 can	
Baked Corn Chips, 2 cups	<1		
Corn chips, 2 cups	2 to 10		

Recipes in **bold italics** can be found in Part III.
The abbreviation *tr.* stands for trace (less than 0.5); the symbol <1 stands for less than one (0.5 to 0.9).

items in bold are our own recipes, which can be found in Part III.

Our goal is to help you adopt a way of eating that progressively delivers less saturated fat, as well as less cholesterol. We will provide CSI guidelines to help you identify the best choice for each food listing. We will provide you with daily CSI goals. We'll tell you what the benefits are for each goal level. As you attain these goals, you will automatically be conforming to an increasingly healthy eating style. The CSI system takes all the guesswork out of it for you. If you "go all the way" to our ultimate goal, you will achieve a way of eating that, if sustained, can lower your risk of heart disease by as much as 40 percent! It is possible to make these dietary changes in as little as four weeks. However, most people choose to change more gradually. They do this by regularly trying new products and recipes and incorporating the ones they like into their eating style. After a while, about half of the foods and recipes they use are lower in CSI, as well as fat and calories. That is the crest of the hill—and from that point on it becomes easier and easier to embrace still more low-CSI choices. Once the goals are achieved, they must, of course, be maintained to secure that substantial 40 percent reduction in risk for coronary heart disease.

HOW DO *WE* RATE/HOW DO *YOU* RATE IN TERMS OF CSI?

With the CSI, we can make comparisons not only among individual foods but also among individual *people* and even individual *countries*. That's right, there's a CSI for the American (U.S.) diet that can be compared with, say, the CSI of the German or Japanese diet. Again, with a single number, we can quickly assess the relative healthiness of different countries and cuisines. All of this can be quite illuminating, as well as exciting.

The CSI of the U.S. diet, per 1,000 Calories, is about 26. That's one of the

world's highest. Right up there with us, "enjoying" similar high-risk eating patterns, are such countries as Australia, New Zealand, the Scandinavian countries, and many Western European countries. Oriental, Mediterranean, Central and South American countries generally have far lower CSIs. Egypt has a national CSI of only 5 per 1,000 Calories! Japan has a CSI of about 13 per 1,000 Calories, which is approximately half of ours. There is a strong correlation between these CSIs and the heart disease mortality rates in these countries, further confirming the validity of the CSI concept. In Japan, for example, the death rate from coronary heart disease is only about 100 males (aged 55–64) per 100,000 population, compared with about 750 males in the same age group per 100,000 U.S. population.

The figures cited above are CSIs for 1,000 Calories. At a more typical (male) intake of 2,800 Calories per day, the CSI of the Western diet is 69. Compare that with a CSI of 12 per 2,800 Calories among the Tarahumara Indians of the Sierra Madre Occidental Mountains of Mexico. We have lived among and extensively studied these remarkable people who are noted for running incredibly long races—some 200 miles! Yet the Tarahumaras live on a diet of mostly beans and corn, which are high in complex carbohydrates and fiber. Not only are the Tarahumaras arguably the world's greatest endurance athletes, they also have a very low mortality rate from coronary heart disease. Their saturated fat and cholesterol intakes are among the lowest on the planet.

But while we may envy the CSI of the Tarahumaras, we needn't achieve scores *that* low in order to significantly lower our risk for heart disease. Table 2 shows you the CSI of the prevailing Western diet at three different caloric levels (1,200; 2,000; 2,800) per day. This is a diet that is a heart-stopping *40 percent fat*, 14 percent saturated fat, and one that contains 200 milligrams cholesterol for every 1,000 Calories. Table 2 shows you how you can improve your overall CSI by gradually changing in three stages. Even a reduction to the CSI Phase One level can save hundreds of thousands of lives. By moving to the CSI Phase Two level, half a million people who will otherwise die of heart disease could be saved every eight years. And by moving to the CSI Phase Three level (CSIs of 10 to 23), as many as a *million* lives could be saved in that same time period. Through a diet consisting of 20 percent fat (with only 5 percent saturated fat and with only 50 milligrams cholesterol for every 1,000 Calories), a full 40 percent reduction in the risk of heart disease can be achieved. But *any* movement in the direction of reduced CSI intake (reduced satu-

TABLE 2
THE CHOLESTEROL–SATURATED FAT INDEX OF THE
PRESENT AMERICAN DIET AND THE CSI PHASE DIET

	CHOLESTEROL (MG/DAY)	SATURATED FAT (GM/DAY)	CSI* (PER DAY)
CSI American Diet (40% fat, 14% saturated fat)			
1,200 Calories	240	19	31
2,000 Calories	400	31	51
2,800 Calories	500	44	69
CSI Phase One (30% fat, 10% saturated fat)			
1,200 Calories	less than 180	13	22
2,000 Calories	less than 300	22	37
2,800 Calories	less than 350	31	49
CSI Phase Two (25% fat, 8% saturated fat)			
1,200 Calories	less than 120	11	17
2,000 Calories	less than 200	18	28
2,800 Calories	less than 220	25	36
CSI Phase Three (20% fat, 5% saturated fat)			
1,200 Calories	less than 60	7	10
2,000 Calories	less than 100	11	16
2,800 Calories	less than 140	16	23

* CSI = 1.01 × grams of saturated fat + 0.05 × milligrams of cholesterol.

rated fat and cholesterol intakes) helps.

Table 3 shows an example of how you can, on approximately 2,200 Calories per day, shift from a high-risk CSI of 51 to a very healthy daily CSI of 17. This is as far as any person will need to go in modifying his or her diet—reducing total fat intake from 40 percent to 21 percent. But even with this very significant reduction in fat intake, one needn't endure any great culinary hardships, as this table makes evident.

In the next chapter we'll provide you with a self-scoring quiz by which you can evaluate your own present daily CSI. We'll tell you what your score means, in terms of health, and we'll provide goals for you to work toward. We feel confident that you will find the CSI the most effective "lever" you've ever used to get you up and moving in the right direction—and to *keep* you there once you've arrived at your dietary destination.

OTHER BENEFITS OF THE CSI AND OF THIS BOOK

In addition to everything else, the CSI can be used to help you with weight control. We'll introduce specially designed weight-control guidelines using CSI goals. You'll find a chapter devoted to this topic. And with the CSI to guide you, you'll learn how to maintain your weight following a period of weight loss.

We also have special chapters on CSI goals for children and on using the CSI

to take some of the risk out of dining at restaurants and fast-food outlets. As nutritional researchers, we've come to appreciate how important it is to instill good eating habits at as early an age as possible—hence our chapter on children. We think you'll find it very useful in launching your kids on the best possible dietary path. And our chapter on dining out will help you get through the restaurants and fast-food dietary mine fields with your health intact and your girth under control. The CSI will enable you to make wise choices even at McDonald's, Wendy's, and the like.

One of the features of this book that we think you'll like best is Part III, our cookbook section, encompassing some delicious, health-promoting recipes. Many of these are low-CSI alternatives to and modifications of high-CSI traditional and "old favorite" recipes. We think you will agree that our low-CSI versions lose very little, if anything, of their taste and texture in the "translation." In fact, we'll *add* tastes and textures to your recipe repertoire. You'll learn from these recipes how little you need "sacrifice" in order to achieve potentially enormous health gains. You'll also soon learn that we never ask you to give up anything without giving you something back in return. "Modification, not deprivation" is one of our mottoes.

We've designed and written this book so that it can be used by *anyone* who wants to change his or her diet and help prevent disease, especially heart disease. But the book is also going to be very helpful, we believe, for dietitians and physicians who are counseling the ever-increasing number of patients being seen as a result, in part, of the recent National Cholesterol Education

TABLE 3
THE CHOLESTEROL–SATURATED FAT INDEX OF SAMPLE INTAKES AT 2,200 CALORIES
FOR THE PRESENT AMERICAN DIET AND THE CSI PHASE THREE DIET

AMERICAN DIET	CSI	CSI PHASE THREE DIET	CSI
Breakfast		*Breakfast*	
½ cup orange juice	tr.	½ grapefruit	tr.
1 slice white toast	tr.	1 cup oatmeal	tr.
1 teaspoon soft margarine	0.7	½ cup skim milk	0.5
1 cup coffee	0	1 slice whole-grain toast	tr.
		1 teaspoon soft margarine	0.7
		Snack	
		1 ***Cereal Bran Muffin***	<1
Lunch		*Lunch*	
sandwich:		1 cup minestrone soup	1
2 ounces ham	6	1 hard roll	tr.
1 ounce Swiss cheese	6	½ cup raw vegetables	tr.
2 slices rye bread	tr.	1 cup grapes	tr.
1 tablespoon mayonnaise	2.1	3 gingersnaps	1
lettuce, tomato	tr.		
½ cup potato chips	1.3		
		Snack	
		3 cups popcorn with 1 teaspoon margarine	<1
Dinner		*Dinner*	
3 pieces fried chicken	16	3 pieces ***Portland Fried Chicken***	8
½ cup potato salad	5	1 cup ***Potato Salad***	1
½ cup baked beans	3	1 cup ***Classic Baked Beans***	tr.
½ cup raw vegetables	tr.	1 cup broccoli	tr.
1 piece apple pie	11	1 whole-grain roll	tr.
		1 teaspoon soft margarine	0.7
		1 cup green salad with 2 tablespoons low-calorie Italian dressing	1
		1 serving ***Apple Crisp***	<1
TOTALS	**51**		**17**

Recipes in ***bold italics*** can be found in Part III.
The abbreviation *tr.* stands for trace (less than 0.5); the symbol <1 stands for less than one (0.5 to 0.9).

Project, in which up to 100 million Americans could be identified as having blood cholesterol levels in the perilous zone—in excess of 200 milligrams per 100 deciliters (mg/dl) of blood. In addition, of course, this book can be of great help to those who have heart disease and want to prevent further damage and even undo some of the damage already done. Such individuals should, of course, be under the ongoing care of a physician and a dietitian. This book will also be useful to people who are working to treat or prevent other diseases— such as cancer of the breast, colon, or prostate, diabetes, gallstones, and obesity—in which fat in the diet is a culprit.

The CSI can be computed for any nutrient data base and can thus be easily incorporated into specific research or clinical situations. The CSI can be computed for fat-modified recipes in cookbooks currently available and for new ones as they are produced in order to provide people many more choices for lower-fat, higher-carbohydrate dishes.

We believe that it would be of great value to health professionals and consumers if the CSI were listed on food labels, thus eliminating the need to consider both cholesterol and saturated fat individually in order to determine the heart-disease causing potential of any given food. We hope that our research, this book, and wide consumer acceptance of the CSI will eventually make CSI labeling a commonplace.

Finally, we wish to note that the CSI is even more important for those hundreds of thousands who are taking cholesterol-lowering drugs. This is because a lower intake of dietary cholesterol and saturated fat can greatly improve the action of the blood-cholesterol-lowering drugs. And, if you can lower your blood cholesterol level 10 to 20 percent by decreasing your CSI intake, it will take fewer drugs to reduce your blood cholesterol level to a low-risk category for heart disease. All of the blood-cholesterol-lowering drugs should be preceded by a low CSI diet. (Of course, no one should take blood-cholesterol-lowering drugs except under the supervision of a physician, because there are side effects associated with *each* of the blood-cholesterol-lowering drugs.)

To better understand how diet can favorably interact with these drugs, consider the case of Joe. Joe has an inherited disorder that results in very high cholesterol; his cholesterol level was 420 milligrams per deciliter (420 mg/dl) at the time that he found out about this problem. His father had died of coronary heart disease at age forty-eight. Joe was only twenty-nine at the time. His doctor prescribed a cholesterol-lowering drug called lovastatin (Mevacor), which increases the LDL receptors we talked about earlier. He also recommended a diet low in cholesterol and saturated fat. The medication cost a lot but got results. Joe took it as prescribed and his cholesterol went down to 331 milligrams per deciliter (331 mg/dl), a 21 percent decrease. That was an improvement but was still quite high. Joe's doctor was considering increasing the dose of lovastatin or adding another medicine when it occurred to him to ask Joe how he was doing on his diet.

"I don't need the diet anymore," Joe said, "because I have this expensive and effective medication." The doctor persuaded Joe that the right diet would still be useful. So Joe agreed to follow a new dietary plan, one that lowers cholesterol, total fat, *and* saturated fat. His cholesterol level soon fell to 270 milligrams per deciliter (270 mg/dl), a further decrease of 18 percent and a very significant improvement. Both the dietary factors and the medication work specifically on the LDL receptor mechanism, increasing LDL receptor activity in the liver, which, in turn, promotes the removal of LDL cholesterol from the blood and lowers the blood cholesterol level.

THE *LIFETIME* FAT/CHOLESTEROL CURE

Congratulations on joining our CSI "revolution." We are confident that you will discover, as we move ahead, that the CSI will give you more control over your eating habits than you've ever enjoyed before. We believe you'll find that it empowers you to take further responsibility for your own health. And we are convinced that the CSI will serve not only as a very effective measuring tool but, more important, as a powerful vehicle for positive change for you and your whole family.

So let's get going. The next step is to find out where we are right now and where we need to go in order to reap the substantial, sometimes life-saving benefits a better diet can deliver.

Take the CSI to heart. It will be your *lifetime* fat/cholesterol cure.

What's *Your* Number?

The following quiz has been designed to enable you to calculate your current CSI. By taking this quiz you will be able to determine where you are now, in terms of diet, and where you need to go to achieve the health benefits described in this book. We'll tell you how to evaluate your quiz results later on in this chapter. Right now let's take the quiz. It's simple and quick. Read the directions below and get started.

Directions: Under each food category listed below, you will find a number of questions, and for each question there are a number of possible answers or choices. Circle the numbers to the left of the choices that *best* describe your eating habits *during the past month*. Put that number in the blank space labeled "score" after each question. If you circle more than one choice for a single question, put the lowest score circled in the blank. For example, if you circle number 1, number 2, and number 3 under question 5 in the Meat, Fish, and Poultry portion of the quiz, your score is 1, which is the score you should enter for question 5. Some questions are worded in such a way that it is likely you will have only one answer; that's the case with question 4, for example, under the Meat, Fish, and Poultry category.

When you have computed the score for each question in a category (such as Meat, Fish, and Poultry), add all of those scores together to arrive at your total score for each category. Once you have done this, we will give you further instructions.

MEAT, FISH, AND POULTRY

For each question, circle as many numbers as apply, but your score for each question is the **lowest** *number circled.*

---

1. Which type of ground beef do you *usually* eat?
    1 Regular hamburger (30% fat)
    2 Lean ground beef (25% fat)
    3 Extra lean/ground chuck (20% fat)
    ✗ 4 Super lean/ground round (15% fat)
    5 Ground sirloin (10% fat) or eat no ground beef

SCORE _____

2. Which *best* describes your typical lunch?
    1 Cheeseburger, typical cheeses, egg dishes (egg salad, quiche, etc.)
    2 Sandwiches (lunch meat, hot dog, hamburger, fried fish, etc.) *or* entrée of meat or chicken (plain or fried)
    ✗ 3 Tuna sandwich, fish entrée (not fried), entrée with small bits of chicken or meat in a soup or casserole
    4 Peanut butter sandwich
    5 Salad, yogurt, cottage cheese, vegetarian dishes (without high-fat cheeses or egg yolk)

SCORE _____

3. Circle all of the choices that characterize the entrées (main courses) at your main meals.
    1 Cheese (Cheddar, Jack, etc.),

eggs, liver, heart, or brains *once a week or more*
    2 Beef, lamb, pork, or ham *once a week or more*
    ✗ 3 Very lean red meat (top round or flank steak), veal, venison, or elk *once a week or more*
    4 Chicken, turkey, rabbit, crab, lobster, or shrimp *twice a week or more*
    5 Fish, scallops, oysters, clams, or meatless dishes containing no egg yolk or high-fat cheese *twice a week or more*

SCORE _____

4. Estimate the number of ounces of meat, cheese, fish, and poultry you eat in a *typical day. Include all meals and snacks.*
    To guide you in your estimate:

4 strips bacon	= 1 oz.
1 small burger patty	= 3–4 oz.
meat in most sandwiches	= 2–3 oz.
1 slice cheese	= 1 oz.
1 chicken thigh	= 2–3 oz.
½ chicken breast	= 3 oz.
1 average T-bone steak	= 8 oz.
1-inch cube cheese	= 1 oz.

    1 Eleven or more ounces *a day*
    2 Nine to ten ounces *a day*
    ✗ 3 Six to eight ounces *a day*

4 Four to five ounces *a day*

5̲ Not more than 1 ounce of cheese, 3 ounces of red meat, poultry, shrimp, crab, lobster, *or* not more than 6 ounces of fish, clams, oysters, scallops *a day*

SCORE _____

5. Which of these have you eaten in the *past month?*

1̲ Bacon, sausage, bologna, and other lunch meats, pepperoni, beef or pork wieners

2 Canadian bacon, turkey wieners

✗3̲ Turkey ham and other poultry lunch meats

4 Soy products (breakfast links)

5̲ None

SCORE _____

TOTAL SCORE ____16____ (Add the scores from the previous five questions.)

DAIRY PRODUCTS AND EGGS

For each question, circle as many numbers as apply. Your score for each question is the low-est number circled.

1. Which kinds of milk do you use for drinking or cooking?

1̲ Whole milk

2̲ Two-percent milk

4̲ One-percent milk, buttermilk

✗5̲ Skim milk, nonfat dry milk, or none

SCORE _____

2. Which toppings do you use at least once a month?

1̲ Sour cream (real or imitation, including IMO*), whipped cream

✗3̲ Nondairy toppings (Cool Whip or Dream Whip)

4 Regular cottage cheese, whole-milk yogurt

✗5̲ Low-fat cottage cheese, low-fat or nonfat yogurt or none

SCORE _____

3. Which frozen desserts do you eat at least once a month?

1̲ Ice cream

2̲ Ice milk, most soft ice cream, Tofutti, frozen yogurt (cream added)

4 Sherbet, low-fat frozen yogurt, Lite Lite Tofutti

✗5̲ Sorbets, ices, nonfat frozen yogurt, Popsicles, or none

SCORE _____

* Certain products are listed to provide examples of food items available. There may be other products of similar composition with different trade names.

4. Which kinds of cheese do you use for snacks or sandwiches?
   - ✗ **1** Cheddar, Swiss, Jack, Brie, feta, American, cream cheese, regular cheese slices, or cheese spreads
   - ✗ **2** Part-skim mozzarella, Lappi, light cream cheese or Neufchâtel, part-skim Cheddar (Kraft Light, Green River, Olympia's Low Fat, or Heidi Ann Low-Fat Ched-Style Cheese)
   - **4** Low-cholesterol "filled" cheese (Scandic Mini Chol [Swedish low cholesterol], or Hickory Farms Lyte)
   - **5** Very-low-fat processed cheese (Dorman's Light, Reduced Calories Laughing Cow, Weight Watchers, or the Lite-line series of cheeses), or no cheese

SCORE _____

5. Which kinds of cheese do you use in cooking (casseroles, vegetables, etc.)?
   - **1** Cheddar, Swiss, Jack, Brie, feta, American, cream cheese, processed cheese (NOTE: Used in most restaurants)
   - ✗ **3** Part-skim mozzarella, Lappi, light cream cheese, part-skim Cheddar (Green River, Olympia's Low Fat, Kraft Light, or Heidi Ann Low-Fat Ched-Style Cheese)
   - **4** Low-cholesterol "filled" cheese (Scandic Mini Chol [Swedish low cholesterol], or Hickory Farms Lyte)
   - **5** Very-low-fat processed cheese (Dorman's Light, Reduced Calories Laughing Cow, Weight Watchers, or the Lite-line series of cheeses), or no cheese

SCORE _____

6. Check the type and number of "visible" eggs you eat.
   - **1** Six or more whole eggs *a week*
   - **2** Three to five whole eggs *a week*
   - ✗ **3** One to two whole eggs *a week*
   - **4** One whole egg *a month*
   - ✗ **5** Egg white, egg substitute such as Egg Beaters, Scramblers, Second Nature, or none

SCORE _____

7. Check the type of eggs usually used in food prepared at home or bought in grocery stores (baked goods, such as cakes and cookies, potato and pasta salads, pancakes, etc.)
   - **1** Whole eggs or mixes containing whole eggs (complete pancake mix, slice-and-bake cookies, etc.)
   - ✗ **3** Combination of egg white, egg substitute, and whole egg
   - **5** Egg white, egg substitute, or none

SCORE _____

TOTAL SCORE ___*23*___ (Add the scores from the previous seven questions.)

FATS AND OILS

For each question, circle as many numbers as apply. Your score for each question is the lowest number circled.

1. Which kinds of fats are used to cook your food (vegetables, meats, etc.)?
   - <u>1</u> Butter, shortening (all brands except Crisco or Food Club) or lard, bacon grease, chicken fat, or eat in restaurants at least *4 times a week*
   - <u>3</u> Soft shortening (Crisco or Food Club) or inexpensive stick margarine
   - ✗ <u>4</u> Tub or soft-stick margarine, vegetable oil
   - ✗ <u>5</u> None or use nonstick pan or spray

SCORE _____

2. Which best describes your *daily* use of these "visible" fats?

Typical Amounts Used:	Your Use in One Day
2 tsp. margarine, butter on toast (each slice)	_____ tsp.
6 tsp. mayonnaise on sandwiches (amount/sandwich)	_____ tsp.
6 tsp. peanut butter on sandwiches (amount/sandwich)	_____ tsp.
2 tsp. margarine, butter on sandwiches (amount/sandwich)	2 tsp.
12 tsp. regular salad dressings on salads	H tsp.
3–6 tsp. margarine, butter on potatoes	_____ tsp.
3 tsp. margarine, butter on vegetables	_____ tsp.
Total	_____ tsp.

   - <u>1</u> Ten teaspoons or more
   - ✗ <u>2</u> Eight to nine teaspoons
   - <u>3</u> Six to seven teaspoons
   - <u>4</u> Four to five teaspoons
   - <u>5</u> Three teaspoons or less

SCORE _____

3. How often do you eat potato chips, corn or tortilla chips, fried chicken, fish sticks, French fries, doughnuts, other fried foods, croissants, or Danish pastries?
   - <u>1</u> Two or more times *a day*
   - <u>2</u> Once *a day*
   - <u>3</u> Two to four times *a week*
   - ✗ <u>4</u> Once *a week*
   - <u>5</u> Less than twice *a month*

SCORE _____

4. Which best describes the amount of margarine, peanut butter, mayonnaise, or cream cheese that you put on breads, muffins, bagels, etc.?
   - <u>1</u> Average (1 teaspoon or more per serving)
   - ✗ <u>2</u> Lightly spread (can see through it)
   - <u>4</u> "Scrape" (can barely see it)
   - <u>5</u> None

SCORE _____

5. Which kind of salad dressings do you use?

    1 Real mayonnaise

    2 Miracle Whip, Ranch, French, Roquefort, blue cheese, and vinegar and oil dressings

    3 Light mayonnaise, Miracle Whip Light, Thousand Island dressing

    4 Russian and Italian dressings, Ranch Salad Dressing made with buttermilk and light mayonnaise or Miracle Whip Light

X 5 Low-calorie dressing, vinegar, lemon juice, Ranch Dressing made with buttermilk and nonfat or low-fat yogurt or use lemon or no salad dressing

SCORE _____

TOTAL SCORE _____17_____ (Add the scores from the previous five questions.)

SWEETS AND SNACKS

For each question, circle as many numbers as apply. Your score for each question is the lowest number circled.

1. How often do you eat dessert or baked goods (sweet rolls, doughnuts, cookies, cakes, etc.)?

    1 Three or more times *a day*

    2 Two times *a day*

    3 Once *a day*

    4 Four to six times *a week*

 X 5 Three or four times *a week or less*

SCORE _____

2. Which of the following are you most likely to select as a dessert choice?

    1 Croissants, pies, cheesecake, carrot cake

    2 Regular cakes, cupcakes, cookies

    4 Low-fat muffins, desserts from low-fat cookbooks, or none

 X 5 Fruits, low-fat cookies (fig bars, va-

nilla wafers, graham crackers, and gingersnaps), angel food cake

SCORE _____

3. Which snack items are you most likely to eat in an average month?

    1 Chocolate

    2 Potato chips, corn or tortilla chips, nuts, party/snack crackers, doughnuts, French fries, peanut butter, cookies

    4 Lightly "buttered" popcorn (1 teaspoon margarine for 3 cups), pretzels, low-fat crackers (soda, graham), "home" baked corn chips, low-fat cookies (gingersnaps, fig bars)

 X 5 Fruit, vegetables, very low-fat snacks, or none

SCORE _____

TOTAL SCORE _____15_____ (Add the scores from the previous three questions.)

How to Compute Your CSI Score

To find out what your category scores mean and how to compute your daily CSI, refer to Table 4. Note that there are two parts to this table. One part is for women and children (who average about 2,000 Calories per day), and the other part is for men and teens (who have an average intake of about 2,800 Calories per day). Select the part that applies to you and fill in the blanks.

First fill in your scores for each of the categories. Let's say, for purposes of illustration, that you are a woman and that you scored 9 for Meat, Fish, and Poultry; 18 for Dairy Products and Eggs; 10 for Fats and Oils; and 6 for Sweets and Snacks. That gives you a combined score for all categories of 43. Enter this in the blank labeled "Combined Score." As you can see from Table 4, that combined score corresponds to a *daily* CSI of 51, characteristic of the present American diet. This is to be expected—but it's not the optimal CSI score. If you are a woman or child who scores a CSI of 51 or more, or a man or teen who scores a CSI of 69 or more, you will want to modify your diet considerably, but gradually.

Look again at Table 4 and note the scores under CSI Phases One, Two, and Three. You'll see where you need to go, with respect to your overall daily CSI. If your combined score places you in CSI Phase One, you're already on your way. If your combined score places you in Phase Two, you're not only on your way, you're doing very well, indeed. Keep up the good work. And if you're in Phase Three, you're a nutritional champion.

You'll want to take this quiz over again from time to time as you gradually make lower CSI food choices and thus adapt to a lower-fat, lower-cholesterol style of eating. Remember, as your CSI goes down, so does your risk of heart disease, stroke, obesity, and some cancers, such as breast and colon cancers.

When you achieve a Phase One CSI,

TABLE 4
COMPUTING YOUR CSI

	YOUR SCORE
Meat, Fish, and Poultry	*16*
Dairy Products and Eggs	*23*
Fats and Oils	*17*
Sweets and Snacks	*15*
COMBINED SCORE	*71*

For Women and Children (2,000 Calories)

QUIZ SCORE =	CSI =	DIET COMPOSITION
57 or less	51	Typical American
58–70	37	CSI Phase One
71–86	(28)	CSI Phase Two
87 or more	16	CSI Phase Three

For Men and Teens (2,800 Calories)

QUIZ SCORE =	CSI =	DIET COMPOSITION
55 or less	69	Typical American
56–68	49	CSI Phase One
69–84	36	CSI Phase Two
85 or more	23	CSI Phase Three

My combined score of _____ gives me a CSI of _____ .

going from 51 to 37, in the case of women and children, and from 69 to 49 for men and teens, you will have reduced your cholesterol intake, on average, from 400–500 milligrams per day to 300–350 milligrams. Fat intake will be reduced from 40 percent of calories to 30 percent (with saturated fat going from 14 percent to 10 percent). On average, these changes will result in up to a 6 percent reduction in your blood cholesterol level and 12 percent reduction in the risk of coronary heart disease.

When you achieve a Phase Two CSI of 28 (women and children) or 36 (men and teens), your cholesterol intake will average about 200 milligrams daily, and the fat content of your diet will be only 25 percent of calories (with just 8 percent of calories in the form of saturated fat). These changes can reduce your blood cholesterol level by up to 13 percent and your risk of coronary heart disease by up to 26 percent.

If you achieve a Phase Three CSI of 16 (women and children) or 23 (men and teens), your diet will consist of 20 percent fat (only 5 percent of the calories will be saturated fat), and your cholesterol intake will average 100 milligrams. Your blood cholesterol level will be reduced up to 20 percent and your risk of coronary heart disease will be reduced by up to 40 percent!

Okay, you're saying, now I know where I am, where I want to go, and why it's well worth the effort. But *how* do I do it?

You've already started. You've begun to learn how the cholesterol and saturated fat *together* begin to add up—and what the CSI score is *right now* in your own case. You're ready and eager to better that score. The following chapters will enable you to do that while you're still learning.

For now, just concentrate on reducing your present CSI score and reaching your first major goal: a daily CSI of 37, if you're a woman or child; a daily CSI of 49, if you are a man or a teen. If you're already at or near those goals, aim for the Phase Two CSI goals. And if you're in Phase Two now and want to go all the way, make the Phase Three daily CSIs your ultimate health destination.

Don't be discouraged if you didn't score as well as you hoped you would. *Very few* people initially have Phase One, let alone Phase Two or Three CSIs. But, with a little work and determination, you'll be surprised at how quickly you can achieve these goals. A few nutritional "marathoners" have attained Phase Three CSIs in as little as four weeks—but a more gradual approach is more typical and, in most cases, is actually preferable. For most, gradualism helps make each positive change in diet a *permanent,* lifelong change, a new habit.

In the Appendix, you'll find the CSI tables for 1,000 foods. In Part II, which immediately follows the chapter you are reading now, you will find sections of the CSI table as they specifically apply to discussions of various food categories, eating situations, and personal considerations (for example, Dairy Products and Eggs *or* Dinner *or* CSI Goals for Children). By consulting these tables, you can quickly determine which food choices add up to your target/goal CSIs. If you make choices that don't exceed 37 (women/children) or 49 (men/teens) for one day, you'll achieve Phase One goals. It's as simple as that!

Table 5 provides an example of what Phase One CSI eating looks like.

TABLE 5
THE CHOLESTEROL–SATURATED FAT INDEX OF CSI PHASE ONE EATING*

	CSI		CSI
Breakfast		Dinner	
Apple juice, ½ cup	tr.	Spaghetti, 1 cup, with	tr.
Oatmeal Buttermilk Pancakes,	1	Marinara Sauce, 1 cup, and	tr.
three 4″		Ground beef (15% fat), 4 oz.	12
Syrup, ¼ cup	0	Lettuce salad, 1 cup	tr.
Soft margarine, 2 tsp.	1.4	Low-cal French dressing, 3 Tbsp.	tr.
Lunch		French bread, 1 piece, (4″ diameter)	tr.
Chili with beef and beans, 1 cup	8	Soft margarine, 2 tsp.	1.4
Corn Bread, 1 piece (2″ × 4″)	<1	Rainbow sherbet, 1 cup	3
Soft margarine, 2 tsp.	1.4		
Orange	tr.		30.2

* 2,180 Calories, 14 percent protein, 32 percent fat, 54 percent carbohydrate
Recipes in **bold italics** can be found in Part III.
The abbreviation *tr.* stands for trace (less than 0.5); the symbol <1 stands for less than one (0.5 to 0.9).

Using the CSI
for a Healthier Heart

CHAPTER

1

How to Use This Part
of the Book

THE COMPREHENSIVE CSI TABLES

In the chapters that comprise this part of the book, you will find CSI tables that collectively include 1,000 foods. Rather than simply run one continuous table, we have broken the tables down and divided them into several chapters to make it much easier for you to find what you're looking for and to properly utilize the CSIs. These chapters include:

- Meats, Poultry, Fish (including shellfish)
- Dairy Products and Eggs
- Fats, Oils, Margarines, Salad Dressings, Nuts
- Fruits, Vegetables, Grains, Beans

These chapters provide CSIs for all major food categories and mixed dishes. They also give you numerous tips and guidelines to help you consistently make lower-CSI choices.

In addition, this part of the book includes special chapters on:

- Breakfast
- Lunch
- Dinner
- Desserts
- Snacks (including beverages and hors d'oeuvres)

These chapters provide CSIs for mixed dishes such as enchiladas, pizzas, and cakes, to name only a few, and CSI goals for *each meal*. They also give you lots of ideas to help you restructure your meals in healthy, delicious new ways.

35

To make it easy for you to find the CSIs of specific foods, each chapter is self-contained. All the tables of foods that pertain to a particular topic can be found in that chapter. For example, the table on breads can be found in five chapters: Fruits, Vegetables, Grains, Beans, Fiber; Breakfast; Lunch; Dinner; and Snacks. Salads can be found in the chapters on Lunch and Dinner. There are other repeats as appropriate. For quick reference, we have also put *all* of the tables in alphabetical order (preceded by a detailed table of contents) in the Appendix.

Finally, Part II includes chapters on:

• How the CSI Can Help You Take the Hazard Out of Dining Out
• Using the CSI for Weight Loss and Control
• CSI Goals for Children
• Putting It All Together: The *Lifetime Cholesterol Cure*

Table 6 (Sandwich Fillings), located at the end of the chapter, is an example of the material included in our comprehensive CSIs. You'll find all of our CSI tables arranged like this one:

1. Within each section of food choices (such as Cold Cuts in Table 6), the items are usually listed in order of CSI from the lowest to the highest.
2. In selected cases, higher-CSI choices immediately follow lower-CSI choices (prepared through modified recipes) to allow for ease of comparison. (See egg salad, for example, in Table 6.)

Many of the CSI tables contain a large number of items. It may not be readily apparent how to tell the desirable CSI choices from the higher (typical) CSI choices. So, in each chapter, we will give you the CSI goal to strive for. For example, in Table 6 those sandwich fillings that have a CSI of 4 or less are desirable. Items that have a CSI of 5 or greater fall into the higher (typical) CSI category. More specific discussion about this table will be found in Chapter 7 on lunch.

Note that, in each table, we provide typical serving sizes for each food. And these serving sizes are described both in familiar household units (such as cups or ounces) and in grams. The CSI is given to the nearest whole number. Total fat is expressed to the nearest gram (there are 5 grams in 1 teaspoon), and calories are listed to the nearest whole number.

Foods with CSI and/or total fat values less than one are indicated in the tables as follow: Values less than 0.5 are listed as trace (tr.); values from 0.5 to 0.9 are listed as less than 1 (indicated by the symbol <1). The CSIs of most breads, grains, cereals, legumes, fruits, and vegetables are less than 0.5 per serving and so appear in the tables as trace. Foods are listed in the state in which they are most commonly consumed (e.g., cooked, raw, smoked, pickled, shelled, etc.). All of the lower-CSI recipes will also be lower in sodium. However, you will find *some* higher-sodium items listed in the tables. Because these are comprehensive tables, some foods with low CSIs will be high in sodium, such as anchovies, jerky, smoked salmon, pickled herring, to name a few. These foods should be consumed infrequently and in small quantities. The items that appear in **bold italics** in the tables are our own fat-modified, lower-CSI recipes (see cookbook section, Part III of this book).

GOING FOR THE GOALS

Remember, the CSI goals we have established in the preceding chapter are based upon a daily intake of 2,800 Calories for men and teens and 2,000 Calories for women and children. We recognize that not everyone has precisely these caloric intakes. These are averages, and serve for *most* people. If you are on a weight-loss diet, however, you will be consuming considerably fewer calories, and your CSI goals will be adjusted accordingly. (See Chapter 12 of Part II.) If you are consuming significantly *more* calories than average, this is usually due to (a) overeating or (b) the need for more calories due to greater-than-average energy expenditure, such as may be experienced by some athletes and by some engaged in strenuous physical work and by very tall and muscular people.

If you are overweight, you are consuming more calories than you require and should cut back. If you are *not* overweight and are consuming greater numbers of calories due to higher energy expenditures, you may make an upward adjustment of your CSI goals. For example, if you are an active man consuming 3,200 Calories per day, that's 400 more calories or approximately 14 percent more calories ($0.14 \times 2,800 = 392$) than average. You may thus adjust your Phase One CSI goal, for example, upward by 14 percent ($0.14 \times 49 = 6.86$, rounded off to 7). That gives you a Phase One CSI goal of 56 ($49 + 7$).

This kind of fine-tuning of CSI goals is strictly optional. Except where calories are being significantly reduced for weight loss, there is no pressing need to adjust the goals.

With respect to calories, we'd like to add that, once you get into a lower-CSI way of eating, you'll find you can fill up without filling out. The lower-CSI foods tend to be those such as fruits, vegetables, grains, and beans that, even though lower in calories, are higher in bulk and thus leave you feeling satisfied and full. It *is* possible to eat more *without* consuming more calories or increasing your CSI.

GUIDELINES NOT DEADLINES

As you proceed through this book, remember also that this is a go-at-your-own-pace program. We believe that, when it comes to nutrition and diet, deadlines are self-defeating. Fail to meet one or two deadlines, and many people feel like failures themselves. We provide *guidelines* instead, guidelines to help you progress at whatever rate *you* choose. If it takes you a year to achieve a consistent Phase One CSI, fine. That's far better than achieving it, fleetingly, in a week or two and then losing it because it was too much change too soon. For most people, it takes a little time to re-educate tastes distorted by years of excess and imbalance (too much fat and too little complex carbohydrate).

As long as you go on adding lower-CSI choices to your regular eating plan, you'll be making important progress—and your own CSI will steadily decline in appreciative response. And along with that steady, gradual decline will come a reduced risk of heart attack and stroke.

TABLE 6
EXAMPLE OF ONE SECTION FROM THE TABLE OF 1,000 FOODS
Sandwich Fillings (Select CSIs of 4 or lower per serving)

	SERVING SIZE	CSI	FAT (GM)	CALORIES
Chicken salad (with mayonnaise)	½ cup (104 gm)	8	32	353
CHEDDAR AND JACK-TYPE CHEESES				
Dorman's Light	1 ounce (28 gm)	<1	5	70
Scandic Mini Chol or Swedish low-fat	1 ounce (28 gm)	2	9	113
Olympia's Low Fat	1 ounce (28 gm)	4	5	72
Green River Part Skim	1 ounce (28 gm)	4	5	72
Heidi Ann Low-Fat Ched-Style Cheese, Kraft Light Naturals Mild Cheddar	1 ounce (28 gm)	4	5	80
Swiss	1 ounce (28 gm)	6	8	107
Cheddar, Monterey Jack, Colby, Havarti, Long Horn	1 ounce (28 gm)	8	9	114
CHEESE SLICES				
Lite-line	1 ounce (28 gm)	2	2	51
Lite 'n' Lively	1 ounce (28 gm)	3	4	74
Kraft Light Naturals (Swiss Reduced Fat)	1 ounce (28 gm)	4	5	90
American	1 ounce (28 gm)	7	9	106
COLD CUTS, BEEF & PORK				
Thin, pressed	6 slices (28 gm)	1	1	35
Pastrami, corned beef	2 ounces (57 gm)	5	5	104
Head cheese	2 ounces (57 gm)	5	9	120

38

Ham	2 ounces	(57 gm)	6	12	159
Salami, beef	2 ounces	(57 gm)	7	11	144
Italian sausage	2 ounces	(57 gm)	7	15	184
Knockwurst	2 ounces	(57 gm)	7	16	174
Bologna	2 ounces	(57 gm)	8	16	180
Polish sausage, kielbasa	2 ounces	(57 gm)	8	16	184
Salami, Genoa (hard)	2 ounces	(57 gm)	9	19	230
Liverwurst	2 ounces	(57 gm)	11	16	184
Braunschweiger	2 ounces	(57 gm)	11	18	204

COLD CUTS, TURKEY & CHICKEN

Ham	2 ounces	(57 gm)	3	3	73
Pastrami	2 ounces	(57 gm)	3	4	80
Bologna	2 ounces	(57 gm)	5	8	113
Salami	2 ounces	(57 gm)	5	8	113
Thin, pressed lunch meats (meat/poultry)	2 slices	(9 gm)	tr.	tr.	12

CHEESE-TYPE SPREADS

Fruit-Nut Sandwich Spread	¼ cup	(52 gm)	1	4	81
Vegetable-Cottage Cheese Sandwich Spread	¼ cup	(42 gm)	<1	<1	34
Reduced Calories Laughing Cow Cheese	1 ounce	(28 gm)	2	3	113
Denver (egg, ham, green pepper)	1 egg	(84 gm)	15	13	165
"Egg" Salad Sandwich Spread	½ cup	(105 gm)	<1	5	110
Tofu "Egg" Salad Sandwich Spread	½ cup	(75 gm)	<1	5	66

The abbreviation *tr.* stands for trace (less than 0.5); the symbol <1 stands for less than one (0.5 to 0.9). Recipes in **bold italics** can be found in Part III.

TABLE 6 (continued)

	SERVING SIZE		CSI	FAT (GM)	CALORIES
Egg salad (with mayonnaise)	½ cup	(111 gm)	24	23	252
FRANKFURTERS					
Chicken or turkey	1 wiener	(45 gm)	5	8	102
Beef	1 wiener	(45 gm)	7	13	145
Corn Dog or Pronto Pup	One	(111 gm)	13	28	344
Hamburger patty (10% fat)	3 ounces	(85 gm)	7	7	170
Hamburger patty (15% fat)	3 ounces	(85 gm)	9	13	215
Hamburger patty (20% fat)	3 ounces	(85 gm)	11	16	246
Hamburger patty (25% fat)	3 ounces	(85 gm)	12	20	278
Ham, baked	2 ounces	(57 gm)	6	12	159
Ham salad	½ cup	(124 gm)	8	28	338
Peanut butter	2 tablespoons	(32 gm)	3	17	190
Roast beef	2 ounces	(57 gm)	6	9	144
Roast turkey (white meat)	2 ounces	(57 gm)	3	2	94
Spam	2 slices (¼")	(85 gm)	12	26	284
SPREADABLES					
Chicken or turkey	½ cup	(104 gm)	5	14	208
Beef or ham	½ cup	(120 gm)	9	20	271
Ham & cheese	½ cup	(120 gm)	14	22	294
Tuna Salad Sandwich Spread	½ cup	(108 gm)	3	2	111
Tuna salad (with light mayonnaise)	½ cup	(102 gm)	4	15	196
Tuna salad (with mayonnaise)	½ cup	(98 gm)	5	25	272

40

VEGETABLE SANDWICH FILLINGS

California Beans	½ cup	(78 gm)	tr.	1	63
Spicy Black Bean Salad	½ cup	(85 gm)	tr.	2	114
Falafel	¼ recipe	(79 gm)	tr.	2	124
Chili Bean Salad	½ cup	(111 gm)	<1	3	128
Southern Caviar	½ cup	(104 gm)	<1	3	136
Chowchow	½ cup	(106 gm)	<1	5	94
Refried Beans	½ cup	(87 gm)	<1	3	113
Refried beans (canned)	½ cup	(121 gm)	<1	2	124
Refried beans (typical restaurant)	½ cup	(122 gm)	6	14	243

SPREADS (SELECT CSIs OF 1.0 OR LOWER)

Mustard, prepared	1 tablespoon	(15 gm)	tr.	<1	11
Horseradish	1 tablespoon	(15 gm)	0	tr.	6
Cranberry sauce	1 tablespoon	(17 gm)	0	tr.	30
Ketchup	1 tablespoon	(17 gm)	tr.	tr.	18
Mayonnaise, light	1 tablespoon	(14 gm)	0.8	5	50
Margarine, soft	1 tablespoon	(14 gm)	2.1	11	101
Mayonnaise, typical	1 tablespoon	(14 gm)	2.1	11	101
Butter	1 tablespoon	(14 gm)	9.3	12	102
Jelly, typical	1 tablespoon	(14 gm)	tr.	tr.	55
Jelly, low-sugar	1 tablespoon	(14 gm)	0	0	28

The abbreviation *tr.* stands for trace (less than 0.5); the symbol <1 stands for less than one (0.5 to 0.9). Recipes in **bold italics** can be found in Part III.

41

Meats, Poultry, Fish

THE MEAT OF THE MATTER

Because meats contribute so much saturated fat and cholesterol to the typical high-CSI American diet, we need to pay special attention to our meat selections. It is *not* necessary to give up red meat in order to have a healthy low-CSI diet—at least not most red meats. We *do* recommend that you not eat organ meats (liver, heart, brains, kidney, gizzards), since they all have such extremely high CSIs. For most people, however, that will be easy since most of you are not eating them anyway. Other meats, fish, and poultry are included through all three phases of our diet. Instead of banning red meat, we seek, instead, to

reduce the amounts consumed gradually and encourage selecting leaner red meats with lower CSIs.

Here are some tips/guidelines to assist you in cutting back on meats as you pursue the CSI Phase One, Two, and Three goals:

Phase One   If, like most Americans, you have been eating red meat regularly, making it the centerpiece of most meals, don't try a "cold turkey" approach to cutting back. Instead, begin by paying attention to the frequency with which you eat red meats and, roughly, the amounts you consume. You'll probably be surprised at just how much meat you are eating. Most people, once they take an informal "meat inventory," realize that *some* cutback is in order and really won't be that difficult to achieve.

The primary goal, remember, is not to

cut out red meats per se but, rather, to reduce your intake of saturated fats and cholesterol. The easiest way to begin is to first trim as much visible fat off meat as possible—*before* cooking. Most people are already doing this. Also remove the skin from poultry before cooking. Much of the fat in chicken and turkey is in and just under the skin.

Next, begin consciously making some lower-CSI choices, using the table you'll find in this chapter. See Figure 1, which compares the CSIs of several meats and other protein choices. You can immediately see how much better it is to choose fish, shellfish, poultry, or very lean (10 percent fat or less) red meats. The more you begin using these meat categories the better. A problem people run into when selecting lower-CSI red meat is that it will be tough and dry if prepared using typical recipes for cooking higher-CSI red meats. Cooking quickly when broiling, barbecuing, or stir-frying, as well as baking with added liquid and stewing are good ways to cook lower-CSI red meats. You will find ideas for other recipes in a later chapter on dinner.

For those of you who are not fish fans, you might start out by trying shellfish, on

CHOLESTEROL–SATURATED FAT INDEX
(3 OUNCES)

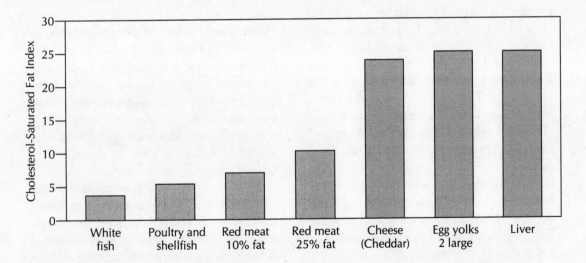

FIGURE 1. The Cholesterol–Saturated Fat Index (CSI) of 3 ounces of fish, poultry, shellfish, meat, cheese, egg yolk, and liver. The CSI for poultry is the average CSI for cooked light and dark chicken without skin. The CSI for shellfish is the average CSI of cooked crab, lobster, shrimp, clams, oysters, and scallops. The CSI for liver is the average for beef or pork liver and chicken liver. A smaller CSI denotes less cholesterol and saturated fat.

occasion, in place of steak or hamburger. Even though shellfish (crab, lobster, and shrimp) have a cholesterol content 1.5 to 2 times higher than that of red meat, their remarkably low saturated fat content gives them an overall CSI as low or lower than even the leanest of red meats (CSIs of 2 to 9 for 3 ounces of shellfish, compared to CSIs of 5 to 28 for 3 ounces of typical red meats). Even many ardent steak fans don't mind giving up their well-marbled (fatty) red meat for a mouth-watering grilled fresh shrimp or scallop dinner.

As for hamburger, that obsession that remains America's most popular meat choice, *modification* is the key word. When it comes to health, not all hamburgers are created equal. To begin with, typical hamburger meat is 30 percent fat (CSI of 15 for 3 ounces). You can make some immediate, easy progress by switching to the 20-percent-fat variety available in most stores (CSI of 11 for 3 ounces). Most people can't tell the difference in terms of taste. Yet, the CSI of the 20-percent-fat meat is about 27 percent lower than that of the typical hamburger. The next step is to try extra-lean ground round (15 percent fat with a CSI of 9 for 3 ounces) and, finally, ground sirloin (10 percent fat with a CSI of 7 for 3 ounces). The CSI of the latter is *less than half* that of regular ground beef. For future reference, the beef industry is developing cattle that are very low in fat (all cuts are 5 to 10 percent fat). These are available in some parts of the country now.

You'll find recipes, by the way, for our *Skinny Burgers* and our *Very Skinny Burgers* using 10-percent-fat ground beef in Part III, the cookbook section. Each of our *Skinny Burgers* has only 375 Calories and a CSI of only 8, while each of our *Very Skinny Burg-*

ers has even fewer calories (288) and a CSI of only 5. Contrast these still-tasty burgers with a Big Mac (570 Calories and a CSI of 16) or a Quarter Pounder with cheese (525 Calories and a CSI of 18).

Another meat Americans consume in great quantities is chicken. Overall, chicken is a much better meat choice than beef or most of the other red meats—*but* chicken prepared using typical recipes and in fast-food outlets and most restaurants can be a very fattening and hazardous item. Two pieces of Kentucky Fried Chicken, for example, contain a breathtaking 431 Calories and pack a CSI of 11. That's *not* something to crow about. Two pieces of our *Portland Fried Chicken* by contrast (see recipe in Part III), have only 187 Calories and a CSI of 5. (We'll have more to say in Chapter 11 about minding your CSIs in restaurants and fast-food stores.)

Phase Two What it generally takes to achieve CSI Phase Two goals is to eat fish, poultry, or meat not more than once a day and to limit consumption to no more than 6 to 8 ounces per day. When you eat cheese (see discussion in next chapter), you should eat even less meat. Of course, the lower your CSI meat choices, the more you can eat and still reach the goal.

Few people have meat at breakfast, but most have meat (and/or cheese) at lunch and dinner. And it quickly adds up. Even a small, single-patty hamburger is 4 ounces of meat. A more typical hamburger is 6 to 8 ounces all by itself. Two slices of lunch meat contribute 2 ounces. A chicken leg and a thigh are 3 ounces; so is a single half of a chicken breast. Many people consume 10 to 22 ounces of meat a day.

When we talk about making ideal lower-

CSI meat choices, we mean those with CSIs of 9 *or lower* for 3 ounces (3 or lower for 1 ounce). Table 7, located at the end of this chapter, shows you the wide range of CSIs per 3-ounce servings: 5 to 110! That heart-stopping 110, by the way, is for a small serving of brains, clearly not the best choice. Obviously, not *all* of your meat selections will have CSIs of 9 or lower, but, to get to Phase Two, you should *generally* make selections in that range. This still leaves you with plenty of variety.

If you choose meats that have CSIs of 9 or lower for 3 ounces, you'll be eating meats that are no greater than 15 percent fat. These include such choices as 10-percent-fat ground beef, roasts (sirloin tip, baron of beef, and heel of round), flank steak, round and cube steak, sirloin steak, game meats, lean lamb stew meat, pork tenderloin, center-cut pork chops, veal cutlet, almost all fish and shellfish, chicken, and turkey.

One of the most useful tips we can offer you with respect to achieving Phase Two meat goals is this: *Buy just the right amount of meat for a given time period.* By purchasing *no more than* the amount you or your family should eat, you won't be tempted to overeat and exceed your CSI; nor will you waste food. For a family of four, for example, the "right" amount of meat, per week, would be: lean red meat, 4½ to 6 pounds boneless; plus 3 to 4 pounds fish; plus 6 to 8 pounds poultry with bone, or 3 to 4 pounds boneless. Thinking in terms of one meal, 2 pounds of fish (32 ounces) cooks down to 24 ounces, making 6-ounce servings for four people.

As you approach the Phase Two goal, you should be using meat in consistently reduced amounts, replacing it with more complex carbohydrates (or you will be hun-

gry from calories lost in selecting leaner and less meat): cereals, grains, legumes, breads, pastas, potatoes, and other vegetables and fruits. You'll find a number of exciting ethnic (Mexican, Oriental, Middle Eastern, and Mediterranean) dishes that exemplify Phase Two eating in our cookbook section, Part III. (See also subsequent discussions in Part II of Fruits, Vegetables, Grains, Beans, Fiber (Chapter 5), Lunch (Chapter 7), and Dinner (Chapter 8), for further ideas.)

As you begin to make progress toward your Phase Two CSI goal, start having *some* meals *without meat* of any kind. In Phase One you learn how to eat breakfast without meat (even on weekends)—and that is a good start. In Phase Two you will begin to experiment with some meatless lunches and a few dinners, too. In place of meats, concentrate on soups, salads, breads, fruits, vegetables, cottage cheese, pasta, rice, tortillas, burritos, etc.

Phase Three To achieve the CSI Phase Three goal typically requires a further reduction in meat and cheese consumption: eating up to 6 ounces of fish, clams, oysters, scallops *or* 3 to 4 ounces of lean red meat, shrimp, crab, lobster, or low-fat cheese per day. The ultimate dinner goal is to have poultry two to three times a week, fish two or three times a week, lean red meat one or two times a week, and meatless dinners once or twice a month (*no* meat or high-fat cheese).

Again, buy meats only in appropriate quantities—just the right amount to cover a given time period. For a family of four, the appropriate amount for a week would be 1 to 2 pounds of boneless lean red meat; plus 4 to 5 pounds of fish; plus 2 to 3 pounds of boneless chicken, or 5 to 6 pounds of chicken with bone.

In Phase Three, you should regard meat not as a main course but rather as a condiment, a "supplement" you use to spice up bean, grain, and other vegetable dishes, as it has been used for centuries in many other, leaner and healthier cuisines of the world.

THE FISH STORY THAT SAVES LIVES

As you go into Phases Two and Three, fish is likely to become a more important part of your diet. When it comes to meat, fish is far and away the best choice you can make. Fish has a low CSI and contains a positive factor that acts against coronary heart disease. For years, medical science has wondered why people who eat large amounts of fish and other marine animals high in fat and cholesterol nevertheless have very low rates of heart disease. Greenland Eskimos and the Japanese, for example, consume large amounts of fish (and also, in the case of the Eskimos, marine mammals such as whale and seal) that are relatively high in fat and cholesterol. Yet, both groups have very low rates of heart disease. Why? What is protecting them?

Recent research has revealed the answer: The protective factor is a special class of polyunsaturated fats called "omega-3 fatty acids." These are found in large quantities in fish, including shellfish. When our own research team fed a pound of salmon a day, along with some extra salmon oil, to two groups of people (one healthy, the other consisting of individuals with elevated blood levels of cholesterol and fat called triglycerides), the results were quite dramatic. After just a few weeks, this fish diet, rich in omega-3 fatty acids, resulted in a 15 percent reduction in cholesterol and a 40 percent reduction in triglycerides in the healthy subjects. The reductions were even greater in those with elevated blood-fat levels.

All fish contain omega-3 fatty acids—and we now know that these substances not only lower blood cholesterol and triglyceride levels but also help prevent the sort of blood clots that are involved in heart attacks and strokes. To take advantage of the omega-3 protective factor, we recommend that you eat fish at least twice a week—but not a pound at a time, as described above. That was strictly for experimental purposes. Servings up to 6 ounces are ideal.

THE CSIs OF MEATS, FISH, AND POULTRY

The CSIs for meats, fish, and poultry are provided in Table 7. Note how low fish is. Most, but not all, of these CSIs are for 3-ounce servings. Serving sizes were selected for foods based on amounts people would typically eat. Pay attention to fat and calories and select your daily CSIs accordingly. Some foods that don't have sky-high CSIs are high in fat and calories—for example, bacon. Again, remember that lower-CSI meat choices refer to CSIs of 9 or lower per 3-ounce serving, or 3 or lower per 1-ounce serving of any given item. But remember, too, that *any* progress you can make toward selecting foods with CSIs *lower than your usual fare* is valuable progress, indeed.

You will note that some meats with low CSIs are high in sodium. Some examples include jerky, chipped beef, bacon and sausage substitutes, ham, and Canadian bacon. These foods should be consumed infrequently and in small quantities.

TABLE 7
THE CSIs OF MEAT, FISH, AND POULTRY

BEEF, LAMB, PORK, TOFU, TVP, ETC. (COOKED, BONELESS)
(SELECT CSIs OF 9 OR LOWER FOR 3 OUNCES, OR 3 OR LOWER FOR 1 OUNCE)

	SERVING SIZE		CSI	FAT (GM)	CALORIES
BEEF					
Jerky	1 ounce (13" x 5/8" x 1/4")	(28 gm)	2	3	53
Chipped beef	3 ounces	(85 gm)	5	5	173
Oxtails	3 ounces	(85 gm)	11	16	246
Brisket (fresh), corned beef, pastrami	3 ounces	(85 gm)	15	26	316
Shank	3 ounces	(85 gm)	15	27	323
Short ribs	3 ounces	(85 gm)	15	27	323
Ground:					
10% fat	3 ounces	(85 gm)	7	7	170
15% fat (extra lean)	3 ounces	(85 gm)	9	13	215
20% fat (most "fast-food" restaurants)	3 ounces	(85 gm)	11	16	246
25% fat (lean)	3 ounces	(85 gm)	12	20	278
30% fat (typical)	3 ounces	(85 gm)	15	27	323

48

Roasts:

Sirloin tip	3 ounces	(85 gm)	9	13	215
Baron of beef	3 ounces	(85 gm)	9	13	215
Heel of round	3 ounces	(85 gm)	9	13	215
Rump	3 ounces	(85 gm)	12	20	278
Blade, chuck, arm	3 ounces	(85 gm)	15	27	323
Tenderloin	3 ounces	(85 gm)	15	27	323
Standing rib	3 ounces	(85 gm)	15	27	323

Steaks:

Flank	3 ounces	(85 gm)	5	5	161
Round, cube	3 ounces	(85 gm)	9	13	215
Sirloin	3 ounces	(85 gm)	9	13	215
T-bone, rib, New York	3 ounces	(85 gm)	15	27	323
Porterhouse, filet mignon	3 ounces	(85 gm)	15	27	323
Stew meat, lean	3 ounces	(85 gm)	11	16	246
Stew meat, typical	3 ounces	(85 gm)	15	27	323

GAME

Venison, rabbit, elk, moose, antelope	3 ounces	(85 gm)	5	5	168
Horsemeat	3 ounces	(85 gm)	5	5	133

The abbreviation *tr.* stands for trace (less than 0.5); the symbol <1 stands for less than one (0.5 to 0.9). Recipes in ***bold italics*** can be found in Part III.

49

TABLE 7 (continued)

	SERVING SIZE		CSI	FAT (GM)	CALORIES
LAMB					
Stew meat, lean	3 ounces	(85 gm)	7	11	189
Chop, rib	3 ounces	(85 gm)	12	17	238
Chop, shoulder	3 ounces	(85 gm)	17	28	323
Ground	3 ounces	(85 gm)	17	28	323
Leg, roast	3 ounces	(85 gm)	10	15	219
Stew meat, typical	3 ounces	(85 gm)	17	28	323
MEAT SUBSTITUTES					
Bacon substitute (Morningstar)	1 ounce	(28 gm)	tr.	3	54
Imitation bacon bits	2 tablespoons	(16 gm)	tr.	3	67
Textured vegetable protein, dehydrated	¼ cup	(24 gm)	tr.	tr.	79
Tofu	2½" x 2½" x 1"	(110 gm)	<1	5	79
Sausage substitute (Morningstar)	1 ounce	(28 gm)	1	5	77
ORGAN MEATS					
Tripe, beef	3 ounces	(85 gm)	5	4	85
Tongue, beef	3 ounces	(85 gm)	9	16	230
Heart, beef	3 ounces	(85 gm)	13	5	160
Chitterlings	3 ounces	(85 gm)	15	24	258
Liver, calf	3 ounces	(85 gm)	16	4	153
Giblets	3 ounces	(85 gm)	18	4	135
Liver, beef or pork	3 ounces	(85 gm)	22	8	161
Liver, chicken	3 ounces	(85 gm)	28	5	133

50

Food	Serving				
Sweetbreads, beef	3 ounces	(85 gm)	28	20	272
Kidney, beef or calf	3 ounces	(85 gm)	39	10	214
Brains, all species	3 ounces	(85 gm)	110	8	117
PORK					
Tenderloin	3 ounces	(85 gm)	5	4	141
Ham, prosciutto	3 ounces	(85 gm)	7	13	192
Chops, center cut	3 ounces	(85 gm)	9	15	227
Ham—center cut, shoulder	3 ounces	(85 gm)	9	18	238
Ham hock	3 ounces	(85 gm)	9	18	238
Pickled pig's feet	3 ounces	(85 gm)	9	14	173
Roast, center cut	3 ounces	(85 gm)	9	15	227
Sausage, link	4 links	(80 gm)	12	25	295
Sausage, patty	3 ounces	(85 gm)	13	26	314
Spareribs, regular and country-style	3 ounces	(85 gm)	13	26	309
Salt pork	3 ounces	(85 gm)	25	60	576
Bacon, Canadian	1 ounce (1½ slices)	(28 gm)	2	2	52
Bacon	1 ounce (4 strips)	(28 gm)	6	14	161
VEAL					
Cutlet	3 ounces	(85 gm)	7	6	176
Roast	3 ounces	(85 gm)	8	8	184
Stew Meat	3 ounces	(85 gm)	8	8	180
Ground	3 ounces	(85 gm)	10	14	229

The abbreviation *tr.* stands for trace (less than 0.5); the symbol <1 stands for less than one (0.5 to 0.9). Recipes in **bold italics** can be found in Part III.

TABLE 7 *(continued)*

	SERVING SIZE		CSI	FAT (GM)	CALORIES
COLD CUTS, BEEF AND PORK					
Thin, pressed	6 slices	(28 gm)	1	1	35
Pastrami, corned beef	2 ounces	(57 gm)	5	5	104
Head cheese	2 ounces	(57 gm)	5	9	120
Salami, beef	2 ounces	(57 gm)	7	11	144
Italian sausage	2 ounces	(57 gm)	7	15	184
Knockwurst	2 ounces	(57 gm)	7	16	174
Bologna	2 ounces	(57 gm)	8	16	180
Polish sausage, kielbasa	2 ounces	(57 gm)	8	16	184
Salami, Genoa (hard)	2 ounces	(57 gm)	9	19	230
Liverwurst	2 ounces	(57 gm)	11	16	184
Braunschweiger	2 ounces	(57 gm)	11	18	204

FISH AND SHELLFISH (COOKED)
(SELECT CSIs OF 9 OR LOWER FOR 3 OUNCES, OR 3 OR LOWER FOR 1 OUNCE)

FISH					
Anchovies, smoked	6 thin fillets	(24 gm)	1	2	50
Herring, pickled	1" x 1" x ½"	(25 gm)	1	5	65
Tuna, canned (water packed)	½ cup	(80 gm)	2	tr.	105
Fish, smoked	3 ounces	(85 gm)	2	4	99

52

Tuna, canned (drained, oil packed)	½ cup	(80 gm)	2	7	158
Salmon, canned	½ cup	(89 gm)	3	5	124
Sashimi (raw tuna)	3 ounces	(85 gm)	3	4	122
White fish (red snapper, halibut, sole, cod etc.)	3 ounces	(85 gm)	3	1	100
Sardines	½ of 3¾-ounce can	(50 gm)	4	6	104
Trout, rainbow	3 ounces	(85 gm)	4	4	128
Salmon, silver (Coho)	3 ounces	(85 gm)	3	6	157
Salmon, Chinook	3 ounces	(85 gm)	7	10	179
Caviar	2 tablespoons	(32 gm)	11	6	81
Squid, octopus	3 ounces	(85 gm)	13	2	103
SHELLFISH*					
Abalone, canned	3 ounces	(85 gm)	2	tr.	68
Scallops	8 one-inch diameter	(80 gm)	2	1	90
Oysters, raw	6 medium	(85 gm)	3	2	61
Clams, canned	½ of 6½-ounce can	(92 gm)	3	2	136
Clams, steamers	25 medium	(85 gm)	3	2	126
Lobster	1½ tails	(85 gm)	3	<1	83
Crabmeat, canned	½ cup	(85 gm)	4	2	87
Oysters, cooked	8 medium	(85 gm)	4	3	81
Crayfish	3 ounces	(85 gm)	8	1	97
Shrimpmeat	⅔ cup	(85 gm)	9	1	84

* Serving size is with shell removed.

The abbreviation *tr.* stands for trace (less than 0.5); the symbol <1 stands for less than one (0.5 to 0.9). Recipes in ***bold italics*** can be found in Part III.

POULTRY (COOKED)
(SELECT CSIs OF 9 OR LOWER FOR 3 OUNCES, OR 3 OR LOWER FOR 1 OUNCE)

	SERVING SIZE		CSI	FAT (GM)	CALORIES
CHICKEN, CORNISH GAME HEN, OR TURKEY					
Light meat (no skin)	3 ounces	(85 gm)	4	3	140
Dark meat (no skin)	3 ounces	(85 gm)	6	7	167
Light meat (with skin)	3 ounces	(85 gm)	6	8	178
Dark meat (with skin)	3 ounces	(85 gm)	7	12	201
Chicken or turkey, ground	3 ounces	(85 gm)	5	5	154
Chicken, canned (boneless)	3 ounces	(85 gm)	5	7	140
Pheasant, wild duck	3 ounces	(85 gm)	8	8	181
Goose, domestic (with skin)	3 ounces	(85 gm)	10	19	259
Duck, domestic (with skin)	3 ounces	(85 gm)	12	24	286
Chicken, giblets	3 ounces	(85 gm)	18	4	135
COLD CUTS, TURKEY & CHICKEN					
Ham	2 ounces	(57 gm)	3	3	73
Pastrami	2 ounces	(57 gm)	3	4	80
Bologna	2 ounces	(57 gm)	5	8	113
Salami	2 ounces	(57 gm)	5	8	113
FRANKFURTER					
Chicken or turkey	1 wiener	(45 gm)	5	8	102

The abbreviation *tr.* stands for trace (less than 0.5); the symbol <1 stands for less than one (0.5 to 0.9). Recipes in **bold italics** can be found in Part III.

CHAPTER

3

Dairy Products and Eggs

SKIM MILK
ICE MILK

Remember those commercials, "Every *body* needs milk?" Well, milk *is* a great food, but *none* of us needs the higher-fat versions that still prevail. Just like the meats that Americans love, milk, cheese, other dairy products, and eggs are also enormously popular components of the present American diet and similarly contribute large amounts of saturated fat and cholesterol to that diet.

Again, there's no need to give up any of these foods entirely. But, to safeguard your health, it is important to make careful and informed choices when it comes to milk, cheeses, ice creams, eggs, and the like.

This chapter will enable you to do precisely that. It's often surprisingly easy to make modifications that will allow you to go on enjoying the taste and texture of dairy products and eggs *without* nearly the amount of risk many of you are now taking.

The following tips and guidelines will help you take the high-CSI "curse" off many of your favorite foods.

Milk, Cream, and Toppings

The whole milk that most Americans drink is 3.5 to 4 percent fat. Some milk cartons proudly claim "3.5 percent fat." To the unwary, that may suggest that much of the fat has been removed or that, at any rate,

55

there's very little fat in the milk; 3.5 percent certainly doesn't sound like much. But, in fact, it's quite a lot: Fully 50 percent of the caloric content of 3.5 percent milk is fat!

Simply by opting for 2 percent milk, you can make some immediate improvement. Consider Figure 2, which graphically illustrates the differences in CSIs of the various milks being sold. The CSI for a cup of whole milk is 7, which translates to a CSI of 11 for the typical 12-ounce glass of milk. Drink three glasses a day and you've racked up a CSI of 33—just from milk alone, not counting any you might use in cooking or on cereal. *Not* a good way to get to Phase One CSI goals (37 for women/children, 49 for men/teens). By switching to milk with 2 percent fat, you reduce your per-cup CSI from 7 to 4.

Once you've adapted to 2 percent, give 1 percent milk a try. Most people can make these changes without great difficulty, but it often takes a week or two to adjust to each reduction. It may help motivate you to learn that, when you go to milk with 1 percent fat, you achieve a per-cup CSI of only 2. If you want to go further yet, consider skim or powdered nonfat milk, both of which have CSIs of less than 1 per cup.

Remember to take this *one step at a time.* People who try to go from whole milk directly to skim or even 1 percent usually go directly *back* to whole milk and then are reluctant to budge. If you are in the habit of using half-and-half on your cereal, go to whole milk before you try any of the lower-fat options. On the other hand, if you're in the habit of using cream on your cereal or, heaven forbid, are drinking the stuff, we advise you to stop that habit *now.* A cup of

typical whipping cream zooms up into the CSI stratosphere with a CSI of 60. And don't be bamboozled by "non-dairy creamers" and the "imitation sour cream" sold in many stores. Even though these may be advertised as "cholesterol-free" or "low in cholesterol," they may contain coconut oil—a highly saturated fat. Some non-dairy creamers have CSIs of 23 per cup. Fortunately, most companies are using soybean oil, so the typical liquid non-dairy creamer has a CSI of 4 per cup, much more accept-

CHOLESTEROL–SATURATED FAT INDEX OF MILK PRODUCTS (1 CUP)

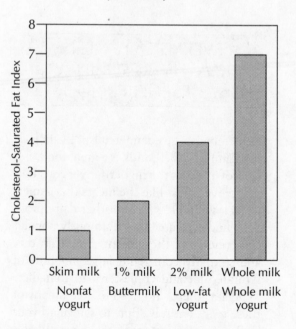

FIGURE 2. The Cholesterol–Saturated Fat Index (CSI) of 1 cup of milk products. A smaller CSI denotes less cholesterol and saturated fat.

able (see Table 8 located at the end of the chapter).

About putting cream in your coffee, the best advise is: *Don't.* But this is not realistic for some people. If you really like a whitener in your coffee, move one step at a time. To give you the facts and help motivate you to make changes, we can tell you that one tablespoon of most liquid non-dairy creamers (now made with soybean oil) has a CSI of 0.3. Doesn't sound like much. However, if you drink 6 cups of coffee a day and add 1 tablespoon of creamer to each cup, your daily intake will provide a CSI of 1.8. If your ultimate goal is to have a daily CSI between 17 and 23, almost 10 percent of your CSI in this case will be taken up with coffee creamer. This means you will have to eat less meat, cheese, ice cream, and chocolate! No wonder we recommend that you use skim or 1 percent fat milk in your coffee. If the cream is still important to you, use one of the liquid non-dairy creamers and make lower CSI choices in other areas.

When it comes to cooking, don't panic if a recipe calls for cream. First try one of the non-dairy creamers with a per-cup CSI of only 4 and then, gradually, substitute 2 percent milk for cream, then 1 percent. Canned evaporated skim milk also works well, because it is more concentrated. You'll be surprised at how well many recipes work without cream. And when you need sour cream (CSI of 18 per half cup) on or in a dish, try light sour cream (CSI of 10 per half cup) or, even better, our *Mock Sour Cream* (see recipe in cookbook section, Part III), which has a CSI of only 2 per half cup.

We all like a little topping on our fruit, other desserts, and baked potatoes. The truth is we like a lot of topping. Our advice is to keep the serving size to no more than ¼ cup and select lower and lower CSI toppings—don't forget nonfat and low-fat plain yogurt. Nonfat or low-fat vanilla yogurt is great on fruit and other desserts, even on strawberry shortcake, and both have very low CSIs.

Say Cheese!

That's right, you can still smile. We're not going to take away the cheese. But making wise choices here is especially crucial. Cheese can be a bit of a challenge and can overwhelm your best intentions if you're not careful. Figure 3 shows you the different CSIs of a variety of cheeses. You may not have heard of some of the lower-CSI choices, but, believe us, they can be your salvation if you're a cheese addict—and many of them are truly delicious. We've found that once people realize there's such a big difference in the fat/cholesterol content of the different cheeses available, they will choose those lower-CSI products more often. Again, gradualism is the key to successful, *permanent* change.

Figure 4 includes the same cheese tips/guidelines we give our patients and participants in our dietary studies. Study these, try them out, and, once you feel you're making progress, try to stick, as much as possible, with those cheeses that have CSIs of *4 or less per ounce.* One ounce of cheese with a CSI of 2 to 4, by the way, is equivalent to 1 ounce of *lean* meat. As previously noted, meat and cheese should be

CHOLESTEROL–SATURATED FAT INDEX OF SELECTED CHEESES (1-OUNCE PORTION)

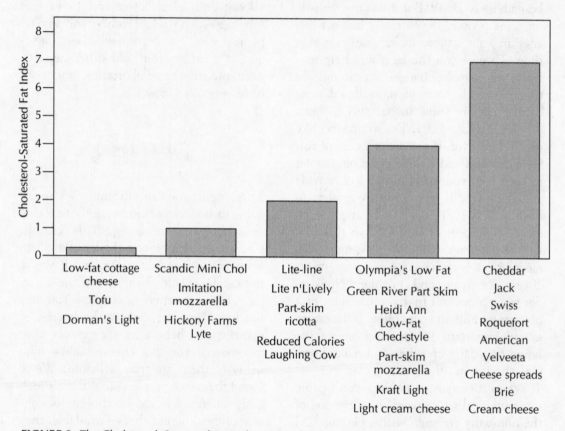

FIGURE 3. The Cholesterol–Saturated Fat Index (CSI) of 1 ounce (28 grams) of selected cheeses. A smaller CSI denotes less cholesterol and saturated fat.

considered *together* in terms of allowable daily intakes. In other words, to attain Phase Two CSI goals, you should consume no more than 6 to 8 ounces of low-CSI meats *and* low-CSI cheeses—combined—daily.

There is great news. Olympia Cheese Company has come out with a very tasty low-fat sharp Cheddar cheese as well as some low-fat flavored cheeses such as jalapeño. (These cheeses may not be available in all sections of the country.) These cheeses have a CSI of 4 per ounce. Because they taste so good, you have to be very careful not to eat too much. These cheeses should be used in small amounts as directed in our recipes, which can be found in Part III.

CHEESE TIPS

1. Cheddar cheese is the cheese of choice for most people. Olympia has a low-fat sharp Cheddar that is very good. There are other somewhat lower-fat choices that are good for cooking but are still too high in fat for snacking. Our favorites include (1) *Olympia's Low Fat Cheese*, (2) *Green River Part Skim Cheese* (we do not recommend the salt-free product), (3) *Kraft Light,* and (4) *Heidi Ann Low-Fat Ched-Style.*

2. *Part-skim mozzarella* is a good cheese to use in place of Cheddar, Jack, or Swiss.

3. *Dorman's Light* or *imitation mozzarella* (made from skim milk and vegetable oil) are even better choices! *Imitation mozzarella* is the cheese that most pizza places have used in Portland, Oregon, for the last fifteen years These cheeses come grated, in slices, and in blocks.

4. *Scandic Mini Chol*—This cheese has the same total *fat* content as Cheddar and Jack but the fat is *soybean oil* so there is much less cholesterol and saturated fat. This is a white cheese that looks very much like Havarti. It melts beautifully! Look for it in the deli section of the supermarket. A low-fat version that we like very much is *Dorman's Light.*

5. *Lite-line* and *Lite n' Lively* are for those who now use cheese slices. We like the Cheddar flavor.

6. For Velveeta lovers, *Scandic Mini Chol* is the choice. It melts very nicely.

7. For those who are looking for a snack or a cheese to spread on bagels or low-fat crackers, *Reduced Calories Laughing Cow* is a must. Our schoolchildren can trade it for anything so it must be good!

8. The *cream cheese* lovers need to know there is no reason ever to buy cream cheese again. Try *Light cream cheese* or *Neufchâtel*—you can't tell the difference. If you want to go even lower in fat try *part-skim ricotta* (not as smooth in texture but is more flavorful. We like it!). Mixed with herbs or fruits it makes a lovely spread for bagels, etc.

9. For cooking: Mix a lower-fat cheese (*Dorman's Light* or *imitation mozzarella*) with higher-fat favorites to get the flavor but not the saturated fat and cholesterol.

10. *Low-fat cottage cheese* is an excellent choice for fillings, or can be whipped in the blender for a mock sour cream. *Tofu* (soybean curd) can also be used as a filling, especially when combined with herbs and seasonings.

11. *Parmesan* is a higher-fat cheese, but since it has a strong flavor it can be used in small amounts for flavoring (1 tsp. to 1 Tbsp. per serving).

12. *Brie, Camembert,* and double-cream *Havarti* are superfatted cheeses that contain more than twice the fat of Cheddar—use these sparingly, if at all!

13. *For the label readers:* For everyday use, consider buying cheeses that contain 6 grams of fat or less per ounce. Cheese made from skim milk and vegetable oil are okay for everyday use even though many contain 6–9 grams of fat per ounce (*Mini Chol, Hickory Farms Lyte*). A *really* low-fat cheese is one that contains 3 grams of fat or less per ounce.

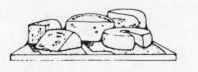

FIGURE 4. Suggestions for selecting cheeses with lower Cholesterol–Saturated Fat Indexes (CSIs).

Ice Cream and Other Frozen Desserts

When the topic of ice cream comes up, most of our patients are *certain* there's not going to be any good news. They're wrong. Yes, many ice creams *do* have some pretty fearsome CSIs, but there *are* better choices among the ice creams; they are not all

equally bad. As usual, the CSI separates the bad guys from the good guys—or at least the better from the worse. (See Figure 5 for a quick overview of the CSIs of frozen desserts.)

The extra-rich gourmet or specialty ice creams (which contain about 18 percent fat) have a per-cup CSI of 30. The cheaper, standard brands are usually about 10 percent fat and have a per-cup CSI of 15.

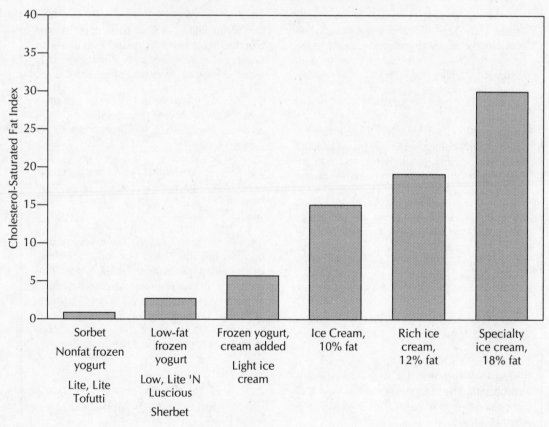

FIGURE 5. The Cholesterol–Saturated Fat Index (CSI) of 1 cup of frozen desserts. A smaller CSI denotes less cholesterol and saturated fat.

Fortunately, there are some gourmet frozen desserts that compare very favorably in taste and texture with even the richest gourmet-brand ice creams. Tofutti is one example and has a per cup CSI of only 3. It is good to use in place of the rich ice creams for special occasions, but not for everyday use because it is high in fat and calories. Light ice cream (ice milk), with a CSI of 6 per cup, is also useful in weaning yourself from higher-fat to lower-fat frozen desserts. Lite Lite Tofutti is an even better choice, with a CSI of less than 1 per cup. (We think the Swiss Almond Tofutti and Chocolate Tofutti are particularly delicious.) Another "lite" frozen dessert is available at Baskin-Robbins. It is called Low, Lite 'N Luscious. It is sugar-free and is sweetened with Nutrasweet. The per-cup CSI is 2.

Word has spread that frozen yogurt is a healthy alternative to ice cream. And, in most cases, it *is*. In some cases, though, cream is being added to the yogurt—so, here too, you must check labels. Some of the cream-added frozen yogurts have CSIs of 6 per cup. You can identify them if the label says a 4-ounce (½ cup) serving contains 4 or more grams of fat. While these are far better choices than ice cream, there are even better choices available. Your best bet is to stick with frozen *nonfat* and *low-fat* yogurts; these have CSIs of almost 0 and 3 per cup. These can be identified if the label says a 4-ounce (½ cup) serving contains 2 or fewer grams of fat. The nonfat frozen yogurt is lower in calories also. It comes in many flavors, including chocolate and vanilla. Our teenager loves it! Ask questions, if you are buying it by the scoop or dish at a frozen yogurt stand. Many are offering nonfat frozen yogurt. The ultimate goal is to select frozen desserts that have a CSI of 3 or lower per cup (8 ounces).

Sherbets and sorbets are other good choices. The typical sherbet has a CSI of 3 per cup, and many sorbets that seem remarkably rich have CSIs of *zero*! You'll find these near or with the gourmet ice creams in your supermarket. Even Haagen-Dazs, the gourmet ice cream maker, is now marketing an excellent raspberry sorbet. Baskin-Robbins has been making a superb line of sorbets for some time. (Try the pineapple and daiquiri flavors.) Vitari is a soft-serve sorbet made from fruit and/or fruit juice. One cup contains 160 Calories and has a per-cup CSI of 0. And there are many other good ones, some imported from Italy, France, and elsewhere. Here again, however, pay attention to labels. There are some sorbets "with cream" that you'll want to avoid. Don't forget that *any* progress you can make toward selecting frozen desserts with CSIs lower than your usual fare is valuable progress.

Eggs and Egg Substitutes

The bad news about eggs is also the good news. As much as 45 percent of all dietary cholesterol for people in the United States used to be derived from eggs alone! That's the bad news. This figure, however, is falling each year. The good news is that if the typical American simply stopped eating egg yolks or products containing them (there's no cholesterol in the whites) he/she could cut cholesterol intake significantly—without making any further dietary change!

The CSI of a single egg yolk is 12. The CSI was computed using the revised lower cholesterol figure for egg yolk (213 milligrams cholesterol per large egg yolk). So if you eat two eggs a day, those alone give you a CSI of 25, leaving very little room for any more fat and cholesterol—from any source—in your diet (that is, if your diet is a healthy one). A typical two-egg omelet without cheese has a CSI of 27, one *with* cheese a CSI of 34 or higher. A half cup of typical egg salad (with mayonnaise) has a CSI of 24. (Refer back to Figure 1 to see how 2 eggs compare with other foods in terms of CSI.)

We don't ask people to give up eggs entirely, only the yolk. We strongly urge you to reduce your intake gradually and to use substitutes as much as possible—and this is one occasion where we suggest you not be *too* gradual. Egg yolks do not fit even into the Phase One CSI goals. When eggs are called for in recipes, do this: *use one and a half or two egg whites in place of each whole egg specified.* This works amazingly well in potato and macaroni salads and in almost all baked goods, including muffins, cakes, cookies, pancakes, and waffles. In most cases, neither you nor your family will be able to tell the difference. And if you don't like the idea of throwing out all those egg yolks, try one of the egg substitutes, which are 99 percent egg white and are very nutritious. Most people would rather consume their CSIs from meat, cheese, and frozen desserts rather than from egg yolk.

THE CSIs OF DAIRY PRODUCTS AND EGGS

Table 8 provides CSIs for all of the individual egg and dairy products.

TABLE 8
THE CSIs OF MILK, CREAM, TOPPINGS; CHEESES; ICE CREAM AND OTHER FROZEN DESSERTS; AND EGGS

Milk, Cream, and Toppings

	SERVING SIZE		CSI	FAT (GM)	CALORIES
MILK (SELECT CSIs OF 2 OR LOWER PER CUP)					
Milk, skim or powdered nonfat	1 cup	(245 gm)	<1	tr.	85
Buttermilk, 1% fat	1 cup	(245 gm)	2	2	98
Milk, 1% fat	1 cup	(244 gm)	2	3	102
Milk, 2% fat	1 cup	(244 gm)	4	5	122
Milk, chocolate, 2% fat	1 cup	(250 gm)	5	7	194
Milk, whole	1 cup	(244 gm)	7	8	149
Milk, skim (evaporated)	1 cup	(256 gm)	<1	<1	200
Milk, whole (evaporated)	1 cup	(252 gm)	15	19	338
Milk, condensed	1 cup	(306 gm)	22	27	982
Coconut milk	1 cup	(240 gm)	46	51	473

The abbreviation *tr.* stands for trace (less than 0.5); the symbol <1 stands for less than one (0.5 to 0.9). Recipes in **bold italics** can be found in Part III.

TABLE 8 (continued)

	SERVING SIZE		CSI	FAT (GM)	CALORIES
OTHER DAIRY BEVERAGES (SELECT CSIs OF 2 OR LOWER PER CUP)					
Cocoa, skim milk, sugar-free	1 cup	(260 gm)	2	2	68
Cocoa, skim milk (Swiss Miss, from vending machine)	1 cup	(264 gm)	2	2	154
Cocoa, whole milk	1 cup	(263 gm)	8	10	217
Instant Breakfast, all flavors, made with skim milk	1 cup	(285 gm)	1	1	215
Instant Breakfast, all flavors, made with whole milk	1 cup	(279 gm)	7	9	279
Egg Nog	1 cup	(246 gm)	tr.	tr.	200
Eggnog, commercial (no alcohol)	1 cup	(254 gm)	16	19	340
YOGURT (SELECT CSIs OF 3 OR LOWER PER CUP)					
Plain:					
Nonfat	1 cup	(227 gm)	<1	tr.	127
Low-fat	1 cup	(227 gm)	3	4	143
Whole Milk	1 cup	(227 gm)	7	8	141
All flavors:					
Nonfat	1 cup	(227 gm)	<1	tr.	200
Low-fat	1 cup	(227 gm)	3	3	250
Whole milk	1 cup	(227 gm)	7	8	275
COTTAGE CHEESE (SELECT CSIs OF 4 OR LOWER PER CUP)					
Dry curd	1 cup	(145 gm)	<1	<1	124
Low-fat (1%)	1 cup	(226 gm)	2	2	163
Low-fat (2%)	1 cup	(226 gm)	4	4	204
Regular	1 cup	(210 gm)	8	9	222

CREAM (SELECT CSIs OF 4 OR LOWER PER CUP)

Evaporated skim milk	1 cup	(256 gm)	<1	<1	200
Liquid non-dairy creamers (soybean oil)	1 cup	(240 gm)	4	24	326
Powdered non-dairy creamer	5⅓ tablespoons*	(32 gm)	11	11	175
Half-and-half	1 cup	(242 gm)	22	28	315
Liquid non-dairy creamers (coconut oil)	1 cup	(240 gm)	23	24	326
Whipping cream	1 cup	(239 gm)	60	74	698

TOPPINGS (SELECT CSIs OF 2 OR LOWER PER ¼ CUP)

Yogurt Dessert Sauce	¼ cup	(57 gm)	<1	<1	61
Low-fat vanilla yogurt	¼ cup	(57 gm)	1	1	50
Dream Whip	¼ cup	(20 gm)	2	3	38
Whipped cream (aerosol can)	¼ cup	(15 gm)	3	4	39
Whipped topping (aerosol can)	¼ cup	(18 gm)	3	4	46
Cool Whip	¼ cup	(19 gm)	4	5	59
Whipped cream, sweetened	¼ cup	(32 gm)	8	9	96
Nonfat plain yogurt	¼ cup	(57 gm)	tr.	tr.	32
Mock Sour Cream	¼ cup	(66 gm)	1	1	55
Sour cream, light (10% fat)	¼ cup	(57 gm)	5	6	90
Sour cream (20% fat)	¼ cup	(60 gm)	9	12	117
Imitation sour cream (store brands, IMO)	¼ cup	(58 gm)	10	11	120

* Equivalent to 1 cup liquid coffee creamer.

The abbreviation *tr.* stands for trace (less than 0.5); the symbol <1 stands for less than one (0.5 to 0.9). Recipes in **bold italics** can be found in Part III.

CHEESES
(SELECT CSIs OF 4 OR LOWER PER OUNCE OR 19 OR LOWER PER CUP GRATED)

	SERVING SIZE		CSI	FAT (GM)	CALORIES
COTTAGE-TYPE CHEESES					
Cottage cheese, dry curd	½ cup	(73 gm)	tr.	tr.	62
Tofu (bean curd)	½ cup	(110 gm)	<1	5	79
Cottage cheese, low-fat (1%)	½ cup	(113 gm)	<1	1	81
Cottage cheese, low-fat (2%)	½ cup	(113 gm)	2	2	102
Cottage cheese, regular (4%)	½ cup	(105 gm)	4	5	111
CHEDDAR AND JACK-TYPE CHEESES					
Dorman's Light*	1 ounce	(28 gm)	<1	5	70
Scandic Mini Chol or Swedish low-fat*	1 ounce	(28 gm)	2	9	113
Olympia's Low-Fat	1 ounce	(28 gm)	4	5	72
Green River Part Skim	1 ounce	(28 gm)	4	5	72
Heidi Ann Low Fat Ched-Style Cheese, Kraft Light Naturals Mild Cheddar	1 ounce	(28 gm)	4	5	80
Swiss	1 ounce	(28 gm)	6	8	107
Cheddar, Monterey Jack, Colby, Havarti, Long Horn	1 ounce	(28 gm)	8	9	114
CHEESE SLICES					
Lite-line	1 ounce	(28 gm)	2	2	51
Lite 'n' Lively	1 ounce	(28 gm)	3	4	74
Kraft Light Naturals (Swiss Reduced Fat)	1 ounce	(28 gm)	4	5	90
American	1 ounce	(28 gm)	7	9	106

VELVEETA-TYPE CHEESES

Mini Chol*	1 ounce	(28 gm)	2	9	113
Velveeta	1 ounce	(28 gm)	5	7	88

CREAM-TYPE CHEESES

Gardenia ricotta, low-fat	2 tablespoons	(30 gm)	<1	1	32
Whipped Honey-Orange Spread	2 tablespoons	(28 gm)	1	2	46
Part-skim ricotta	2 tablespoons	(30 gm)	2	2	39
Light Philadelphia cream cheese	1 ounce	(28 gm)	4	5	60
Neufchâtel (lower-fat cream cheese)	1 ounce	(28 gm)	5	7	74
Cream cheese including whipped	1 ounce	(28 gm)	8	10	99

PIZZA-TYPE CHEESES

Imitation mozzarella*	1 ounce	(28 gm)	1	6	80
Lite part-skim mozzarella	1 ounce	(28 gm)	2	2	60
Part-skim mozzarella	1 ounce	(28 gm)	4	5	72

SNACK AND PARTY-TYPE CHEESES

Hickory Farms Lyte*	1 ounce	(28 gm)	1	6	90
Scandic Mini Chol or Swedish low-fat*	1 ounce	(28 gm)	2	9	113
Reduced Calories Laughing Cow	1 ounce	(28 gm)	2	3	45
String, Lappi	1 ounce	(28 gm)	4	5	72
Cheese spread (jars)	1 ounce	(28 gm)	5	7	88

The abbreviation tr. stands for trace (less than 0.5); the symbol <1 stands for less than one (0.5 to 0.9). Recipes in *bold italics* can be found in Part III.

CHEESES (continued)

	SERVING SIZE		CSI	FAT (GM)	CALORIES
Brie	1 ounce	(28 gm)	6	8	95
Gruyère	1 ounce	(28 gm)	6	8	107
Edam, Limburger, Port du Salut	1 ounce	(28 gm)	8	9	114
Roquefort or blue	1 ounce	(28 gm)	8	9	114
Feta	1 ounce	(28 gm)	8	9	114
GRATED					
Dorman's Light*	1 cup	(114 gm)	2	20	285
Imitation mozzarella*	1 cup	(110 gm)	5	23	310
Scandic Mini Chol*	1 cup	(114 gm)	6	36	454
Kraft Light Naturals Cheddar	1 cup	(114 gm)	16	20	322
Part-skim mozzarella	1 cup	(114 gm)	15	18	290
Green River Part Skim or Olympia's Low-Fat	1 cup	(140 gm)	18	22	356
Parmesan	2 tablespoons	(10 gm)	2	3	46
Parmesan	1 cup	(80 gm)	19	24	365
Cheddar or Monterey Jack	1 cup	(140 gm)	37	46	564

* Cheese made with skim milk and vegetable oil, thus the fat is less saturated than in regular cheeses.

ICE CREAM AND OTHER FROZEN DESSERTS
(SELECT CSIs OF 3 OR LOWER PER CUP)

Soft-serve sorbet (Vitari)	1 cup	(153 gm)	0	0	160
Cranberry Sherbet	1 cup	(160 gm)	0	tr.	162
Sno-cone, Slushie, fruit ice, sorbet	1 cup	(193 gm)	0	0	255
Strawberry Ice	1 cup	(190 gm)	0	<1	240
Frozen yogurt, nonfat	1 cup	(184 gm)	tr.	tr.	224
Pumpkin Frozen Yogurt	1 cup	(234 gm)	tr.	tr.	208
Lite Lite Tofutti	1 cup	(238 gm)	<1	<1	180
Low, Lite 'n' Luscious (Baskin-Robbins)	1 cup	(208 gm)	2	3	214
Frozen yogurt, low-fat	1 cup	(150 gm)	3	4	227
Sherbet	1 cup	(193 gm)	3	4	270
Tofutti*	1 cup	(170 gm)	3	24	420
Ice Milk, typical soft-serve	1 cup	(175 gm)	4	5	224
Mocha Mix Frozen Dessert*	1 cup	(158 gm)	4	14	280
Frozen yogurt, cream added	1 cup	(167 gm)	6	7	240
Light ice cream (ice milk)	1 cup	(150 gm)	6	8	236
Ice cream, store brands (10% fat)	1 cup	(163 gm)	15	18	329
Ice cream, rich (12% fat)	1 cup	(208 gm)	19	24	480
Ice cream, extra rich (18% fat)	1 cup	(208 gm)	30	38	580
Popsicle	One	(75 gm)	0	0	99
Fudgesicle	One	(73 gm)	tr.	tr.	91

* Made with vegetable oil instead of butterfat.

The abbreviation *tr.* stands for trace (less than 0.5); the symbol <1 stands for less than one (0.5 to 0.9). Recipes in **bold italics** can be found in Part III.

69

DESSERTS (continued)

	SERVING SIZE		CSI	FAT (GM)	CALORIES
Jell-O Pudding Pops	One	(1.8 fl. oz.)	2	2	80
Dreamsicle	One	(66 gm)	2	3	104
Ice cream sandwich	One	(62 gm)	4	5	173
Drumstick, Nutti-Buddie	One	(61 gm)	6	10	189
Ice cream bar (chocolate covered)	One	(85 gm)	12	13	224
Ice cream cone (cone only)	One	(12 gm)	tr.	tr.	45

EGGS AND EGG DISHES
(SELECT CSIs OF 2 OR LOWER PER SERVING)

	SERVING SIZE		CSI	FAT (GM)	CALORIES
EGGS					
Whites	Two	(66 gm)	0	0	32
Whole	One	(50 gm)	12	6	79
Yolks	Two	(34 gm)	25	11	125
EGG SUBSTITUTES					
Egg Beaters	¼ cup	(60 gm)	0	0	30
Second Nature	¼ cup	(60 gm)	0	2	49
Scramblers	¼ cup	(60 gm)	0	4	68
Homemade Egg Substitute	¼ cup	(60 gm)	<1	4	70

70

EGG DISHES

Scrambled whites	½ cup	(99 gm)	0	0	48
Scrambled egg substitute	½ cup	(114 gm)	2	8	127
Scrambled eggs, typical	½ cup, 2 eggs	(124 gm)	27	20	244
Egg McMuffin	One	(138 gm)	16	16	340
Sausage McMuffin with egg	One	(165 gm)	24	33	517
Egg, poached or fried with margarine	One	(55 gm)	13	9	113
Spanish Omelet	⅙ recipe	(183 gm)	tr.	1	93
Vegetable Frittata	½ recipe	(272 gm)	2	7	232
Egg omelet, plain	2 eggs	(128 gm)	27	20	244
Egg omelet, cheese	2 eggs	(154 gm)	34	28	349
Egg omelet, ham & cheese	2 eggs	(190 gm)	36	32	413
Deviled egg, made with *"Egg" Salad Sandwich Spread*	½ egg, 2 teaspoons filling	(26 gm)	tr.	tr.	17
Deviled egg, typical	½ egg	(28 gm)	8	6	65

EGG SANDWICHES

"Egg" Salad Sandwich Spread	½ cup	(105 gm)	<1	5	110
Tofu "Egg" Salad	½ cup	(75 gm)	<1	5	66
Egg salad (with mayonnaise)	½ cup	(111 gm)	24	23	252

The abbreviation *tr.* stands for trace (less than 0.5); the symbol <1 stands for less than one (0.5 to 0.9). Recipes in *bold italics* can be found in Part III.

71

Fats, Oils, Margarines, Salad Dressings, Nuts

THE FATS OF LIFE

In this chapter we're going to help you sort out some of the fatty foods that can complicate your life and, in excess, imperil your health. *All* fats, when overused, are bad for you. They pack a lot of calories without much bulk and are thus prime contributors to weight gain and obesity. They are also implicated in some cancers. And, as we've already discussed, the saturated fats, along with cholesterol, are principal culprits in the most pervasive form of heart disease, coronary heart attacks.

It astonishes most people to learn that they consume *tons* of fat over their lifetimes. The typical woman in the United States and Western Europe consumes about 5,000 pounds of fat (two and one-half tons); her male counterpart eats even more—about 7,000 pounds (three and one-half tons). Some eat *twice* this amount. Obviously, there's plenty of room to cut back when it comes to fat. The CSIs will help you do that, but before we get to them, let's review, briefly, the various types of fats:

Cholesterol This special type of fat is usually, but not always, associated with saturated fats of animal origin. Cholesterol in the diet shuts down the LDL receptors in the liver. Less LDL is removed by the liver, thus raising the levels of total cholesterol and LDL cholesterol in the blood. This contributes to blockage of arteries. You've

72

probably heard of "good cholesterol" and "bad cholesterol" that circulate in the blood. These are lipoproteins, composed of fat (lipid) and protein, that carry cholesterol through the water-soluble blood. HDL (high-density lipoprotein) cholesterol is the "good cholesterol" because it helps carry cholesterol *out* of the tissues and out of the body. LDL (low-density lipoprotein) cholesterol, on the other hand, is the "bad cholesterol" because it carries cholesterol *into* the cells of the body, and especially in the arteries. When the LDL cholesterol level is high, cholesterol can build up in the cells of the arterial wall. There are, of course, no lipoproteins in food (no LDL or HDL)—only free cholesterol.

Saturated Fats These are fats that are generally solid at room temperature. These dietary fats can increase the amount of cholesterol that accumulates in the blood. They do this in the same way dietary cholesterol raises the blood cholesterol: by interfering with the action of the liver LDL receptor, which has the chief job of removing LDL cholesterol from the blood. When there is more saturated fat in the diet, less LDL is removed by the liver, thus increasing the LDL cholesterol level in the blood. Some saturated fats also increase the tendency of blood to form clots. Blood clots can block completely an artery that has already narrowed due to atherosclerosis and thus precipitate a heart attack or stroke.

Most animal fats are very highly saturated. Fish and shellfish are the exceptions. They contain a special class of polyunsaturated fats (omega-3) to be discussed later in this chapter. Vegetable oils, for the most part, are much less saturated—but there are exceptions, notably coconut oil, cocoa butter (the fat of chocolate), and palm oil, which are highly saturated. When you see a label that says "contains only vegetable fat" or "contains no cholesterol," be wary. Read the label carefully to see if any of the above listed saturated vegetable oils are included. *The CSIs of these oils, even though they contain no cholesterol, are as high or higher than even those of butter and lard!* Avoid them.

You should also know that when many normally polyunsaturated vegetable oils undergo a process known as *hydrogenation,* they can become highly saturated. But today, most margarines and peanut butters are only lightly hydrogenated, do not contain a lot of saturation, and can be used in moderation. Also, many baked goods, snack crackers, and the like use partially hydrogenated vegetable oils. It is very difficult to tell by the label if these fats have been lightly or highly hydrogenated. We have provided as much specific information as possible about products that are made using partially hydrogenated vegetable oils. This information can be found in the tables at the end of each chapter. There is growing public interest in having the food industry *not* use highly hydrogenated vegetable oils and naturally occurring highly saturated vegetable oils (coconut oil and palm oil) in food products. Having the saturated fat content and the CSI on the label would be helpful.

Monounsaturated Fats The monounsaturated fatty acids are found in both animal and vegetable fats. Olive oil and peanut oil, as well as avocado, are particularly rich sources. Again, the body makes all the monounsaturates it needs; they are not essential in diet. Monounsaturates have long been regarded as "neutral" in terms of their effects on blood cholesterol concentrations, neither raising nor lowering them. Recent studies have indicated, however, that large amounts of dietary monounsaturates in the diet lower blood cholesterol levels in comparison to saturated fats. And there have been reports that people living in the Mediterranean basin, where olive oil is consumed in rather large quantities, have fewer heart attacks than people in the United States and many other countries.

All of this has led some to believe that olive oil should be used in greater amounts. Is this a valid belief? Probably *not*. Olive oil is very low in saturated fatty acids and, to the extent that it is used *in place of* saturated fats, this can be expected to result in lower cholesterol concentrations—but that does not mean the monounsaturates themselves are causing reductions in cholesterol levels. And there are other likely reasons for the lower incidence of heart attacks in the Mediterranean area. The diet there emphasizes fish, beans, fruit, and vegetables and is, overall, low in both saturated fats and cholesterol. It is a low-CSI diet.

All fats need to be limited in the diet, including the monounsaturates and polyunsaturates. The saturated fats, in particular, need to be restricted, but when it comes to fat, of any kind, more is *never* better. We recommend that you use olive oil, if you like it, for salad dressings, and peanut oil for stir-fried dishes. You will probably prefer to use the blander polyunsaturated oils for most of your cooking needs.

Polyunsaturated Fats Unlike the other types of fats we've been discussing, the polyunsaturates are *essential* fatty acids. This means the body can't synthesize them and so they must be obtained directly from the diet. Even though these fats are essential, they should not be consumed in large quantities. The body's need for polyunsaturates can actually be met without adding fat to the diet—by eating low-fat animal products and fruits, vegetables, grains, and beans, which contain the polyunsaturates. So polyunsaturate deficiencies are almost unheard of. Among the most common oils that are high in polyunsaturates are soybean, rapeseed (canola), corn, sunflower, and safflower oils.

Fish Oils See Chapter 2 in Part II for information about the omega-3 fatty acids, a special class of polyunsaturates unique to fish and marine mammals. These fats help reduce blood concentrations of triglyceride and cholesterol. More important, they lessen the body's tendency to form blood clots. Blood clots can block completely the flow of blood through a narrowed artery and cause a heart attack or stroke. But, once again, more is not better. Follow the guidelines for consumption of fish and shellfish and you will get the right amount of oils rich in omega-3 in your diet: Eat fish at least twice a week (serving sizes are 6 ounces of fish, clams, oysters, scallops, *or* 3 to 4 ounces of shrimp, crab, lobster). Note that the fatter fish (e.g., salmon, sardines, etc.) are great to use.

Let's turn now to some of the fatty foods themselves and learn how to keep the lid on them—and our CSIs.

Oils

Vegetable oils tend to be much less saturated than animal fats—except for palm oil and coconut oil (CSIs of 54 and 95 per half cup). So we recommend you use vegetable oils in your cooking—in small amounts because, as you can tell by Table 9 at the end of the chapter, they do contain some saturated fat. We recommend vegetable oils that have CSIs of 9 to 18 per half cup. If you wish to use the oils with the lowest CSIs, that is fine. Of all the vegetable oils, rapeseed oil is especially low in saturated fat. However, if you stick to the amount we recommend for cooking and baking, any of the lower-CSI oils fit into a low-CSI eating style. We feel most people will prefer to use a variety of the oils with CSIs of 9 to 18 per half cup in order to add to their eating pleasure. Check Table 9 at the end of the chapter to determine the CSI of the various vegetable oils. There are many good choices.

Butter and Margarine

One of the easiest ways to reduce your daily CSI is to substitute *soft* margarine for butter. Every teaspoon of butter has a CSI of 3.1. Even the "worst" (hard-stick) type of margarine, by contrast, has a per-teaspoon CSI of only 0.8. The diet, soft-stick, and tub margarines are better choices, with CSIs of 0.3 to 0.7 per teaspoon. Our recent experience is that most margarines have good CSIs, unless they contain butterfat, lard, coconut oil, or palm oil. It is easy to tell—just leave the margarine on the counter overnight. If it is very soft in the morning, the oil has not been highly hydrogenated and the CSI will be between 0.3 and 0.7 per teaspoon.

Start paying attention to the amount of butter you use each day, not only as a spread but also in your cooking and in prepared foods. Butter CSIs add up very quickly. Half a cup of butter has a CSI of 71, compared with a CSI of 15 for half a cup of typical tub or soft-stick margarine. Many people, incidentally, would never think of consuming lard in the quantities that they consume butter. They think of lard as being "pure fat" and butter as healthy and nutritious. But, in reality, a half cup of lard, with a CSI of 46, would actually be less risky than a half cup of butter with a CSI of 71—not that we recommend either one!

The best way to cut back on butter is to use margarine in its place whenever butter is called for in a recipe. Most people are already doing this. Once you've mastered that, start cutting back on the amount of butter you spread on bread and other foods. Then switch to margarine. And once you've eliminated the butter, start limiting the margarine, as well. *Scrape* it on your toast and sandwiches rather than "lard" it on. If you use margarine to brown garlic, onions, other vegetables, or meats, gradually reduce the amounts until you are using only 1 teaspoon to 1 tablespoon.

Some people like to use Butter Buds, which is butter with the fat removed—so the CSI is 0. It is a powder that can be sprinkled on or dissolved in a small amount of water and put on potatoes, other vegetables, or on popcorn (the powder only.)

Mayonnaise and Miracle Whip

We've found that as some people cut back on butter and margarine, they increase their intake of mayonnaise or Miracle Whip by spreading it liberally on sandwiches. That is self-defeating. "Hold the mayo" is still good advice. Those old favorites are both *more than two-thirds fat* and have CSIs of 1.3 and 2.1 per tablespoon. These CSIs may not seem large but they add up very quickly. Fortunately, there are lower-CSI alternatives for both products— CSIs of 0.6 (Miracle Whip Light) and 0.8 (light mayonnaise) per tablespoon. Spread these light mayos very thinly on bread. Try mustard (CSI of almost 0) on your sandwiches. We like hot or Dijon mustard on turkey and tuna sandwiches.

Peanut Butter

Here's another American favorite. The good news is that peanut butter contains absolutely no cholesterol. The bad news is that peanut butter is about 50 percent fat and some of it is saturated. The wise use of peanut butter is for a sandwich—as part of a meal—not as a snack food. The bad use of peanut butter is to eat it off the end of a spoon or a knife (yes, most of us have been guilty of this!). A tablespoon of typical, lightly hydrogenated, peanut butter has a CSI of 1.4, compared with a CSI of 2.1 for a tablespoon of typical soft margarine. Natural peanut butter, the kind in which the

oil comes to the top, has a CSI of 1.1 per tablespoon. The difference in CSI for the two types of peanut butter is minimal, so choose the kind you like. Whether the peanut butter is chunky or smooth doesn't matter; the CSIs are identical.

Shortening, Lard, Bacon Grease

Whenever a recipe calls for shortening (CSI of 26 to 34 per half cup), lard (CSI of 46 per half cup), or bacon grease (CSI of 40 per half cup), substitute a vegetable oil (CSIs of 9 to 18 per half cup) or a soft vegetable shortening (CSI of 26 per half cup). Be aware, however, that some vegetable shortenings are made of *highly hydrogenated* vegetable oils and are, therefore, higher in saturated fat (CSIs of 34 per half cup). Check labels, although the information is not always given. If in doubt, two vegetable shortenings we can recommend are Crisco and Food Club.

Salad Dressings

As people eat more salads, they also *increase* their intake of fatty salad dressings. In order to have more "spread" for your bread, you need to select very low–CSI and very low–fat salad dressings. Fortunately there are a growing number of delicious alternatives that are much healthier. Figure 6 lets you visualize the considerable CSI differences among the various salad dressings. A more detailed listing is given in Table 9 at the end of this chapter.

Mayonnaise and Miracle Whip warrant special consideration because they are often used "as is" in large quantities (several cups at a time) in potato salad, coleslaw, and macaroni or other pasta salads. One cup of mayonnaise has a CSI of 33, and one cup of Miracle Whip has a CSI of 20. One cup of light mayonnaise has a CSI of 12 and one cup of Miracle Whip Light has a CSI of 10—a considerable improvement.

You can do even better by adding increasing amounts of plain nonfat yogurt to dilute the fat. For an example of the ideal combination, see our *Tangy Salad Dressing* recipe in Part III—the CSI is 5 per cup.

Chocolate

Here's a fat—and that's essentially what chocolate is—that many Americans and Western Europeans say they can't live

CHOLESTEROL–SATURATED FAT INDEX OF SALAD DRESSINGS (¼ CUP)

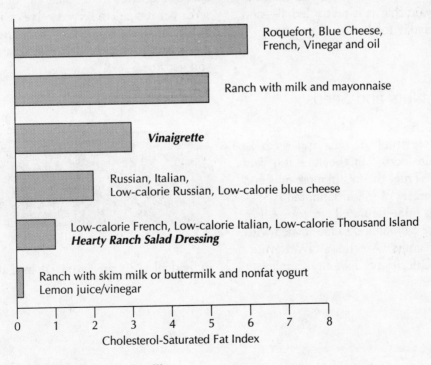

Recipes in **bold italic** can be found in Part III.

FIGURE 6. The Cholesterol–Saturated Fat Index (CSI) of ¼ cup of selected salad dressings.

without. Well, it's not as bad as eating lard, for example, but a single cup of chocolate chips packs a hefty CSI of 36. Many people find carob a satisfying substitute. A cup of carob chips has a CSI of 5, which is *one-seventh* that of chocolate chips. Don't be fooled by butterscotch chips—they have a CSI of 43 per cup.

For baking, we recommend that you use cocoa powder plus oil (CSI of 5 per three tablespoons cocoa plus one tablespoon oil) in place of baking chocolate (CSI of 9 per ounce). Also use chocolate syrup (CSI of less than 1 per quarter cup). But note that chocolate syrup contains a lot of sugar and calories. There will be more about chocolate in the chapter on snacks (Chapter 10) later in Part II. We want you to start becoming aware that it is pretty lethal—and *not* an everyday food.

Nuts and Seeds

Many people think of nuts and seeds as high protein foods, but they are also very high in fat. True, the fats in most nuts and seeds are largely of the unsaturated type— but there is some saturated fat, too. All in all, nuts are *half fat* and so are loaded with calories. Peanuts, America's favorite nut, have 423 Calories per half cup. Sunflower seeds contain 410 Calories per half cup and macadamia nuts 470 Calories per half cup! These facts and the CSIs will help you see the need to use nuts and seeds sparingly— to add crunch to your casseroles, breads, and desserts. The CSI of most nuts is from 3 to 6 per half cup. Chestnuts, which are used in dressings at holiday times, have a CSI of only 1 per half cup. Brazil nuts, with a CSI of 11 per half cup, should be used infrequently. Nuts and seeds are *not* good snack foods. Start using them as a condiment, to spice up salads and vegetable dishes, such as in our recipes for *Crunchy Vegetable Salad* and *Cashew Chicken* (see Part III for recipes). When nuts are called for in a recipe, use *small* amounts—*no more than* one-quarter to one-half cup of nuts or seeds per recipe (to serve twelve or more). Put them on top where they show and leave them in bigger pieces—a real treat when you get one.

THE CSIs OF FATS/OILS/SALAD DRESSINGS/CHOCOLATE/NUTS

Individual CSIs are provided in Table 9.

TABLE 9
THE CSIs OF FATS; SALAD DRESSINGS; CHOCOLATE; AND NUTS

FATS AND SPREADS

	SERVING SIZE		CSI	FAT (GM)	CALORIES
OILS (SELECT CSIs OF 18 OR LOWER PER ½ CUP)					
Rapeseed (Puritan-Canola)	½ cup	(109 gm)	9	109	981
Safflower (Saffola)	½ cup	(109 gm)	10	109	981
Walnut	½ cup	(109 gm)	10	109	981
Sunflower (Sunlite)	½ cup	(109 gm)	11	109	981
Corn (Mazola)	½ cup	(109 gm)	14	109	981
Olive	½ cup	(108 gm)	15	108	972
Sesame	½ cup	(109 gm)	16	109	981
Soybean (Crisco, My-te-Fine, Western Family, Wesson)	½ cup	(109 gm)	16	109	981
Cottonseed/Soybean Mix	½ cup	(109 gm)	17	109	981
Avocado	½ cup	(109 gm)	18	109	981
Peanut (Planter's)	½ cup	(108 gm)	18	108	972
Palm	½ cup	(109 gm)	54	109	981
Coconut	½ cup	(109 gm)	95	109	981
MARGARINE AND BUTTER (SELECT CSIs OF 15 OR LOWER PER ½ CUP, OR 0.7 OR LOWER PER TEASPOON)					
Margarine, diet (40% fat, not recommended for baking)	½ cup	(115 gm)	7	45	400
Margarine, table spread (60% fat, Country Crock)	½ cup	(115 gm)	11	70	621
Margarine, liquid (squeeze type)	½ cup	(113 gm)	15	91	812

The abbreviation *tr.* stands for trace (less than 0.5); the symbol <1 stands for less than one (0.5 to 0.9). Recipes in **bold italics** can be found in Part III.

79

TABLE 9 *(continued)*

	SERVING SIZE		CSI	FAT (GM)	CALORIES
Margarine, tub or soft stick (Saffola, Mazola, Fleischmann's)		(114 gm)	15	91	809
Margarine, hard stick (inexpensive store brands)		(114 gm)	19	91	809
Butter		(114 gm)	71	92	817
Margarine, diet (40% fat)	1 teaspoon	(5 gm)	0.3	2	17
Margarine, table spread (60% fat)	1 teaspoon	(5 gm)	0.5	3	27
Margarine, liquid (squeeze type)	1 teaspoon	(5 gm)	0.7	4	35
Margarine, tub or soft stick	1 teaspoon	(5 gm)	0.7	4	35
Margarine, hard stick (inexpensive store brands)	1 teaspoon	(5 gm)	0.8	4	35
Butter	1 teaspoon	(5 gm)	3.1	4	36
Peanut butter	1 tablespoon	(16 gm)	1.4	8	95

MAYONNAISE AND MIRACLE WHIP (SELECT CSIs OF 0.8 OR LOWER PER TABLESPOON)

Miracle Whip, Light Salad Dressing	1 tablespoon	(14 gm)	0.6	4	45
Miracle Whip Salad Dressing, Cholesterol-free	1 tablespoon	(14 gm)	1.1	7	70
Miracle Whip Salad Dressing, Regular	1 tablespoon	(14 gm)	1.3	7	70
Mayonnaise, Light (Heart Beat)	1 tablespoon	(14 gm)	0.5	4	40
Mayonnaise, Light (Best Foods, Kraft)	1 tablespoon	(14 gm)	0.8	5	50
Mayonnaise (Best Foods, Kraft, Saffola), Cholesterol-free	1 tablespoon	(14 gm)	1.7	11	101
Mayonnaise (Best Foods, Kraft, Saffola), Regular	1 tablespoon	(14 gm)	2.1	11	101

OTHER FATS (SELECT CSIs OF 26 OR LOWER PER ½ CUP)

Peanut Butter	½ cup	(129 gm)	11	66	762

Shortening (Crisco)	½ cup	(103 gm)	26	103	927
Shortening (Fluffo, Snowdrift)	½ cup	(102 gm)	34	103	927
Bacon grease	½ cup	(102 gm)	40	103	927
Lard	½ cup	(102 gm)	46	102	918
Suet (beef fat)	½ cup	(102 gm)	55	102	869

SALAD DRESSINGS AND MAYONNAISE

RANCH-TYPE SALAD DRESSINGS (SELECT CSIs OF 3 OR LOWER PER 4 TABLESPOONS-QUARTER CUP)

Ranch with skim milk or buttermilk and nonfat yogurt	4 tablespoons	(59 gm)	tr.	tr.	28
Hearty Ranch Salad Dressing	4 tablespoons	(62 gm)	<1	3	51
Western Salad Dressing	4 tablespoons	(62 gm)	1	3	51
Ranch-type salad dressing (typical)	4 tablespoons	(59 gm)	5	23	213
Russian, low-calorie	4 tablespoons	(65 gm)	2	3	92
Russian Salad Dressing	4 tablespoons	(60 gm)	1	9	100
Russian salad dressing, typical	4 tablespoons	(59 gm)	2	12	180
Fresh Ginger Salad Dressing	4 tablespoons	(58 gm)	<1	4	76

The abbreviation *tr.* stands for trace (less than 0.5); the symbol <1 stands for less than one (0.5 to 0.9). Recipes in **bold italics** can be found in Part III.

SALAD DRESSINGS AND MAYONNAISE (continued)

	SERVING SIZE		CSI	FAT (GM)	CALORIES
Vinaigrette Salad Dressing					
Oil & vinegar salad dressing	4 tablespoons	(55 gm)	3	21	196
French salad dressing, low-calorie	4 tablespoons	(62 gm)	6	32	287
Red French Salad Dressing	4 tablespoons	(65 gm)	<1	4	87
French salad dressing, typical	4 tablespoons	(62 gm)	1	8	148
Thousand Island Salad Dressing	4 tablespoons	(63 gm)	6	25	267
Thousand Island salad dressing, low-calorie	4 tablespoons	(56 gm)	1	3	68
Thousand Island salad dressing, typical	4 tablespoons	(61 gm)	1	7	97
Blue cheese, low-calorie	4 tablespoons	(59 gm)	4	20	240
Roquefort/blue cheese salad dressing, typical	4 tablespoons	(61 gm)	2	4	46
Italian salad dressing, low-calorie	4 tablespoons	(61 gm)	6	32	280
Italian salad dressing, typical	4 tablespoons	(60 gm)	1	6	63
	4 tablespoons	(59 gm)	2	16	180

MAYONNAISE AND MIRACLE WHIP (SELECT CSIs OF 12 OR LOWER PER CUP)

	SERVING SIZE		CSI	FAT (GM)	CALORIES
Tangy Salad Dressing	1 cup	(240 gm)	5	11	224
Mayonnaise, Light (Heart Beat)	1 cup	(224 gm)	7	64	640
Miracle Whip, Light Salad Dressing	1 cup	(224 gm)	10	64	720
Mayonnaise, Light (Best Foods, Kraft)	1 cup	(224 gm)	12	80	800
Miracle Whip Salad Dressing, Cholesterol-free	1 cup	(224 gm)	17	112	1,120
Miracle Whip Salad Dressing, Regular	1 cup	(224 gm)	20	112	1,120
Mayonnaise (Best Foods, Kraft, Saffola), Cholesterol-free	1 cup	(224 gm)	26	175	1,584
Mayonnaise (Best Foods, Kraft, Saffola), Regular	1 cup	(224 gm)	33	175	1,584

CHOCOLATE (BAKING)
(SELECT CSIs OF 5 OR LOWER PER SERVING)

	SERVING SIZE		CSI	FAT (GM)	CALORIES
BAKING CHIPS					
Carob chips	1 cup	(170 gm)	5	10	695
Chocolate chips	1 cup	(170 gm)	36	60	898
Butterscotch chips	1 cup	(170 gm)	43	53	903
BAKING CHOCOLATE					
Carob powder	¼ cup	(28 gm)	0	tr.	106
Cocoa powder, unsweetened	¼ cup	(28 gm)	4	7	84
Cocoa powder plus oil (to equal one ounce chocolate)	3 Tbsp. cocoa & 1 Tbsp. oil	(35 gm)	5	19	187
Chocolate, baking (sweet/German)	1 ounce	(28 gm)	6	10	148
Chocolate, baking (unsweetened)	1 ounce	(28 gm)	9	15	143
CHOCOLATE SAUCE					
Syrup type (canned)	¼ cup	(76 gm)	<1	2	211
Fudge type	¼ cup	(76 gm)	7	10	251

The abbreviation *tr.* stands for trace (less than 0.5); the symbol <1 stands for less than one (0.5 to 0.9). Recipes in **bold italics** can be found in Part III.

83

NUTS AND SEEDS
(SHELLED)

	SERVING SIZE	CSI	FAT (GM)	CALORIES
Chestnuts	½ cup (72 gm)	1	3	269
Poppyseeds	½ cup (67 gm)	3	30	357
Filberts	½ cup (68 gm)	3	43	430
Pecans	½ cup (54 gm)	3	37	360
Walnuts	½ cup (50 gm)	3	31	321
Almonds	½ cup (71 gm)	4	37	418
Pistachios	½ cup (64 gm)	4	31	369
Sunflower seeds	½ cup (72 gm)	4	36	410
Sesame seeds	½ cup (64 gm)	5	35	376
Peanuts	½ cup (73 gm)	5	36	423
Cashews	½ cup (65 gm)	6	31	374
Mixed nuts	½ cup (72 gm)	6	41	444
Pine nuts	½ cup (60 gm)	6	37	341
Pumpkin seeds	½ cup (69 gm)	6	32	373
Macadamia	½ cup (67 gm)	7	49	470
Brazil	½ cup (70 gm)	11	46	459

The abbreviation *tr.* stands for trace (less than 0.5); the symbol <1 stands for less than one (0.5 to 0.9). Recipes in **bold italics** can be found in Part III.

Fruits, Vegetables, Grains, Beans, Fiber

THE NO-CSI, LOW-CSI, HIGH-FIBER FOODS

As you begin cutting back on higher-CSI foods, and using lower-CSI meat, cheese, eggs, and dairy products, you'll be getting fewer calories and will need something to fill the void. That something is what this chapter is about: the no-CSI and very low–CSI foods—fruits, vegetables, grains, and beans. These are foods rich in complex carbohydrates and fiber, excellent choices for disease prevention, overall good health, energy and weight control.

That's right—weight control. Many people still think of carbohydrates as fattening, but this is a mistaken assumption. How did innocent carbohydrates get this bad reputation? For the most part, it's been guilt by association: homespun pasta, simple rice, pure potatoes corrupted by reckless sour cream and butter sauces, naive beans and grains led blindly into high-fat crimes by cheesy cons such as Cheddar and Swiss.

Clearly, it will do no good to switch to carbohydrates if you bury them in fat. But take a little care and even the most criminal carbohydrate dish can be rehabilitated. You'll find many examples of "cleaned-up" carbs in our cookbook section, Part III. The trick is simply to use low-fat cheeses, yogurt, and smaller amounts of leaner meats in traditional carbohydrate dishes, such as macaroni salad, spaghetti, lasagna. These dishes—we guarantee you—will still be delicious, and they will be far more healthful.

One of our major goals, as we cut the

fat, is to increase carbohydrate intake from 45 percent of calories (typical of the current American diet) to 60 to 65 percent of all calories. There are three general types of carbohydrate: sugars (the "simple" carbohydrates), starches (the "complex" carbohydrates, so called because they are much larger molecules than the sugars), and fiber (similar to starches but not digestible by humans). Your goal is to eat more of the complex starches and fibers and less of the sugars. Fiber is what gives complex carbohydrates bulk, enabling you to fill up without filling out. Fiber, which has no calories (because it is not metabolized by the body), absorbs water in the intestinal tract and becomes bulkier yet. (It is a good cure for constipation.)

High–complex carbohydrate foods, by the way, are excellent sources of protein—of plant rather than animal origin. Foods rich in plant proteins are, in many ways, superior to foods rich in animal proteins since they contain no cholesterol, are very low in fat, and contribute all of the vital amino acids that the body needs and many vitamins, minerals, and fiber. They are excellent sources of long-lasting energy. Athletes take note!

Meeting the Carbohydrate Goals

Here are some goals to aim for; *don't* try to meet these all at once. Take your time and adapt gradually.

Whole Grains, Breads, Potatoes Most Americans presently eat only one food containing significant amounts of complex car-

bohydrates per meal—a potato, a slice of bread, a bowl of cereal, etc. To attain your CSI goals, we advise you to eat *at least two* such foods per meal. This is not as difficult as it may sound. For example, you can eat whole-grain toast *and* cereal at breakfast; a sandwich *and* bean soup at lunch; bread *and* pasta at dinner; popcorn, muffins, bagels, low-fat crackers for snacks. Women and children need fewer calories, so should eat smaller-sized servings. Men and teens will need to eat larger-sized servings to obtain enough energy (calories).

Most of us are unaware of the many grains used in the cuisines of the world. Rice and wheat are staples of the U.S. cuisine. Begin to add "new" grains to your diet, and your eating style will become more interesting—bulgur, barley, couscous, cornmeal, wild rice, acini, and orzo. If these sound like names from a word game to you and you have no idea how to use them, don't worry. We will give you many ideas for using these grains in later chapters, and the recipes can be found in Part III. We even have a delicious recipe for *Cornmeal Pancakes*.

Beans and Peas Gradually increase your intake to 3 to 5 cups of cooked beans, lentils, and peas *each week*. (The lower amounts apply to women/children, the higher to men/teens.) Here, in particular, you need to go slowly. Almost everyone can adapt to beans if they give their digestive systems a chance to get used to them. One way to start out is to add 2 to 4 tablespoons of garbanzo or kidney beans to green salads several times a week. Put a few beans in the soup. Add a few beans to the casserole. Get a bean burrito. Small amounts of beans eaten almost daily will get you to

TABLE 10
HOW TO MEET YOUR WEEKLY BEAN QUOTA

	CUPS OF BEANS PER WEEK	
	Women/Children	Men/Teens
Appetizers		
Bean Dip with **Baked Corn Chips**	¼	½
Hummous with **Pita Chips**	¼	½
Soups		
Split pea soup	½	¾
Rick's Chili	½	¾
Salads		
Tossed salad with		
Kidney beans	⅛	¼
Garbanzo beans	⅛	¼
Spicy Black Bean Salad	⅓	⅔
Main Dishes		
Your Basic Bean Burrito	½	1
Bean Hot Dish	⅓	⅔
TOTAL (cups of beans)	3	5⅓

Recipes in **bold italics** can be found in Part III.

your goal. It's definitely worth the effort because beans are among the most nutritious foods on the planet and are used in the cooking of nearly all cultures. Table 10 shows you how you can easily meet your weekly bean quota.

Vegetables   In a sound dietary program to prevent heart disease and cancer, vegetables are of great importance. Vegetables have always been a predominant part of the human diet, dating back to prehistoric times. The earliest humans were hunter/gatherers, seeking out and eating plant foods as they became ripe. Tens of thousands of different species of plants grow on the land and in the oceans, forming the base of the food chains for all animal and human life. Plants manufacture carbohydrates through photosynthesis, make amino acids and proteins, and are also the major sources of vitamins, minerals, and many other nutrients the body requires.

There are many reasons why plants and vegetables help prevent heart disease, cancer, and other disorders of overconsumption. Vegetables are nearly always low in calories and can be consumed in almost any amount that matches the appetite. They are filling but not fattening. They can be prepared in innumerable ways and need never become boring or monotonous. In addition to being rich sources of all known nutrients, vegetables contain other valuable health-protecting ingredients, more and more of which are being discovered all the time. Among these constituents, recently coming into prominence, are the saponins. Saponins are widespread in the plant kingdom and have the ability to inhibit absorption of dietary cholesterol from the intestinal tract. In this capacity they lower blood LDL cholesterol levels and help prevent atherosclerosis.

Vegetables also contain large quantities of substances that inhibit the development of cancer. The cruciferous vegetables, of which there are some four thousand species, including cauliflower, broccoli and turnips, are particularly important in this regard. Broccoli is rapidly becoming America's favorite vegetable. The protective factors in the cruciferous vegetables have not yet all been identified. Beta carotene is one substance found in vegetables (especially carrots) that definitely helps protect against some cancers. Ascorbic acid (vitamin C) and folic acid are similarly found in large amounts in many vegetables, and these, too, have been found to inhibit some cancers.

Thomas Jefferson, who favored rich French cooking when he was younger, modified his culinary tastes as he aged, noting "Like my friend the Doctor [i.e., Benjamin Rush] I have lived temperately, eating little animal food and that not as an aliment [main course], so much as a condiment for the vegetables which constitute my principal diet." Modern science is bearing out the wisdom of Jefferson's diet, a diet that prolongs life and productivity.

Women and children should eat 1½ to 2½ cups of vegetables per day. Men and teens need 2½ to 4 cups per day. These can be fresh, frozen, or canned. Be creative with your vegetables. Mix them into pastas, rice, and bean dishes, use them in soups, make kabobs of them, get into stir-frying. And, remember, *don't* take one step forward and two backward by smothering your vegetables in fatty salad dressings, sour

TABLE 11
HOW TO MEET YOUR DAILY VEGETABLE GOALS

	WOMEN/CHILDREN	MEN/TEENS
Lunch	Salad bar— 1 cup lettuce ½ cup vegetables	Salad Bar— 2 cups lettuce ¾ cup vegetables
Dinner	Broccoli— 1 cup	Broccoli— 1¼ cups
TOTAL	2½ cups	4 cups

cream, and other high-CSI outlaws. Table 11 provides just one way you can meet your vegetable goals.

Fruits This one is simple. Eat 3 to 5 pieces of fruit a day. Dried, fresh, and frozen are fine, but if you go for the canned variety, avoid those in high-calorie sweetened syrups (or, if you must use these, drain and rinse them before eating). Most fruits have CSIs of almost zero. Three exceptions are avocados (CSI of 1 per ¼ avocado or 4 per avocado), olives (CSI of 1 per ½ cup), and coconut (with a shocking CSI of 12 per ½ cup).

Fiber One of the most effective ways of reducing your daily CSI is to increase your fiber intake. Most Americans consume only 15 to 20 grams of dietary fiber daily. You should be consuming 35 to 50 grams per day. (On the basis of new scientific findings, we decreased the fiber goal slightly from our previous book, *The New American Diet*.) Dietary fibers, found only in plant foods, are indigestible carbohydrates (some soluble, some insoluble) that add bulk to the diet without calories and thus help prevent weight gain. Dietary fibers also help prevent certain cancers, diverticulosis, constipation, and some other disorders. There is also good evidence that soluble fibers—for example, oat bran and beans—help lower blood cholesterol levels.

We recommend gradually increasing both soluble and insoluble fibers. Soluble fibers help lower the blood cholesterol level, insoluble fibers help prevent constipation. Most people can adjust to increased fiber intakes. The key is to increase your intake *slowly and drink plenty of water*. As first steps, put a few beans in soups, find new dessert recipes using fruit, and eat oatmeal for breakfast several times a week.

There are other ways to get the daily recommended 35 to 50 grams of fiber from foods:

- Adding 3 or 4 cups of oat bran or 1 to 2 cups of beans to the daily diet (this can quickly become monotonous, so read on).
- Eating oat muffins (but at 3½ to 5 grams of fiber per muffin, one would need to consume 7 to 14 muffins a day in addition to other foods, so this isn't too practical, either).

- *Eating a large variety of foods that all contain soluble fiber*: fruits, vegetables, grains, and beans. This is the most enjoyable way, and also the best way to secure the benefits of the many types of fibers.

Approximately one-third of our recipes contain 3 or more grams of dietary fiber per serving. Many contain much more than that. It makes sense to consume a variety of foods as part of an overall low-CSI eating style as shown in the two sample menus in Table 12. You don't have to make a special effort to eat a high-fiber diet if you eat from the food groups containing whole grains, fruits (not juice), vegetables, and beans.

THE CSIs OF FRUITS, VEGETABLES, GRAINS, BEANS

Table 13 (page 11) provides you with the CSIs of individual foods.

TABLE 12
HOW TO INCREASE YOUR FIBER INTAKE: TWO SAMPLE MENUS

Sample Menu One

		FIBER (gm)
Breakfast		
Vegetable Frittata	½ recipe	6
Blueberries	½ cup	3
Snack		
Pumpkin-Oat Muffin	1	4
Lunch		
Lasagna Primavera	1/12 recipe	4
Whole Wheat French Bread	1/5 loaf	3
Banana	1	2
Dinner		
Hot and Sour Soup	1 cup	<1
Cashew Chicken	¼ recipe	4
White rice	1½ cups	3
Baked Apple	1	4
Snack		
Popcorn	3 cups	1
	TOTAL	**35**

Sample Menu Two

		FIBER (gm)
Breakfast		
Oatmeal Buttermilk Pancakes	3	6
Grapefruit	½	2
Snack		
Cereal Bran Muffin	1	4
Lunch		
Navy Bean Soup	1 cup	6
Soda crackers	6	1
Carrot sticks	½ cup	1
Apple	1	3
Snack		
Bean Dip	¼ cup	6
Baked Corn Chips	1 cup	2
Dinner		
Lively Lemon Roll-ups	1/5 recipe	5
Sunshine Spinach Salad	1½ cups	3
Whole Wheat French Bread	1/5 loaf	3
Depression Cake	3" x 3" piece	3
Snack		
Popcorn	3 cups	1
	TOTAL	**46**

Recipes in **bold italics** can be found in Part III. The symbol <1 stands for less than one (0.5 to 0.9). The first menu above contains approximately 1,600 Calories; the other approximately 1,900 Calories. Both contain substantial amounts of fiber. You should add drinks, low-fat dairy products, small amounts of margarine, etc., to complete the menus and reach the appropriate calorie levels optimal for your daily diet.

TABLE 13
THE CSIs OF BEANS; BREADS AND TORTILLAS; FRUITS; GRAINS; AND VEGETABLES

BEANS (LEGUMES) COOKED
(SELECT CSIs OF 1 OR LOWER)

	SERVING SIZE		CSI	FAT (GM)	CALORIES
Beans, no fat added (navy, pinto, kidney, black, etc.)	½ cup	(90 gm)	tr.	1	106
Lentils, split peas, no fat added	½ cup	(100 gm)	tr.	1	115
Garbanzo (chick peas), black-eyed peas	½ cup	(124 gm)	tr.	3	212
Soybeans	½ cup	(90 gm)	<1	5	117
Tofu (bean curd)	½ cup	(110 gm)	<1	5	79
Pork and beans (canned)	½ cup	(128 gm)	1	4	155
BAKED					
Rancher's Beans	½ cup	(119 gm)	tr.	tr.	171
Classic Baked Beans	½ cup	(95 gm)	tr.	1	115
Baked beans with ham	½ cup	(128 gm)	3	6	192
REFRIED					
Black Beans with 1000 Uses	½ cup	(106 gm)	tr.	tr.	63
Refried Beans	½ cup	(87 gm)	<1	3	113
Refried beans (canned)	½ cup	(121 gm)	<1	2	124
Refried beans (typical restaurant)	½ cup	(122 gm)	6	14	243

The abbreviation *tr.* stands for trace (less than 0.5); the symbol <1 stands for less than one (0.5 to 0.9). Recipes in *bold italics* can be found in Part III.

91

BEANS (LEGUMES) COOKED *(continued)*

	SERVING SIZE		CSI	FAT (GM)	CALORIES
DIPS					
Bean Dip	¼ cup	(64 gm)	tr.	1	59
Jalapeño dip	¼ cup	(69 gm)	2	4	83
SOUPS					
Greek Lentil	1 cup	(255 gm)	tr.	1	149
Greek-Style Garbanzo	1 cup	(217 gm)	tr.	4	156
Navy Bean	1 cup	(163 gm)	tr.	<1	79
Split Pea	1 cup	(240 gm)	tr.	1	106
Black Bean Chili	1 cup	(244 gm)	<1	4	277
Minestrone	1 cup	(244 gm)	1	3	83
Rose Bowl Chili	1 cup	(267 gm)	2	5	213
Split pea, lentil, etc.	1 cup	(250 gm)	2	6	170

BREADS AND TORTILLAS
(SELECT CSIs OF 1 OR LOWER PER SERVING)

YEAST BREADS					
White	1 slice	(25 gm)	tr.	<1	68

92

Whole wheat	1 slice	(29 gm)		tr.		<1	70
Raisin	1 slice	(23 gm)		tr.		<1	61
Rye	1 slice	(29 gm)		tr.		tr.	70
Pumpernickel	1 slice	(25 gm)		tr.		tr.	62
English muffin	One	(57 gm)		tr.		1	135
Whole Wheat French Bread	1/5 loaf	(38 gm)		tr.		<1	125
Grape-nut Bread	1 slice or roll	(42 gm)		tr.		1	99
French, Italian, sourdough	4¼" x 2¾" x 1"	(30 gm)		tr.		tr.	83
Pita or pocket	One	(64 gm)		tr.		<1	180
Boston brown	1 slice	(48 gm)		tr.		<1	101
Cinnamon swirl	1 slice	(22 gm)		tr.		<1	59
Egg	1 slice	(33 gm)		2		2	89
Cheese	1 slice	(29 gm)		2		3	87
Challah	1 slice	(33 gm)		2		2	89
Focaccia	1/8 loaf	(60 gm)		1		5	190
Boboli	1/8 loaf	(60 gm)		2		8	183
YEAST ROLLS							
Hard	1 small	(25 gm)		tr.		<1	77
Kaiser	One	(50 gm)		tr.		2	153
Caraway Dinner Roll	One	(48 gm)		tr.		<1	108
Pan or dinner-type	One	(28 gm)		<1		2	83
Poor boy or submarine	3" x 11½"	(135 gm)		1		4	385
Crescent	One	(28 gm)		3		6	101

The abbreviation *tr.* stands for trace (less than 0.5); the symbol <1 stands for less than one (0.5 to 0.9). Recipes in **bold italics** can be found in Part III.

BREADS AND TORTILLAS *(continued)*

	SERVING SIZE		CSI	FAT (GM)	CALORIES
Croissant	One	(55 gm)	9	12	167
TORTILLAS					
Corn, plain	5¾" diameter	(23 gm)	tr.	<1	52
Taco or tostada shell, fried	5½" diameter	(14 gm)	1	3	63
Flour, plain	7½" diameter	(38 gm)	1	3	118
Flour, fried	7½" diameter	(43 gm)	3	8	162
BAGELS					
Plain or flavored	One	(75 gm)	tr.	2	225
Egg	One	(75 gm)	2	4	225
MUFFINS AND SCONES					
Blueberry Bran Muffin	One	(89 gm)	tr.	<1	146
Cereal Bran Muffin	One	(59 gm)	<1	4	116
A Barrel of Muffins	One	(43 gm)	<1	4	105
Poppyseed Muffin	One	(62 gm)	<1	5	163
Nutty Orange Muffin	One	(63 gm)	<1	5	167
Mexican Cornbread Muffin	One	(74 gm)	<1	4	165
Pumpkin Oat Muffin	One	(82 gm)	<1	4	177
Applesauce Oatmeal Muffin	One	(59 gm)	<1	5	157
Dutchy Crust Muffins or Coffee Cake	One	(64 gm)	<1	5	181
Cinnamon Rhubarb Muffin	One	(50 gm)	<1	4	140
Typical plain muffin	One	(55 gm)	2	6	149
Oatmeal Raisin Muffin	One	(47 gm)	<1	4	137

	Serving	Weight			
Oatmeal raisin muffin, typical	One	(61 gm)	2	6	164
Yogurt Scone	One	(60 gm)	<1	3	136
Fruit Scone	One	(39 gm)	<1	4	107
QUICK BREADS					
Grandma Kirschner's Date Nut Bread	½" slice	(61 gm)	tr.	4	209
Pumpkin Harvest Loaf	½" slice	(38 gm)	<1	4	163
Lemon Nut Bread	½" slice	(58 gm)	<1	5	153
Cornbread	2" x 4" x 2"	(78 gm)	<1	6	180
Fruit Bread	½" slice	(55 gm)	<1	4	151
Orange Walnut Bread	½" slice	(55 gm)	<1	4	166
Banana Nut Bread	½" slice	(66 gm)	<1	4	142
Whole Wheat Quick Bread	½" slice	(36 gm)	<1	2	93
Nut bread	½" slice	(58 gm)	2	10	199
Zucchini bread (no nuts)	½" slice	(45 gm)	3	9	172
Pumpkin bread (no nuts)	½" slice	(45 gm)	4	5	161
Cornbread, typical	3" x 3" x 1"	(59 gm)	5	8	190
MISCELLANEOUS					
Breadstick, plain	One 7½"	(11 gm)	tr.	tr.	30
Hamburger or hot dog bun	One	(40 gm)	<1	2	114
Breadcrumbs, commercial	½ cup	(50 gm)	<1	2	195
Lefse	1 serving	(38 gm)	1	3	78
Croutons, commercial	½ cup	(18 gm)	3	4	89
Popover	One	(40 gm)	5	4	92

The abbreviation *tr.* stands for trace (less than 0.5); the symbol <1 stands for less than one (0.5 to 0.9). Recipes in **bold italics** can be found in Part III.

95

FRUITS
(SELECT CSIs OF LESS THAN 1)

	SERVING SIZE	CSI	FAT (GM)	CALORIES
Fruits, most varieties:	1 medium piece, 1 cup melon or berries, ½ cup grapes, ½ cup canned fruit, ½ cup juice, ¼ cup dried	tr.	tr.	60
Avocado	¼ (50 gm)	1	8	84
Olives, green	½ cup (70 gm)	1	9	81
Olives, black	½ cup (70 gm)	1	10	97
Coconut, raw	½ cup (40 gm)	12	13	142

GRAINS (COOKED)
(SELECT CSIs OF 1 OR LOWER PER CUP)

RICE				
White	1 cup (205 gm)	tr.	tr.	223
Brown	1 cup (150 gm)	tr.	<1	179
Wild	1 cup (212 gm)	tr.	<1	189

WHEAT

Couscous	1 cup	(146 gm)	tr.	tr.	164
Bulgur	1 cup	(135 gm)	<1	tr.	227
Macaroni or spaghetti	1 cup	(130 gm)	<1	tr.	192
Lasagna or manicotti noodles	1 cup	(87 gm)	tr.	tr.	129
Egg noodles	1 cup	(160 gm)	2	3	200

MISCELLANEOUS

Barley	1 cup	(150 gm)	<1	tr.	203
Millet	1 cup	(135 gm)	2	tr.	262
Chow mein noodles	1 cup	(45 gm)	11	4	220

FLOUR

Wheat, white	1 cup	(115 gm)	1	tr.	419
Whole wheat	1 cup	(120 gm)	2	tr.	400
Rye	1 cup	(88 gm)	2	tr.	308
Cornmeal	1 cup	(138 gm)	2	tr.	491

VEGETABLES
(SELECT CSIs OF 1 OR LOWER PER SERVING)

Vegetables (carrots, celery, green beans, tomatoes, broccoli, cauliflower, etc.) cooked	½ cup	(93 gm)	tr.	tr.	25
raw	1 cup	(123 gm)	tr.	tr.	25
Vegetables (peas, corn, potatoes, winter squash, hominy, etc.)	½ cup	(80 gm)	tr.	tr.	65
Leafy vegetables (lettuce, spinach, etc.), raw	1 cup	(55 gm)	tr.	tr.	10

The abbreviation *tr.* stands for trace (less than 0.5); the symbol <1 stands for less than one (0.5 to 0.9). Recipes in **bold italics** can be found in Part III.

CHAPTER

6

Breakfast

THE CSI OF CHAMPIONS

So far we've been talking about major food groups and daily CSI goals. Another way to approach dietary change is meal-by-meal. Table 14 shows you one way you might distribute your CSIs among the three daily meals and snacks. This is just one possible distribution. Obviously, if you like a big breakfast and usually have only a very light lunch, then your distribution will be different. But the pattern suggested in Table 14 is one that approximates the eating habits of many people—those who favor a light breakfast, moderate lunch, and heavier dinner.

Of course, even a breakfast that is "light" by some standards can deliver a

staggering CSI. The CSI of a breakfast that includes eggs and bacon, for example, can easily exceed 30—a far cry from the CSI of 1 to 5½ that we are suggesting for breakfast. Are we daft? How can someone eat a breakfast worthy of the name and come up with a total CSI that is between 1 and 4 for women and children and between 1½ and 5½ for men and teens?

Easy. Table 15 provides several examples. These are truly the breakfasts of champions. (These sample breakfasts provide amounts for women and children. Men and teens need about one-third more than the amounts listed.)

Actually, many Americans have learned, over the last twenty years, how to have breakfast *without* "eggs and bacon." They eat cereal, toast, pancakes, fruit, and so on. You will probably find our breakfast

TABLE 14
THE CHOLESTEROL–SATURATED FAT INDEX (CSI) DAILY GOALS*

	BREAKFAST	LUNCH	DINNER	SNACKS	TOTAL
Women/Children	(2,000 Calories)				
CSI American Diet	5	12	28	6	51
CSI Phase One	4	9	20	4	37
CSI Phase Two	2	5	18	3	28
CSI Phase Three	1	3	11	2	17
Men/Teens	(2,800 Calories)				
CSI American diet	8	18	35	8	69
CSI Phase One	5½	12½	24½	5½	48
CSI Phase Two	3	7	22	4	36
CSI Phase Three	1½	4	15½	3	24

* This is only one of many possible daily CSI distributions.

suggestions more familiar than our lunch and dinner suggestions—and may find your way to Phase Three breakfast eating pretty quickly. Also, you will be surprised to see that a breakfast can go from a CSI of 1, using a cup of skim milk, to a CSI of 2— just by using a cup of 1-percent-fat milk instead of skim milk. The CSI goes to a big CSI of 4 by selecting a cup of 2-percent-fat milk. Likewise, the CSI goes up 0.7 for every teaspoon of soft margarine you use— now you know why we recommend that you learn the "art of scraping" (¼ to ½ teaspoon per slice of toast).

If you take a close look at the three weeks of breakfasts, you will discover very subtle differences among Phase One, Phase Two, and Phase Three breakfasts. Phase One breakfasts mean that you cook with low-CSI recipes. The only unmodified recipe included in these weekly meal plans is the French toast, which is eaten in a restaurant—and only once during the week. If you are eating Phase One breakfasts and eat out more often, you will need to select fruit, juice, toast, and cereal with 2-percent-fat milk. All of the milk used in these Phase One breakfasts is 2-percent fat in amounts of ½- to ¾-cup servings. The serving size for soft margarine is 1 or 2 teaspoons, and margarine is always used on toast and muffins. If you choose butter (CSI of 3.1 per teaspoon), you will have to reduce your CSI for lunch or dinner.

Phase Two breakfasts probably won't look much different to you. The milk used in Phase Two is 1-percent fat. The serving size for margarine is 1 teaspoon, and on 3 days *no* margarine is used on toast and muffins; jams and honey are okay. A number of low-CSI recipes were selected to show you how much variety these goals still allow: *Blueberry Bran Muffins, Spanish Omelet, Crepes,* and *Orange Waffles.* There are *no* breakfasts with higher-CSI foods, which means that in Phase Two you will want to order very carefully when eating breakfast in a restaurant—and that includes weekends.

In Phase Three, only skim milk is used.

TABLE 15
CSI PHASE ONE, PHASE TWO, AND PHASE THREE WEEK OF BREAKFASTS

DAY 1	DAY 2	DAY 3	DAY 4	DAY 5	DAY 6	DAY 7
			CSI Phase One Breakfast Plans			
Orange juice, ¾ cup Wheaties, 1 cup Sugar, 1 tsp. 2% milk, ¾ cup Rye toast, 1 slice Soft margarine, 1 tsp.	Pink grapefruit, ½ *"Eggs" Benedict*	Grape juice, ½ cup Oatmeal, ½ cup with raisins, ½ Tbsp. 2% milk, ½ cup *Pumpkin Oat Muffin* Soft margarine, 1 tsp.	Orange juice, ¾ cup Cornflakes, 1 cup 2% milk, ¾ cup Sugar, 1 tsp. Whole wheat toast, 1 slice Soft margarine, 1 tsp.	Apple juice, ½ cup *Oatmeal Buttermilk Pancakes*, three 4" Syrup, ¼ cup Soft margarine, 2 tsp.	*Orange Waffle*, with fresh strawberries, ¾ cup Soft margarine, 2 tsp. Syrup, ¼ cup	Breakfast Out: Orange juice, ¾ cup French toast, 1 serving Syrup, ¼ cup Soft margarine, 1 tsp.
			CSI Phase Two Breakfast Plans			
Pink grapefruit, ½ Oatmeal, 1 cup Brown sugar, 1 tsp. 1% milk, ¾ cup *Blueberry Bran Muffins*, 2	Cantaloupe, ½ *Spanish Omelet* English muffin, 1 Strawberry jam, 2 tsp.	Orange juice, ¾ cup Granola, low-fat, ½ cup 1% milk, ¾ cup	Strawberries, ½ cup Cream of Wheat, 1 cup Sugar, 2 tsp. 1% milk, ¾ cup Raisin bread toast, 2 slices Soft margarine, 1 tsp.	Fruit cup: Banana slices, ½ cup Orange sections, ½ cup Bran Flakes, 1 cup 1% milk, ¾ cup Whole wheat toast, 2 slices Grape jelly, 2 tsp.	Orange juice, ¾ cup Apple crepes: *Crepes*, 2 Apple pie filling, ½ cup Nonfat plain yogurt, 2 Tbsp.	*Cinnamon Waffle*, 1 Blackberries, ⅔ cup Blackberry syrup, ¼ cup Soft margarine, 1 tsp.
			CSI Phase Three Breakfast Plans			
Orange juice, ¾ cup Applesauce unsweetened, ½ cup *Cornmeal Pancakes*, 2 Soft margarine, 2 tsp. Syrup, ¼ cup	Cantaloupe, ½ Puffed Wheat, 1 cup Skim milk, ¾ cup Whole wheat English muffin, 1 Strawberry preserves, 2 tsp.	Fresh raspberries, ½ cup Shredded Wheat, 1 cup Skim milk, ¾ cup Whole wheat raisin toast, 2 slices Soft margarine, 1 tsp.	Sliced banana in Plain nonfat yogurt, 6 oz. *Cereal Bran Muffin*, 2 Orange marmalade, 1 Tbsp.	Pink grapefruit, ½ *Skinny Hash Browns* Whole wheat toast, 2 slices Blackberry preserves, 2 tsp.	Honeydew melon, ½ Oatmeal, 1 cup Skim milk, ¾ cup Whole wheat English muffin, ½ Honey, 2 tsp.	Orange juice, ¾ cup *German Oven Pancake*, ½, with Blueberries, ½ cup, Peaches, ½ cup & Powdered sugar, 1 tsp.

Recipes in **bold italics** can be found in Part III. The food amounts shown are for women and children; men and teens need about one-third more.

Notice that margarine (in 1-teaspoon servings) is used on only two days. For the other five mornings, preserves, marmalade, and honey are used as spreads on English muffins, muffins, and toast. The amazing thing about Phase Three breakfasts is that a number of delicious low-CSI recipes can be used: for example, *Cornmeal Pancakes*, *Cereal Bran Muffins*, *Skinny Hash Browns*, and *German Oven Pancake* (all found in the cookbook section).

For those who can't imagine starting the morning without cereal, don't despair. Almost all ready-to-eat and cooked cereals (see Table 16 at the end of this chapter) have an ideal CSI of almost zero. Add a cup of 1 percent milk to that and you'll have a breakfast with a CSI of 2. Supplement this, if you like, with other nearly zero–CSI foods, such as fruit or juice. If you also want toast with 1 teaspoon margarine (CSI of 0.7), you need to use skim milk in order to keep your breakfast CSI at 2. Note that most commercial granolas have CSIs, per cup, of anywhere from 3 to 17, with the majority being closer to 17—just like eating a high-fat cookie! One exception is Golden Temple granola (CSI of less than 1 per cup). Be sure that any commercial granola does not contain coconut oil. Another good choice is muesli, which has a CSI of almost zero per cup.

If you're in the habit of starting off your day with a rich, gooey pastry, some definite modification is called for. A maple bar has a CSI of 6, a Danish roll has a CSI of 8, a croissant 9, and a sticky nut roll 13. A Poptart has a CSI of 2, an unfrosted doughnut 4, and the frosted variety anywhere from 5 to 7. But check out our recipes (Part III) for *Sunrise Cake* (CSI of < 1 per serving) and *Baked Doughnut Holes* (CSI of almost 0 for two). A typical plain muffin is another possibility (CSI 2), as are our own *Blueberry Bran Muffin* (CSI tr.) and our *Cereal Bran Muffin* (CSI <1).

If you are a lover of breakfast dishes that contain eggs, you are in luck. We have many wonderful recipes. *German Oven Pancake* is easy to make. *"Eggs" Benedict* and *Spanish Omelet* are popular, you won't want to miss our *Vegetable Frittata* and our *French Toast*.

As you compute your breakfast CSIs, remember to consult the "Other Breakfast Foods" section of Table 16 to include any butter, margarine, yogurt, milk (see cereals), cream, bacon, sausage, or other foods you consume. For those of you who eat breakfast on the run—at restaurants or at fast-food outlets—see Chapter 11 later in Part II for further tips and guidelines.

BREAKFAST CSIs

Table 16 shows the CSIs of individual food choices.

TABLE 16
THE CSIs OF BREAKFAST CHOICES
Cereals
(Select CSIs of 2 or lower per cup)

	SERVING SIZE		CSI	FAT (GM)	CALORIES
READY-TO-EAT					
Wheat Bran, unprocessed	1 tablespoon	(4 gm)	tr.	<1	7
All-Bran	1 cup	(85 gm)	tr.	2	212
Bran Buds	1 cup	(84 gm)	tr.	2	217
Branflakes	1 cup	(39 gm)	tr.	<1	127
Branflakes with Raisins	1 cup	(57 gm)	tr.	1	175
Cheerios/Wheaties	1 cup	(29 gm)	tr.	tr.	101
Chex, Corn & Rice	1 cup	(28 gm)	tr.	tr.	110
Corn Flakes/Rice Krispies	1 cup	(23 gm)	tr.	tr.	89
Grape-nuts	1 cup	(112 gm)	tr.	tr.	403
Grape-nut Flakes	1 cup	(32 gm)	tr.	tr.	115
Kashi	1 cup	(22 gm)	tr.	<1	74
Presweetened, variety of brands	1 cup	(28 gm)	tr.	<1	110
Puffed Rice	1 cup	(14 gm)	0	tr.	56
Puffed Wheat	1 cup	(12 gm)	tr.	tr.	44
Shredded Wheat	1 biscuit/25 bite-size	(24 gm)	tr.	<1	86
Special K	1 cup	(21 gm)	tr.	tr.	82
Captain Crunch	1 cup	(37 gm)	2	3	156
Muesli	1 cup	(84 gm)	tr.	2	280

102

	SERVING SIZE		CSI	FAT (GM)	CALORIES
Granola, low-fat commercial (Golden Temple)	1 cup	(57 gm)	<1	6	250
Granola, commercial with soy oil (Vita Crunch)	1 cup	(113 gm)	3	18	495
Granola, commercial with coconut oil	1 cup	(113 gm)	17	20	503
COOKED					
Farina, Cream of Wheat, Ralston, Roman Meal, Malt-O-Meal	1 cup	(233 gm)	tr.	tr.	126
Oat bran	1 cup	(240 gm)	tr.	2	103
Oatmeal, regular	1 cup	(234 gm)	tr.	2	145
Oatmeal, instant	1 cup	(207 gm)	tr.	3	217

MILK

	SERVING SIZE		CSI	FAT (GM)	CALORIES
MILK (SELECT CSIs OF 2 OR LOWER PER CUP)					
Milk, skim or powdered nonfat	1 cup	(245 gm)	<1	tr.	85
Buttermilk, 1% fat	1 cup	(245 gm)	2	2	98
Milk, 1% fat	1 cup	(244 gm)	2	3	102
Milk, 2% fat	1 cup	(244 gm)	4	5	122
Milk, chocolate, 2% fat	1 cup	(250 gm)	5	7	194
Milk, whole	1 cup	(244 gm)	7	8	149

The abbreviation tr. stands for trace (less than 0.5); the symbol <1 stands for less than one (0.5 to 0.9). Recipes in **bold italics** can be found in Part III.

BREADS AND TORTILLAS
(SELECT CSIs OF 1 OR LOWER PER SERVING)

	SERVING SIZE		CSI	FAT (GM)	CALORIES
YEAST BREADS					
White	1 slice	(25 gm)	tr.	<1	68
Whole wheat	1 slice	(29 gm)	tr.	<1	70
Raisin	1 slice	(23 gm)	tr.	<1	61
Rye	1 slice	(29 gm)	tr.	tr.	70
Pumpernickel	1 slice	(25 gm)	tr.	tr.	62
English muffin	One	(57 gm)	tr.	1	135
Whole Wheat French Bread	1/5 loaf	(38 gm)	tr.	<1	125
Grape-nut Bread	1 slice or roll	(42 gm)	tr.	1	99
French, Italian, sourdough	4¼" x 2¾" x 1"	(30 gm)		tr.	83
Pita or pocket	One	(64 gm)	tr.	<1	180
Boston brown	1 slice	(48 gm)	tr.	<1	101
Cinnamon swirl	1 slice	(22 gm)	tr.	<1	59
Egg	1 slice	(33 gm)	2	2	89
Cheese	1 slice	(29 gm)	2	3	87
Challah	1 slice	(33 gm)	2	2	89
Focaccia	1/8 loaf	(60 gm)	1	5	190
Boboli	1/8 loaf	(60 gm)	2	8	183

104

YEAST ROLLS

Hard	1 small	(25 gm)	tr.	<1	77
Kaiser	One	(50 gm)	tr.	2	153
Caraway Dinner Roll	One	(48 gm)	tr.	<1	108
Pan or dinner-type	One	(28 gm)	<1	2	83
Poor boy or submarine	3" x 11½"	(135 gm)	1	4	385
Crescent	One	(28 gm)	3	6	101
Croissant	One	(55 gm)	9	12	167

TORTILLAS

Corn, plain	5¾" diameter	(23 gm)	tr.	<1	52
Taco or tostada shell, fried	5½" diameter	(14 gm)	1	3	63
Flour, plain	7½" diameter	(38 gm)	1	3	118
Flour, fried	7½" diameter	(43 gm)	3	8	162

BAGELS

Plain or flavored	One	(75 gm)	tr.	2	225
Egg	One	(75 gm)	2	4	225

MUFFINS AND SCONES

Blueberry Bran Muffin	One	(89 gm)	tr.	<1	146
Cereal Bran Muffin	One	(59 gm)	<1	4	116
A Barrel of Muffins	One	(43 gm)	<1	4	105
Poppyseed Muffin	One	(62 gm)	<1	5	163
Nutty Orange Muffin	One	(63 gm)	<1	5	167

The abbreviation *tr.* stands for trace (less than 0.5); the symbol <1 stands for less than one (0.5 to 0.9). Recipes in **bold italics** can be found in Part III.

BREADS AND TORTILLAS *(continued)*

	SERVING SIZE		CSI	FAT (GM)	CALORIES
Mexican Cornbread Muffin	One	(74 gm)	<1	4	165
Pumpkin Oat Muffin	One	(82 gm)	<1	4	177
Applesauce Oatmeal Muffin	One	(59 gm)	<1	5	157
Dutchy Crust Muffins or Coffee Cake	One	(64 gm)	<1	5	181
Cinnamon Rhubarb Muffin	One	(50 gm)	<1	4	140
Typical plain muffin	One	(55 gm)	2	6	149
Oatmeal Raisin Muffin	One	(47 gm)	<1	4	137
Oatmeal raisin muffin, typical	One	(61 gm)	2	6	164
Yogurt Scone	One	(60 gm)	<1	3	136
Fruit Scone	One	(39 gm)	<1	4	107
QUICK BREADS					
Grandma Kirschner's Date Nut Bread	½" slice	(61 gm)	tr.	4	209
Pumpkin Harvest Loaf	½" slice	(38 gm)	<1	4	163
Lemon Nut Bread	½" slice	(58 gm)	<1	5	153
Cornbread	2" x 4" x 2"	(78 gm)	<1	6	180
Fruit Bread	½" slice	(55 gm)	<1	4	151
Orange Walnut Bread	½" slice	(55 gm)	<1	4	166
Banana Nut Bread	½" slice	(66 gm)	<1	4	142
Whole Wheat Quick Bread	½" slice	(36 gm)	<1	2	93
Nut bread	½" slice	(58 gm)	2	10	199
Zucchini bread (no nuts)	½" slice	(45 gm)	3	9	172
Pumpkin bread (no nuts)	½" slice	(45 gm)	4	5	161
Cornbread, typical	3" x 3" x 1"	(59 gm)	5	8	190

BAKERY GOODS
(SELECT CSIs OF 2 OR LOWER PER SERVING)

BISCUITS

Old-style Wheat Biscuit	One	(34 gm)	<1	4	86
Canned	One 2"	(21 gm)	<1	3	68
Baking powder	One 2"	(28 gm)	2	5	118
Scone	One 4"	(56 gm)	6	12	294

BISCUIT OR BAKING MIX

Baking Mix, modified	1 cup	(121 gm)	4	17	491
Typical (Bisquick)	1 cup	(113 gm)	10	17	475

SWEET ROLLS

Poptart	One	(50 gm)	2	6	196
Brioche	One	(30 gm)	4	6	119
Sweet roll, cinnamon	One 4"	(69 gm)	5	11	276
Maple bar	One	(42 gm)	6	12	192
Danish	One 4"	(58 gm)	8	18	235
Croissant	One	(55 gm)	9	12	167
Sunday Morning Sticky Buns	⅑ recipe	(60 gm)	<1	3	214
Sticky nut roll	One 4"	(102 gm)	13	20	444

The abbreviation *tr.* stands for trace (less than (0.5); the symbol <1 stands for less than one (0.5 to 0.9). Recipes in **bold italics** can be found in Part III.

107

BAKERY GOODS (continued)

	SERVING SIZE		CSI	FAT (GM)	CALORIES
DOUGHNUTS					
Baked Doughnut Holes	Two	(40 gm)	tr.	3	118
Doughnut, cake (unfrosted)	One 3"	(36 gm)	4	6	153
Doughnut, cake (frosted)	One 3"	(67 gm)	5	10	279
Doughnut, cake (frosted, with coconut)	One 3"	(73 gm)	7	12	309
COFFEE CAKES					
Sunrise Cake	1/16 of cake	(68 gm)	<1	4	161
Coffee cake, streusel topping	3" x 3" x 2"	(94 gm)	6	12	316

BREAKFAST DISHES
(SELECT CSIs OF 4 OR LOWER PER SERVING)

	SERVING SIZE		CSI	FAT (GM)	CALORIES
PANCAKES					
Cornmeal Pancakes	Two 5"	(136 gm)	<1	3	178
Cornmeal pancakes, typical	Two 5"	(139 gm)	7	9	228
Oatmeal Buttermilk Pancakes	Three 4"	(162 gm)	1	3	228
Modified pancakes (made with oil, skim milk, no yolks)	Three 4"	(143 gm)	1	6	212
Typical pancakes (made from mix)	Three 4"	(138 gm)	8	10	258
German Oven Pancake	1/2 pancake	(369 gm)	2	10	373*
Dutch Baby (typical)	1/2 pancake	(183 gm)	29	22	402

*Contains fruit.

Item	Serving				
Crepe Blintz	One	(216 gm)	4	7	239
Blintz, typical	One	(115 gm)	12	14	227
Crepe	One	(35 gm)	tr.	2	62
Crepe, typical	One	(68 gm)	5	4	116
WAFFLES					
Orange Waffles	One 7"	(111 gm)	1	8	197
Cinnamon Waffles	One 7"	(111 gm)	2	8	197
Modified waffles (made with oil, no yolks, skim milk)	One 7"	(113 gm)	2	8	192
Typical waffles	One 7"	(113 gm)	8	13	249
FRENCH TOAST					
French Toast	¼ recipe	(56 gm)	tr.	1	95
Modified (made with skim milk, egg substitute)	One	(75 gm)	<1	4	116
Typical	One	(72 gm)	5	6	131
OMELETS					
Spanish Omelet	⅙ recipe	(183 gm)	tr.	1	93
Vegetable Frittata	½ recipe	(272 gm)	2	7	232
Omelet, plain	2 eggs	(128 gm)	27	20	244
Omelet, cheese	2 eggs	(154 gm)	34	28	350
Omelet, ham & cheese	2 eggs	(190 gm)	36	32	413

The abbreviation *tr.* stands for trace (less than 0.5); the symbol <1 stands for less than one (0.5 to 0.9). Recipes in **bold italics** can be found in Part III.

BREAKFAST DISHES *(continued)*

	SERVING SIZE	CSI	FAT (GM)	CALORIES
EGGS				
Whites	Two (66 gm)	0	0	32
Whole	One (50 gm)	12	6	79
Yolks	Two (34 gm)	25	11	125
EGG SUBSTITUTES				
Egg Beaters	¼ cup (60 gm)	0	0	30
Second Nature	¼ cup (60 gm)	0	2	49
Scramblers	¼ cup (60 gm)	0	4	68
Homemade Egg Substitute	¼ cup (60 gm)	<1	4	70
OTHER EGG DISHES				
Scrambled Whites	½ cup (99 gm)	0	0	48
Scrambled Egg Substitute	½ cup (114 gm)	2	8	127
Scrambled Eggs, typical	½ cup, 2 eggs (124 gm)	27	20	244
Egg McMuffin	One (138 gm)	16	16	340
Sausage McMuffin with egg	One (165 gm)	24	33	517
Egg, fried with margarine	One (55 gm)	13	9	113
Two fried eggs and four slices bacon	One serving (138 gm)	32	32	387
"Eggs" Benedict	One (193 gm)	4	11	238
Eggs Benedict, typical	One (132 gm)	30	25	721

OTHER BREAKFAST FOODS

Fruits, most varieties:	1 medium piece, 1 cup melon or berries, ½ cup grapes, ½ cup canned fruit, ½ cup juice, ¼ cup dried	(100 gm)	60	tr.	tr.

YOGURT (SELECT CSIs OF 3 OR LOWER PER CUP)

Plain:					
Nonfat	1 cup	(227 gm)	127	tr.	<1
Low-fat	1 cup	(227 gm)	143	4	3
Whole Milk	1 cup	(227 gm)	141	8	7
All flavors:					
Nonfat	1 cup	(227 gm)	200	tr.	<1
Low-fat	1 cup	(227 gm)	250	3	3
Whole milk	1 cup	(227 gm)	275	8	7

MARGARINE AND BUTTER (SELECT CSIs OF 0.7 OR LOWER PER TEASPOON)

Margarine, diet (40% fat, not recommended for baking)	1 teaspoon	(5 gm)	17	2	0.3
Margarine, table spread (60% fat, Country Crock)	1 teaspoon	(5 gm)	27	3	0.5
Margarine, liquid (squeeze type)	1 teaspoon	(5 gm)	35	4	0.7

The abbreviation *tr.* stands for trace (less than 0.5); the symbol <1 stands for less than one (0.5 to 0.9). Recipes in **bold italics** can be found in Part III.

111

OTHER BREAKFAST FOODS *(continued)*

	SERVING SIZE		CSI	FAT (GM)	CALORIES
Margarine, tub or soft stick (Saffola, Mazola, Fleischmann's)	1 teaspoon	(5 gm)	0.7	4	35
Margarine, hard stick (inexpensive store brands)	1 teaspoon	(5 gm)	0.8	4	35
Butter	1 teaspoon	(5 gm)	3.1	4	36
OTHER SWEETS					
Honey	½ cup	(168 gm)	0	0	511
Honey	1 tablespoon	(21 gm)	0	0	64
Jam, jelly, typical	½ cup	(160 gm)	tr.	tr.	437
Jam, jelly, typical	1 tablespoon	(20 gm)	tr.	tr.	55
Jam, Jelly, low-sugar	½ cup	(160 gm)	0	0	223
Jam, Jelly, low-sugar	1 tablespoon	(20 gm)	0	0	30
Sugar, brown	½ cup	(110 gm)	0	0	410
Sugar, powdered	½ cup	(64 gm)	0	0	247
Sugar, granulated	½ cup	(96 gm)	0	0	370
Syrup, maple-flavored	½ cup	(168 gm)	0	0	487

112

BACON AND SAUSAGE (SELECT CSIs OF 2 OR LOWER PER OUNCE)

Bacon substitute (Morningstar)	1 ounce	(28 gm)	tr.	3	54
Bacon Canadian	1 ounce (1½ slices)	(28 gm)	2	2	52
Bacon	1 ounce (4 strips)	(28 gm)	6	14	161
Sausage substitute (Morningstar)	1 ounce	(28 gm)	1	5	77
Sausage, link	1 link	(20 gm)	3	6	74
Sausage, patty	3 ounces	(28 gm)	4	9	105
HASH BROWNS					
Skinny Hash Browns	1 cup	(155 gm)	<1	5	174
Hash browns	1 cup	(155 gm)	5	17	375

The abbreviation tr. stands for trace (less than (0.5); the symbol <1 stands for less than one (0.5 to 0.9). Recipes in **bold italics** can be found in Part III.

CHAPTER

7

Lunch

POWER CSI-ING

Remember "power lunching"? The so-called power lunch, popularized in fitness magazines and the like, was said to keep you trim, alert, and energized and was supposed to give you a competitive edge, whether you were an athlete about to run a race or a businessperson about to cut a deal. It turns out there was some validity to this idea, because, at its best, the power lunch was usually rich in energy-sustaining complex carbohydrates and was generally low-CSI fare.

If you want to design your own power lunches, first aim for those that pack CSIs of no more than 9 (women/children) or 12½ (men/teens). See Table 17 for an ex-

ample of meal-by-meal CSI distributions. The suggested lunch CSIs of 9 and 12½ are Phase One. Eventually, you'll want to get to 3 (women/children) or 4 (men/teens).

Start by Building a Better Sandwich

When it comes to rehabilitating lunch, one of the best ways to start is by remodeling that Western World fixture, the sandwich. This is an excellent place to cut back on meat and cheese. It has to be done somewhere, and many find it easier to make those cuts at lunch than at dinner—at least in the beginning. (We'll talk about fast-

TABLE 17
THE CHOLESTEROL–SATURATED FAT INDEX (CSI) DAILY GOALS*

	BREAKFAST	LUNCH	DINNER	SNACKS	TOTAL
Women/Children	(2,000 Calories)				
CSI American Diet	5	**12**	28	6	51
CSI Phase One	4	**9**	20	4	37
CSI Phase Two	2	**5**	18	3	28
CSI Phase Three	1	**3**	11	2	17
Men/Teens	(2,800 Calories)				
CSI American Diet	8	**18**	35	8	69
CSI Phase One	5½	**12½**	24½	5½	48
CSI Phase Two	3	**7**	22	4	36
CSI Phase Three	1½	**4**	15½	3	24

* This is only one of many possible distributions.

food and restaurant lunches later in Chapter 11, but the same principles apply.)

Eventually you will want to try some meatless, cheeseless sandwiches, such as *Chili Bean Salad* in pita bread or a bean burrito. But start out by simply modifying the kind of sandwiches you normally eat so that they contain *less* and leaner meat, cheese, and spreads. Here are some ways to do this:

Breads: Generally, use breads made from *whole grains*. These contain more nutrients and more fiber than the white breads and are more flavorful. Most people make this transition without difficulty, but if you find the taste or texture of whole-grain bread a bit alien, start out by using a slice of white and a slice of dark when you construct your sandwiches. The sandwiches we encourage always have two slices of bread—none of this open-faced business. This will provide more complex carbohydrate and fiber. Most breads have a CSI of almost 0, which means the filling and spread is where all the

important CSI choices are made. Don't forget about croissants—each one has a CSI of 9! See Table 19 located at the end of this chapter, for the CSIs of all your sandwich (and other lunch) needs.

Hamburgers and Lunch Meats: As you can also tell from Table 19, typical hamburgers (with a CSI of 25) do not fit into a lower CSI lunch. In the very beginning, however, our *Very Skinny Burgers* (CSI of 5) or our *Skinny Burgers* (CSI of 8) *can* fit into a lunch with a CSI goal of 9 (women and children) or 12½ (men and teens). With an ultimate lunch goal of a CSI of 3 or 4, hamburger only fits if you plan to have a meatless dinner. Most people will probably prefer to forgo the hamburger for lunch, particularly after they discover other delicious lower-CSI options. You'll also want to drop the high-fat varieties of lunch meat, such as salami, bologna, and typical wieners. Try thinly sliced breast of chicken or turkey instead. Look at the differences in CSIs for 2-ounce servings—bologna is 8, roast beef or ham is 6, and roast turkey is 3. Other improved choices include turkey wieners, turkey pastrami, and turkey ham. You won't be able to tell many of these from the "real thing." Even better (lower CSI) selections include *very thinly sliced* pressed turkey and other lunch meats. Use first six and gradually decrease to two of these paper-thin slices for sandwiches and supplement with a variety of vegetables such as cucumbers, tomatoes, sprouts, etc. Six slices of these very thin lunch meats have CSIs of 1, and two slices have a CSI of almost zero!

Cheeses: Ideally only the very low–CSI cheeses fit as sandwich fillers—CSIs of 2 or lower per 1-ounce serving. On your way to this goal you could use one of the part-skim cheeses (CSIs of 4 per ounce) and hold the amount to ½ ounce. Reduced Calories Laughing Cow cheese (CSI of 2 per ounce) spreads well on bagels and low-fat crackers.

Sandwich Spreads: No matter how careful you are with your meat allocation, you can undo all your good work if you aren't equally wise about your sandwich spreads. A single tablespoon of butter, after all, has a CSI of more than 9. Peanut butter, on the other hand, is actually quite a good choice. A tablespoon of peanut butter has a CSI of 1.4. Add jam and jelly (nearly zero CSIs) for more filling, if desired. (But beware of the added calories.) Mustard, horseradish, and ketchup are also good choices—all have zero or trace CSIs. If you use mayonnaise, use the "light," low-fat variety. Try to eliminate butter entirely, and if you use margarine, use it sparingly. When you try almost zero–CSI sandwiches filled

with vegetables, you'll be surprised how tasty they are when you spice them up with a little mustard or horseradish. Also, try some of our low-CSI spreads (see recipes in Part III), such as our yolkless *"Egg" Salad Sandwich Spread* and our *Tuna Salad Sandwich Spread.* Then think of moving on to still different types of sandwiches, such as those made with pocket or pita bread. Try filling a pita bread with our *Spicy Black Bean Salad* or *Chili Bean Salad*—or do what the Middle Easterners do and put *Falafel* in it. You can roll these same sandwich fillings in flour tortillas or be a little more traditional and stick with *Refried Beans* or *Your Basic Bean Burrito* or *Burritos With Black Beans.* And don't forget pizza—at least the kind you can make at home. Try our *Quick-and-Easy Pan Bread Pizza* and *Pita Pizza* recipes. These can be wrapped in foil and travel well in a sack for lunch. For a high-fiber filler try our *Baked Bean Special Sandwich.*

Once again, don't try to restructure the sandwich in one heroic swoop. If you've been in the habit of making mega-CSI sandwiches, laden with butter or margarine, mayonnaise, cheese, *and* meat, behead these monsters one fat at a time. (Just to show you how monstrous these can be, a ham-and-cheese croissant sandwich has a CSI of 35, and contains 64 grams of fat [13 teaspoons] and 756 Calories!) And as you take out old flavorings, add new ones, such as horseradish, mustard, onions, olive slices, or pickles. Browse through Part III for some additional sandwich ideas. Try, for example, our *Fruit-Nut Sandwich Spread,* which is excellent on graham crackers, and our *Vegetable–Cottage Cheese Sandwich Spread,* which is very good on tiny rye rounds. As you've been scaling down on the fat in these sandwiches, the calories are also being reduced—so other foods need to be added or the hunger bells will go off at 3 P.M.! Crunchy vegetables, two fruits, or a fruit yogurt can do the trick.

The Soup CSI Rescue

When in doubt, soup can be your salvation at lunch. Table 19 lists the CSIs of many commercially available soups, in addition to many of our own soup recipes. Soups are a great vehicle for increasing your vegetable/grain/bean/pasta intake. Next time you're torn between a cheeseburger and a ham sandwich, try a soup instead. It won't be long before you're making soup a healthy habit. If you don't own a wide-mouth thermos, this is the time to buy one—if you carry your lunch to work.

Even with soups, however, you've got to use common sense. There are *cream* soups with CSIs, per cup, of 14. And there's a mock turtle soup you can buy that will make a tortoise out of you with a per-cup CSI of 34! But, overall, even the store-bought soups are among the lower-CSI lunch choices. Unfortunately most of these still have a salt problem. You'll find several of our soups, which don't have a salt problem, listed in Table 19 and the recipes for them in Part III. Most of these have CSIs per cup of 2 or less, and many have CSIs of almost zero. Among the latter are our *Navy Bean, Greek-Style Garbanzo, Potato Leek* (a "cream" soup), *Minestrone,* and *Black Bean Chili.* And remember that soup provides a

very easy way to increase your consumption of beans. Low-fat soda crackers, oyster crackers, hard rolls, etc., are all good additions to the "soup scene."

Leftover CSIs

Another good solution for what to have at lunch is what was left over from dinner—provided you're making the kind of dinner selections we recommend in the following chapter. These include a lot of potato, vegetable, bean, grain, and rice dishes, all deliciously seasoned, sometimes with small amounts of meat and cheese. So as you read Chapter 8 on dinner later in Part II, think lunch, as well.

SAMPLE LOW-CSI LUNCHES

Table 18 provides you with 21 sample lunches, seven for each of the three CSI phases. These should make it evident that you can "power-CSI" and still enjoy enormously varied and tasty luncheon fare. In fact, for many of you, especially those previously addicted to a monotonous series of meat-and-cheese sandwiches, these sample menus *should* considerably broaden your luncheon horizons (but not your behinds).

Remember that we said many of you have already learned how to eat meatless,

TABLE 18

CSI PHASE ONE, PHASE TWO, AND PHASE THREE WEEK OF LUNCHES

Day 1	Day 2	Day 3	Day 4	Day 5	Day 6	Day 7
CSI Phase One Lunch Plans						
Tostada: Corn tortilla (fried), one 6" **Refried Beans**, ¼ cup Ground beef (20% fat), 1 oz. Low-fat cheese, 1½ oz. Lettuce, ¼ cup Chopped tomato, 1 Tbsp. Brownie, from mix Apple	In a restaurant: Calzone with 2 oz. part-skim mozzarella cheese and vegetables Green salad, 1 cup French dressing, 2 Tbsp. Nectarine	Sandwich: Whole wheat bread, 2 slices Tuna salad made with light mayonnaise, ½ cup Light mayonnaise, 2 Tbsp. Lettuce leaf Carrot sticks Apple Gingersnaps, 3	Chili with beef and beans, 1 cup **Corn Bread**, 1 piece (2" x 4") Soft margarine, 2 tsp. Orange	Hot Dog: Bun Turkey wiener Mustard, 2 tsp. Coleslaw, ½ cup Low-fat fruited yogurt, 1 cup	**Tomato Soup**, 1 cup Ham and cheese sandwich: Whole wheat bread, 2 slices Turkey ham, 1 oz. Kraft Light Natural Cheddar, 1½ oz. Light mayonnaise, 2 Tbsp. Green salad, 1 cup Italian dressing, 2 Tbsp. Fresh pear	**French Onion Soup**, 1 cup **Chicken Salad with Yogurt-Chive Dressing**, 1½ cups
CSI Phase Two Lunch Plans						
Thick Crust Pizza with mozzarella cheese, green peppers, onions, mushrooms, ¼ of 14" pizza Apple **Oatmeal Cookies**, 2	**Moroccan Vegetable Stew**, 2 cups Soda crackers (unsalted tops), 6 Green salad, 1 cup Low-cal French dressing, 2 Tbsp. Fresh pear	**Rick's Chili**, 1½ cups Soda crackers (unsalted tops), 10 Carrot sticks, ½ cup Celery sticks, ½ cup Fresh green grapes, ½ cup	**Gazpacho**, 1 cup Sandwich: Whole wheat bread, 2 slices Thin, pressed lunch meat (turkey), 6 slices Alfalfa sprouts, ¼ cup Light mayonnaise, 1 Tbsp. Mustard, 2 tsp. Tomato, 2 slices Fresh pear 1% milk, 1 cup	Sandwich: Whole wheat bread, 2 slices Peanut butter, 2 Tbsp. Vegetable sticks: Carrots, ½ cup Celery, ½ cup Fig bars, 3 Orange	Lunch in a Cafeteria Baked potato, 1 large with 2 pats margarine Chives, 1 Tbsp. Three-bean salad, ¾ cup French bread, 2 pieces (4" diameter) Soft margarine, 2 tsp. Apricots canned in own juice, ½ cup	Stuffed tomato: Tomato, 1 **Alphabet Seafood Salad**, 1 cup Bagel, 1 Reduced Calories Laughing Cow, ¾ oz. Honeydew melon, ½ cup
CSI Phase Three Lunch Plans						
Greek Lentil Soup, 1 cup Melba rounds, 6 Reduced Calories Laughing Cow, ¾ oz. Green grapes, 1 cup	Burrito: Flour tortilla (7½") **Refried Beans**, ½ cup **Chowchow**, ½ cup Plain nonfat yogurt, 2 tsp. Strawberries, 1 cup	**Chili Bean Salad**, 1 cup served in Whole wheat pita bread **Potato Leek Soup**, 1 cup Orange	Leftover **Four-Star Pasta Salad**, 1 cup Corn on the cob, 1 piece Soft margarine, 1 tsp. Wheatberry roll Apple	**Minestrone Soup**, 1 cup Salad Bar: Lettuce, 1 cup Cherry tomatoes, 4 Radishes, 4 slices Cucumber slices, ¼ cup Kidney beans, ¼ cup Garbanzo beans, ¼ cup Low-calorie French dressing, 4 Tbsp. Hard roll	**Navy Bean Soup**, 1 cup Sandwich: Whole wheat bread, 2 slices Thin, pressed lunch meat (turkey), 2 slices Mustard, 2 tsp. Lettuce, 1 leaf Tomato, 2 slices Banana	In a restaurant: Crab Louis: Crab, ½ cup Egg white, 1 Lettuce, 1½ cups Carrot (grated), ¼ cup Cucumber, ¼ cup Tomato, ½ Black olive **Thousand Island Salad Dressing**, ¼ cup (brought from home) Whole wheat rolls, 2 Fresh fruit cup, 1 cup

Recipes in **bold italics** can be found in Part III. The food amounts shown are for women and children; men and teens need about one-third more.

cheeseless breakfasts. That is not true for lunch. The goal is to move toward meatless and cheeseless, to use only nonfat dairy products, to include beans on many days, and to always eat vegetables and fruit for lunch, with only an occasional sweet dessert. These sample lunches will take you gradually from Phase One to Phase Two and on to Phase Three. The amounts listed are for women and children. Men and teens need about one-third more than the amounts listed.

Phase One lunches: There are a number of features that characterize Phase One lunches. There is meat or cheese (of the leaner varieties) in all seven lunches. Nothing is fried or in batter. Sandwiches are made using turkey lunch meats and part-skim cheeses—both in smaller amounts (less than 3 ounces total)—and using a light mayonnaise or Miracle Whip Light in serving sizes of no more than 2 tablespoons. Lower-CSI regular salad dressings can be used, such as Italian or Russian in 2-tablespoon amounts. Low-fat yogurt is also used. Twenty-percent-fat ground beef is used instead of the usual 30 percent fat, as in the tostada for Day 1. Beans are included on two days. A brownie made from a mix is included. This brownie is made with oil and egg whites, contains no nuts, and is not frosted. It tastes great. Cookies are included in lunch on three days—they are no longer an everyday food. CSI recipes are used, such as *Refried Beans* in the tostada, *Cornbread, Tomato Soup, French Onion Soup,* and *Chicken Salad with Yogurt-Chive Dressing.*

Note that milk is *not* included as a drink in any of these lunches. If you decide to drink a glass (1½ cups) of 2-percent-fat milk, this will increase the CSI by 6 on any day. It is easy to see that drinking 2-percent-fat milk and keeping the CSI at 9 per day means you would have to choose *very low*–CSI foods. If you are a milk drinker, you will want to select a 1-percent-fat milk (CSI of 3 per glass) or skim milk (CSI of 1½ per glass) and save your CSIs for other foods.

Phase Two lunches: In Phase Two lunches, the sandwich has less meat—6 slices of *thin, pressed* lunch meat (1 ounce) and 1 tablespoon light mayonnaise, producing a CSI of around 2 for the entire sandwich. More vegetables are used—¼ cup alfalfa sprouts and 2 tomato slices—to bulk up the sandwich. Mustard is added to enhance the flavor. Peanut butter sandwiches contain 2 tablespoons peanut butter and no margarine. This gives a CSI of 3. Jam or jelly could be added since their CSIs are almost 0, but don't forget they *do* contain calories. You will know you have a Phase Two sandwich if the CSI adds up to 2 or 3. In Phase One, there was meat and cheese (of the leaner varieties) in all seven of the lunches. In Phase Two, four of the seven lunches contain no meat or cheese. This means selecting a vegetarian pizza, a bean burrito (not fried), or vegetable soup if you eat out for lunch. Beans are included in three lunches. Low-calorie salad dressings in 2-tablespoon amounts are used on salads. Nonfat yogurt and 1 teaspoon margarine per slice of bread are Phase Two choices. A low-CSI cheese (Reduced Calories Laughing Cow) is spread on bagels instead of cream cheese. Notice that fruit and vegetables are included in each of the seven lunches. Low-CSI cookies are used—fig bars and *Oatmeal Cookies*. Also, low-CSI recipes greatly enhance the variety of these lunches—*Moroccan Vegetable Stew*, *Rick's Chili*, *Gazpacho*, and *Alphabet Seafood Salad*. A small amount of 1-percent-fat milk fits in Phase Two lunches. However, if you are a milk drinker, a glass (1½ cups) of 1-percent-fat milk will add another 3 to each daily CSI, making the average 8 instead of 5. This essentially turns a Phase Two lunch into a Phase One lunch. You will have to select even lower-CSI foods if you decide to drink a glass of 1-percent-fat milk regularly and still expect to meet Phase Two lunch goals. Consider switching to skim.

Phase Three lunches: The sandwich in Phase Three is even leaner and is essentially meatless—two-slices of thin, pressed lunch meats are used to impart flavor. No mayonnaise is used. The bulk of the sandwich consists of vegetables, and mustard adds the zip (many like the Dijon type). You will notice that we suggest a hearty *Navy Bean Soup* and a banana to go with this low-calorie but tasty sandwich. Six of the seven lunches are now meatless and cheeseless. Crab is included on the Day 7 lunch. When you get to the next chapter on dinner, you will notice that the Day 7 dinner is meatless and cheeseless, so meat is included only *once* during the day—a basic Phase Three goal. Beans are part of five of the lunches in Phase Three (*Greek Lentil Soup*, *Refried Beans* in a burrito, *Chili Bean Salad*, beans on the salad, and *Navy Bean Soup*). Light mayonnaise is not used as a spread but is

used in small quantities in some of the mixed dishes, such as the *Four-Star Pasta Salad*. Another big difference in Phase Three is that *no* spread is used on bread—we saved it for the corn on the cob. Nonfat yogurt is also a feature of Phase Three lunches. And doesn't that crab Louis sound good? Unfortunately a quarter cup of the restaurant's Thousand Island dressing would add another 4 to the already high CSI of 6 for this special lunch. This means you will want to bring your low-CSI *Thousand Island Salad Dressing* from home—not so much trouble if it means eating this delicious salad and having a great time with your friends and family. If the *Four-Star Pasta Salad* sounds like more work than you'll ever put into a lunch item, don't fret, it's a leftover from the Day 3 dinner. And leftover meatless dishes make great tasting and convenient lunches. By now we all know that skim milk is a Phase Three choice. See—you can "power-lunch" and eat low-CSI at the same time.

THE CSIs OF LUNCH CHOICES

Table 19 lists the CSIs of individual lunch choices, covering breads, sandwich fillings and spreads, sandwiches and pizzas, soups, crackers, salads, cookies and bars, and other lunch foods.

TABLE 19
THE CSIs OF LUNCH CHOICES
Breads and Tortillas (Select CSIs of 1 or lower per serving)

	SERVING SIZE		CSI	FAT (GM)	CALORIES
YEAST BREADS					
White	1 slice	(25 gm)	tr.	<1	68
Whole wheat	1 slice	(29 gm)	tr.	<1	70
Raisin	1 slice	(23 gm)	tr.	<1	61
Rye	1 slice	(29 gm)	tr.	tr.	70
Pumpernickel	1 slice	(25 gm)	tr.	tr.	62
English muffin	One	(57 gm)	tr.	1	135
Whole Wheat French Bread	⅓ loaf	(38 gm)	tr.	<1	125
Grape-nut Bread	1 slice or roll	(42 gm)	tr.	1	99
French, Italian, sourdough	4¼" x 2¾" x 1"	(30 gm)	tr.	tr.	83
Pita or pocket	One	(64 gm)	tr.	<1	180
Boston brown	1 slice	(48 gm)	tr.	<1	101
Cinnamon swirl	1 slice	(22 gm)	tr.	<1	59
Egg	1 slice	(33 gm)	2	2	89
Cheese	1 slice	(29 gm)	2	3	87
Challah	1 slice	(33 gm)	2	2	89
Focaccia	⅛ loaf	(60 gm)	1	5	190
Boboli	⅙ loaf	(60 gm)	2	8	183
YEAST ROLLS					
Hard	1 small	(25 gm)	tr.	<1	77

The abbreviation *tr.* stands for trace (less than 0.5); the symbol <1 stands for less than one (0.5 to 0.9). Recipes in **bold italics** can be found in Part III.

121

TABLE 19 *(continued)*

	SERVING SIZE		CSI	FAT (GM)	CALORIES
Kaiser	One	(50 gm)	tr.	2	153
Caraway Dinner Roll	One	(48 gm)	tr.	<1	108
Pan or dinner-type	One	(28 gm)	<1	2	83
Poor boy or submarine	3" x 11½"	(135 gm)	1	4	385
Crescent	One	(28 gm)	3	6	101
Croissant	One	(55 gm)	9	12	167
TORTILLAS					
Corn, plain	5¾" diameter	(23 gm)	tr.	<1	52
Taco or tostada shell, fried	5½" diameter	(14 gm)	1	3	63
Flour, plain	7½" diameter	(38 gm)	1	3	118
Flour, fried	7½" diameter	(43 gm)	3	8	162
BAGELS					
Plain or flavored	One	(75 gm)	tr.	2	225
Egg	One	(75 gm)	2	4	225
MUFFINS AND SCONES					
Blueberry Bran Muffin	One	(89 gm)	tr.	<1	146
Cereal Bran Muffin	One	(59 gm)	<1	4	116
A Barrel of Muffins	One	(43 gm)	<1	4	105
Poppyseed Muffin	One	(62 gm)	<1	5	163
Nutty Orange Muffin	One	(63 gm)	<1	5	167
Mexican Cornbread Muffin	One	(74 gm)	<1	4	165
Pumpkin Oat Muffin	One	(82 gm)	<1	4	177
Applesauce Oatmeal Muffin	One	(59 gm)	<1	5	157

122

	Serving	Weight			Calories
Dutchy Crust Muffins or Coffee Cake	One	(64 gm)	<1	5	181
Cinnamon Rhubarb Muffin	One	(50 gm)	<1	4	140
Typical plain muffin	One	(55 gm)	2	6	149
Oatmeal Raisin Muffin	One	(47 gm)	<1	4	137
Oatmeal raisin muffin, typical	One	(61 gm)	2	6	164
Yogurt Scone	One	(60 gm)	<1	3	136
Fruit Scone	One	(39 gm)	<1	4	107
QUICK BREADS					
Grandma Kirschner's Date Nut Bread	½" slice	(61 gm)	tr.	4	209
Pumpkin Harvest Loaf	½" slice	(38 gm)	<1	4	163
Lemon Nut Bread	½" slice	(58 gm)	<1	5	153
Cornbread	2" x 4" x 2"	(78 gm)	<1	6	180
Fruit Bread	½" slice	(55 gm)	<1	4	151
Orange Walnut Bread	½" slice	(55 gm)	<1	4	166
Banana Nut Bread	½" slice	(66 gm)	<1	4	142
Whole Wheat Quick Bread	½" slice	(36 gm)	<1	2	93
Nut bread	½" slice	(58 gm)	2	10	199
Zucchini bread (no nuts)	½" slice	(45 gm)	3	9	172
Pumpkin bread (no nuts)	½" slice	(45 gm)	4	5	161
Cornbread, typical	3" x 3" x 1"	(59 gm)	5	8	190

The abbreviation *tr.* stands for trace (less than 0.5); the symbol <1 stands for less than one (0.5 to 0.9). Recipes in **bold italics** can be found in Part III.

123

TABLE 19 (continued)

	SERVING SIZE	CSI	FAT (GM)	CALORIES
MISCELLANEOUS				
Breadstick, plain	One 7½" (11 gm)	tr.	tr.	30
Hamburger or hot dog bun	One (40 gm)	<1	2	114
Breadcrumbs, commercial	½ cup (50 gm)	<1	2	195
Lefse	1 serving (38 gm)	1	3	78
Croutons, commercial	½ cup (18 gm)	3	4	89
Popover	One (40 gm)	5	4	92

SANDWICH FILLINGS
(SELECT CSIs OF 4 OR LOWER PER SERVING)

	SERVING SIZE	CSI	FAT (GM)	CALORIES
Chicken salad (with mayonnaise)	½ cup (104 gm)	8	32	353
CHEDDAR AND JACK-TYPE CHEESES				
Dorman's Light	1 ounce (28 gm)	<1	5	70
Scandic Mini Chol or Swedish low-fat	1 ounce (28 gm)	2	9	113
Olympia's Low Fat	1 ounce (28 gm)	4	5	72
Green River Part Skim	1 ounce (28 gm)	4	5	72
Heidi Ann Low-Fat Ched-Style Cheese, Kraft Light Naturals Mild Cheddar	1 ounce (28 gm)	4	5	80
Swiss	1 ounce (28 gm)	6	8	107
Cheddar, Monterey Jack, Colby, Havarti, Long Horn	1 ounce (28 gm)	8	9	114

CHEESE SLICES

Lite-line	1 ounce	(28 gm)	2	2	51
Lite 'n' Lively	1 ounce	(28 gm)	3	4	74
Kraft Light Naturals (Swiss Reduced Fat)	1 ounce	(28 gm)	4	5	90
American	1 ounce	(28 gm)	7	9	106

COLD CUTS, BEEF & PORK

Thin, pressed	6 slices	(28 gm)	1	1	35
Pastrami, corned beef	2 ounces	(57 gm)	5	5	104
Head cheese	2 ounces	(57 gm)	5	9	120
Ham	2 ounces	(57 gm)	6	12	159
Salami, beef	2 ounces	(57 gm)	7	11	144
Italian sausage	2 ounces	(57 gm)	7	15	184
Knockwurst	2 ounces	(57 gm)	7	16	174
Bologna	2 ounces	(57 gm)	8	16	180
Polish sausage, kielbasa	2 ounces	(57 gm)	8	16	184
Salami, Genoa (hard)	2 ounces	(57 gm)	9	19	230
Liverwurst	2 ounces	(57 gm)	11	16	184
Braunschweiger	2 ounces	(57 gm)	11	18	204

COLD CUTS, TURKEY & CHICKEN

Ham	2 ounces	(57 gm)	3	3	73
Pastrami	2 ounces	(57 gm)	3	4	80
Bologna	2 ounces	(57 gm)	5	8	113
Salami	2 ounces	(57 gm)	5	8	113
Thin, pressed lunch meats (meat/poultry)	2 slices	(9 gm)	tr.	tr.	12

The abbreviation *tr.* stands for trace (less than 0.5); the symbol <1 stands for less than one (0.5 to 0.9). Recipes in **bold italics** can be found in Part III.

SANDWICH FILLINGS (continued)

	SERVING SIZE		CSI	FAT (GM)	CALORIES
CHEESE-TYPE SPREADS					
Fruit-Nut Sandwich Spread	¼ cup	(52 gm)	1	4	81
Vegetable-Cottage Cheese Sandwich Spread	¼ cup	(42 gm)	<1	<1	34
Reduced Calories Laughing Cow Cheese	1 ounce	(28 gm)	2	3	113
Denver (egg, ham, green pepper)	1 egg	(84 gm)	15	13	165
"Egg" Salad Sandwich Spread	½ cup	(105 gm)	<1	5	110
Tofu "Egg" Salad Sandwich Spread	½ cup	(75 gm)	<1	5	66
Egg salad (with mayonnaise)	½ cup	(111 gm)	24	23	252
FRANKFURTERS					
Chicken or turkey	1 wiener	(45 gm)	5	8	102
Beef	1 wiener	(45 gm)	7	13	145
Corn Dog or Pronto Pup	One	(111 gm)	13	28	344
Hamburger patty (10% fat)	3 ounces	(85 gm)	7	7	170
Hamburger patty (15% fat)	3 ounces	(85 gm)	9	13	215
Hamburger patty (20% fat)	3 ounces	(85 gm)	11	16	246
Hamburger patty (25% fat)	3 ounces	(85 gm)	12	20	278
Ham, baked	2 ounces	(57 gm)	6	12	159
Ham salad	½ cup	(124 gm)	8	28	338
Peanut butter	2 tablespoons	(32 gm)	3	17	190
Roast beef	2 ounces	(57 gm)	6	9	144
Roast turkey (white meat)	2 ounces	(57 gm)	3	2	94
Spam	2 slices (¼")	(85 gm)	12	26	284

SPREADABLES

Chicken or turkey	½ cup	(104 gm)	5	14	208
Beef or ham	½ cup	(120 gm)	9	20	271
Ham & cheese	½ cup	(120 gm)	14	22	294
Tuna Salad Sandwich Spread	½ cup	(108 gm)	3	2	111
Tuna salad (with light mayonnaise)	½ cup	(102 gm)	4	15	196
Tuna salad (with mayonnaise)	½ cup	(98 gm)	5	25	272

VEGETABLE SANDWICH FILLINGS

California Beans	½ cup	(78 gm)	tr.	1	63
Spicy Black Bean Salad	½ cup	(85 gm)	tr.	2	114
Falafel	¼ recipe	(79 gm)	tr.	2	124
Chili Bean Salad	½ cup	(111 gm)	<1	3	128
Southern Caviar	½ cup	(104 gm)	<1	3	136
Chowchow	½ cup	(106 gm)	<1	5	94
Refried Beans	½ cup	(87 gm)	<1	3	113
Refried beans (canned)	½ cup	(121 gm)	<1	2	124
Refried beans (typical restaurant)	½ cup	(122 gm)	6	14	243

SPREADS (SELECT CSIs OF 1.0 OR LOWER)

Mustard, prepared	1 tablespoon	(15 gm)	tr.	<1	11
Horseradish	1 tablespoon	(15 gm)	0	tr.	6
Cranberry sauce	1 tablespoon	(17 gm)	0	tr.	30
Ketchup	1 tablespoon	(17 gm)	tr.	tr.	18

The abbreviation *tr.* stands for trace (less than 0.5); the symbol <1 stands for less than one (0.5 to 0.9). Recipes in **bold italics** can be found in Part III.

127

SANDWICH FILLINGS (continued)

	SERVING SIZE	CSI	FAT (GM)	CALORIES
Mayonnaise, light	1 tablespoon (14 gm)	0.8	5	50
Margarine, soft	1 tablespoon (14 gm)	2.1	11	101
Mayonnaise, typical	1 tablespoon (14 gm)	2.1	11	101
Butter	1 tablespoon (14 gm)	9.3	12	102
Jelly, typical	1 tablespoon (14 gm)	tr.	tr.	55
Jelly, low-sugar	1 tablespoon (14 gm)	0	0	28

SANDWICHES AND PIZZA
(SELECT CSIs OF 5 OR LOWER PER SERVING)

	SERVING SIZE	CSI	FAT (GM)	CALORIES
Baked Bean Special Sandwich	¼ recipe (280 gm)	<1	3	374
HAMBURGERS				
Very Skinny Burgers	One (156 gm)	5	10	288
Skinny Burgers	One (212 gm)	8	15	375
Hamburger, typical	One (236 gm)	25	50	763
Ham-and-cheese croissant sandwich	One (196 gm)	35	64	756
BURRITOS (NOT DEEP-FRIED)				
Burritos with Black Beans	One (217 gm)	2	4	242
Your Basic Bean Burrito	One 8" (202 gm)	2	5	269
Bean burrito	One 8" (161 gm)	7	16	384
Beef burrito	One 8" (125 gm)	9	16	353

THIN CRUST PIZZA

Spicy Cheese Pizza	¼ of 14″ pizza	(357 gm)	5	9	390
Green pepper-mushroom-onion	¼ of 14″ pizza	(292 gm)	9	14	419
Canadian bacon	¼ of 14″ pizza	(229 gm)	10	16	446
Pepperoni	¼ of 14″ pizza	(229 gm)	13	23	509
Cheese	¼ of 14″ pizza	(257 gm)	16	24	552
Combination	¼ of 14″ pizza	(279 gm)	20	38	676

THICK CRUST PIZZA

Spicy Cheese Pizza	¼ of 14″ pizza	(417 gm)	4	7	565
Green pepper-mushroom-onion	¼ of 14″ pizza	(360 gm)	6	9	574
Canadian bacon	¼ of 14″ pizza	(334 gm)	7	12	611
Pepperoni	¼ of 14″ pizza	(334 gm)	10	19	674
Cheese	¼ of 14″ pizza	(343 gm)	11	16	664
Combination	¼ of 14″ pizza	(384 gm)	17	33	842
Quick-and-Easy Pan Bread Pizza	⅙ of recipe	(251 gm)	2	11	339
Pita Pizza	1 pizza	(149 gm)	3	5	255
Veggie Pockets with Creamy Dressing	2 small pockets or 1 large pocket	(186 gm)	<1	3	234

The abbreviation *tr.* stands for trace (less than 0.5); the symbol <1 stands for less than one (0.5 to 0.9). Recipes in **bold italics** can be found in Part III.

SOUPS
(SELECT CSIs OF 3 OR LOWER PER SERVING)

		SERVING SIZE		CSI	FAT (GM)	CALORIES
BEAN SOUPS						
Greek Lentil	1 cup	(255 gm)		tr.	1	149
Greek-Style Garbanzo	1 cup	(217 gm)		tr.	4	156
Navy Bean	1 cup	(163 gm)		tr.	<1	79
Split Pea	1 cup	(240 gm)		tr.	1	106
Lentil	1 cup	(238 gm)		<1	4	145
Split pea, lentil, etc.	1 cup	(250 gm)		2	6	170
Beer-cheese soup	1 cup	(251 gm)		14	23	308
Broth, beef, diluted	1 cup	(243 gm)		0	0	29
Broth, chicken, diluted	1 cup	(243 gm)		tr.	1	39
Black Bean Chili	1 cup	(244 gm)		<1	4	277
Rick's Chili	1 cup	(215 gm)		<1	3	126
Chicken chili with beans	1 cup	(213 gm)		1	4	190
Rose Bowl Chili	1 cup	(267 gm)		2	5	213
Chili con carne with beans	1 cup	(255 gm)		8	14	282
Chili con carne without beans	1 cup	(255 gm)		11	18	282
Creamy Chicken Noodle Soup	1 cup	(250 gm)		3	3	185
Chicken noodle soup	1 cup	(240 gm)		3	5	170
Clam chowder (tomato base)	1 cup	(251 gm)		1	4	153

130

Clam chowder (New England style) diluted with skim milk	1 cup	(245 gm)	1	3	131
Clam chowder (New England style) diluted with whole milk	1 cup	(244 gm)	4	7	162
Consommé	1 cup	(243 gm)	0	0	29
CREAM SOUPS					
Potato Leek	1 cup	(212 gm)	tr.	1	61
Potato	1 cup	(248 gm)	3	10	169
Mushroom, diluted with skim milk	1 cup	(248 gm)	3	10	173
Mushroom, diluted with whole milk	1 cup	(248 gm)	6	14	204
Broccoli	1 cup	(299 gm)	14	18	230
Egg drop soup	1 cup	(268 gm)	8	4	79
French Onion Soup with bread and low-fat cheese	1 cup	(183 gm)	2	4	109
French onion soup with bread and regular cheese	1 cup	(284 gm)	4	6	212
Gazpacho	1 cup	(267 gm)	1	6	99
Gazpacho, typical	1 cup	(255 gm)	3	17	188
Hearty Fish Soup	1 cup	(228 gm)	2	3	106
Hot and Sour Soup	1 cup	(227 gm)	<1	3	68
Hot and Sour Soup, typical	1 cup	(238 gm)	5	6	124
Minestrone	1 cup	(231 gm)	tr.	2	81
Minestrone, typical	1 cup	(244 gm)	1	3	83
Mock turtle soup	1 cup	(244 gm)	34	16	247

The abbreviation *tr.* stands for trace (less than 0.5); the symbol <1 stands for less than one (0.5 to 0.9). Recipes in **bold italics** can be found in Part III.

SOUPS (continued)

	SERVING SIZE		CSI	FAT (GM)	CALORIES
Oyster stew made with skim milk	1 cup	(245 gm)	3	9	162
Oyster stew made with whole milk	1 cup	(240 gm)	9	16	234
Tomato Soup	1 cup	(117 gm)	tr.	tr.	55
Tomato soup (canned) diluted with skim milk	1 cup	(248 gm)	1	2	128
Tomato soup (canned), diluted with whole milk	1 cup	(248 gm)	4	6	160
Top Raamen	1 cup	(227 gm)	2	8	161
Turkey-Vegetable Chowder	1 cup	(209 gm)	2	3	140
Fish and Leek Chowder	1 cup	(240 gm)	2	2	142
Turtle soup	1 cup	(248 gm)	2	4	92
Moroccan Vegetable Stew	1 cup	(193 gm)	tr.	2	81
Vegetable Beef Soup	1 cup	(257 gm)	1	2	80
Vegetable beef soup (canned)	1 cup	(240 gm)	3	5	170
Mulligatawny Stew	1 cup	(244 gm)	3	5	174
Hungarian Mushroom Soup	1 cup	(255 gm)	<1	3	116
Hungarian mushroom soup, typical	1 cup	(300 gm)	12	16	212
SOUPS FOR CASSEROLES, ETC.					
Homemade Cream Soup Mix	Equivalent of 1 can	(230 gm)	<1	1	131
Cream of celery (condensed, undiluted)	1 can	(305 gm)	5	14	220
Cream of chicken (condensed, undiluted)	1 can	(305 gm)	6	18	284
Cream of mushroom (condensed, undiluted)	1 can	(305 gm)	6	23	314

SALADS
(SELECT CSIs OF 3 OR LOWER PER SERVING)

GREEN SALADS

Green salad (1 cup, 55 gm) with: low-calorie blue cheese dressing	2 tablespoons	(31 gm)	1	2	30
Blue cheese dressing	2 tablespoons	(30 gm)	3	16	147
Blue cheese dressing	¼ cup	(59 gm)	6	32	287
Green salad (1 cup, 55 gm) with: low-calorie French dressing	2 tablespoons	(33 gm)	tr.	2	51
Red French Dressing	2 tablespoons	(31 gm)	<1	5	87
Russian Salad Dressing	2 tablespoons	(30 gm)	<1	4	57
French dressing	2 tablespoons	(32 gm)	3	13	140
French dressing	¼ cup	(63 gm)	6	25	274
Green salad (1 cup, 55 gm) with: low-calorie Italian dressing	2 tablespoons	(30 gm)	1	3	39
Italian dressing	2 tablespoons	(30 gm)	1	8	97
Italian dressing	¼ cup	(59 gm)	2	16	187
Green salad (1 cup, 55 gm) with: 3 Tbsp. vinegar + 1 Tbsp. olive oil	¼ cup	(59 gm)	2	14	129
2 Tbsp. vinegar + 2 Tbsp. olive oil	¼ cup	(57 gm)	4	27	250
Green salad (1 cup, 55 gm) with: *Western Salad Dressing*	2 tablespoons	(29 gm)	tr.	1	31
Ranch dressing (typical restaurant)	2 tablespoons	(30 gm)	2	11	114

The abbreviation *tr.* stands for trace (less than 0.5); the symbol <1 stands for less than one (0.5 to 0.9). Recipes in *bold italics* can be found in Part III.

SALADS (continued)

	SERVING SIZE		CSI	FAT (GM)	CALORIES
Green salad (1 cup, 55 gm) with: **Thousand Island Salad Dressing**	2 tablespoons	(28 gm)	tr.	1	37
low-calorie Thousand Island dressing	2 tablespoons	(31 gm)	1	3	56
Thousand Island dressing	2 tablespoons	(30 gm)	2	10	127
Thousand Island dressing	¼ cup	(59 gm)	4	20	247
Sunshine Spinach Salad	1 cup	(105 gm)	tr.	2	51
Snowbird Salad	1 cup	(120 gm)	<1	5	58
Vinaigrette Salad Dressing with Greens	1 cup	(61 gm)	tr.	2	31
Caesar salad	1 cup	(87 gm)	6	20	207
CHEF-TYPE SALADS					
Crab Louis without egg, with ¼ cup **Thousand Island Salad Dressing**	1 salad	(389 gm)	7	7	232
Crab Louis without egg, with ½ cup low-calorie Thousand Island salad dressing	1 salad	(455 gm)	8	18	348
Crab Louis with egg, ½ cup low-calorie Thousand Island salad dressing	1 salad	(505 gm)	20	24	427
Crab Louis with egg, ½ cup Thousand Island salad dressing	1 salad	(501 gm)	26	51	714
Shrimp Louis without egg, with ¼ cup **Thousand Island Salad Dressing**	1 salad	(389 gm)	8	7	232
Shrimp Louis without egg, with ½ cup low-calorie Thousand Island salad dressing	1 salad	(455 gm)	10	17	364
Shrimp Louis with egg, ½ cup low-calorie Thousand Island salad dressing	1 salad	(505 gm)	22	23	443
Shrimp Louis with egg, ½ cup Thousand Island salad dressing	1 salad	(501 gm)	28	50	730

Food	Amount	Weight			Calories
Chef's salad without egg, with Cheddar cheese, ham, turkey, ½ cup low-calorie Thousand Island dressing	1 salad	(466 gm)	19	34	545
Chef's salad with egg, with Cheddar cheese, ham, turkey, ½ cup low-calorie Thousand Island dressing	1 salad	(516 gm)	31	40	624
Chef's salad with egg, with Cheddar cheese, ham, turkey, ½ cup Thousand Island salad dressing (typical restaurant)	1 salad	(512 gm)	40	67	910
MISCELLANEOUS SALADS					
Confetti Appleslaw	1 cup	(105 gm)	tr.	1	55
Orange Yogurt Fruit Slaw	1 cup	(144 gm)	tr.	2	96
Sesame Slaw	1 cup	(114 gm)	tr.	3	91
Sesame slaw, typical	1 cup	(145 gm)	4	30	331
Cole slaw with salad dressing	1 cup	(120 gm)	4	19	201
Cole slaw with mayonnaise	1 cup	(120 gm)	6	29	282
Potato Salad	1 cup	(255 gm)	1	4	206
German potato salad	1 cup	(188 gm)	2	5	163
Potato salad, typical	1 cup	(240 gm)	10	26	392
California Beans	1 cup	(155 gm)	tr.	2	126
Summer Bean Salad	1 cup	(178 gm)	<1	4	199
Spicy Black Bean Salad	1 cup	(170 gm)	<1	4	228
Chili Bean Salad	1 cup	(221 gm)	<1	5	255
Three-bean salad	1 cup	(167 gm)	4	23	287
Curried Chicken with Peanut Salad	1 cup	(123 gm)	2	5	119

The abbreviation *tr.* stands for trace (less than 0.5); the symbol <1 stands for less than one (0.5 to 0.9). Recipes in **bold italics** can be found in Part III.

135

SALADS (continued)

	SERVING SIZE		CSI	FAT (GM)	CALORIES
Chicken Salad with Yogurt-Chive Dressing	1 cup	(172 gm)	3	3	169
Simply Wonderful Turkey Salad	1 cup	(171 gm)	1	4	156
Chicken salad with mayonnaise	1 cup	(209 gm)	17	64	705
Orange Bulgur Salad	1 cup	(397 gm)	tr.	1	252
Tabouli	1 cup	(220 gm)	1	8	178
Tabouli, typical	1 cup	(219 gm)	3	19	269
Carrot Raisin Salad	1 cup	(136 gm)	<1	2	166
Carrot raisin salad, typical	1 cup	(108 gm)	6	9	152
Waldorf Salad	1 cup	(147 gm)	2	10	196
Waldorf salad, typical	1 cup	(155 gm)	6	36	382
Greek Salad	1 cup	(114 gm)	<1	3	55
Aspic with mayonnaise, crab, asparagus	1 cup	(209 gm)	3	12	162
Absolutely Delicious Molded Salad	1/15 recipe	(185 gm)	tr.	tr.	150
Holiday Wreath Salad	1 cup	(262 gm)	2	5	274
Fruit salad with marshmallows and whipped cream	1 cup	(152 gm)	7	9	180
Crunchy Vegetable Salad	1 cup	(191 gm)	1	5	136
Crunchy vegetable salad, typical	1 cup	(257 gm)	13	47	561
Cheese and pea salad	1 cup	(187 gm)	15	13	247
Moroccan Salad	1 cup	(163 gm)	<1	4	229
Montana Pasta Salad	1 cup	(196 gm)	<1	4	169
Four-Star Pasta Salad	1 cup	(137 gm)	<1	3	154
Alphabet Seafood Salad	1 cup	(181 gm)	2	3	242

Macaroni (with mayonnaise)	1 cup (184 gm)	7	36	510
Salad Athene	1 cup (69 gm)	1	4	103
Salad Athene, typical	1 cup (137 gm)	3	14	195
Crunchy Confetti Salad	1 cup (186 gm)	<1	6	170
Curried Rice and Artichoke Salad	1 cup (250 gm)	<1	3	206
Fruit and Rice Salad	1 cup (155 gm)	tr.	3	169
Lemony Beets	⅙ recipe (58 gm)	<1	5	66
Green Bean, Mushroom, and Tomato Salad	⅙ recipe (109 gm)	1	4	67

CHIPS, CRACKERS, AND POPCORN
(SELECT CSIs OF 2 OR LOWER PER SERVING)

CRACKERS					
Very Low–Fat Varieties:	(average nutrient values)	(40 gm)	tr.	tr.	134
Armenian Crackerbread	1 large				
Breadsticks, plain	3½ sticks				
Cracklesnax	24				
Crispy Cakes (Squared Rice Cakes)	7 squares				
Crokine	8 slices				
Kavli	4 slices				
Matzo	1⅓				
Rice Cakes	4				

The abbreviation *tr.* stands for trace (less than 0.5); the symbol <1 stands for less than one (0.5 to 0.9). Recipes in **bold italics** can be found in Part III.

CHIPS, CRACKERS, AND POPCORN (continued)

	SERVING SIZE	CSI	FAT (GM)	CALORIES
Ry Krisp, Natural	6			
Siljans Knacke (Swedish Crispbread)	½			
"Sunshine" Krispy (soda crackers)	14			
Wasa Lite Rye	5			
Low-Fat Varieties:	(average nutrient values) (40 gm)	2	5	172
Soda crackers (most brands)	13			
Stoned Wheat Thins	6			
Ak Mak	7			
Melba Rounds	13			
Ry Krisp, Seasoned	6			
Carr's Table Water Crackers	12			
Bremner	17			
Pretzel Goldfish	60			
Harvest Crisps	18			
High-Fat Varieties:	(average nutrient values) (40 gm)	3	9	192
Wheat Thins	20			
Triscuits	9			
Ritz	12			
Chicken in a Biskit	20			
Most "party" varieties	12–20			
Pretzels	20 twists/ 1 cup sticks (40 gm)	1	2	156

COOKIES AND BARS
(SELECT CSIs OF 3 OR LOWER PER SERVING)

HOMEMADE COOKIES

Modified:					
Forgotten Kisses	3 cookies	(21 gm)	tr.	2	70
Lace Cookies	3 cookies	(14 gm)	tr.	2	60
Lebkuchen	2 cookies	(36 gm)	tr.	1	115
Gingies	1 large	(33 gm)	tr.	2	110
Carob	2 large	(41 gm)	1	8	166
Crispy Spice	3 large	(44 gm)	1	8	187
Oatmeal	2 medium	(24 gm)	1	5	124
Typical:					
Oatmeal	2 cookies	(53 gm)	2	9	186
Peanut butter	2 cookies	(37 gm)	4	9	166
Sugar	2 cookies	(33 gm)	4	6	134
Chocolate chip	2 cookies	(40 gm)	6	11	186

COMMERCIAL COOKIES

Fortune cookies	3 cookies	(23 gm)	1	2	103
Gingersnaps	Six 2"	(42 gm)	2	4	176
Animal	16 small	(43 gm)	2	4	181
Graham crackers	6 squares	(42 gm)	2	4	176
Vanilla wafers	Twelve 1½"	(45 gm)	3	4	189
Fig bars	Three 1½"	(47 gm)	3	4	197

The abbreviation *tr.* stands for trace (less than 0.5); the symbol <1 stands for less than one (0.5 to 0.9). Recipes in **bold italics** can be found in Part III.

COOKIES AND BARS (continued)

	SERVING SIZE		CSI	FAT (GM)	CALORIES
Pecan shortbread	Three 2"	(43 gm)	4	10	204
Oatmeal	Three 3"	(41 gm)	4	10	204
Oreos	Four 2"	(44 gm)	5	10	219
Chocolate chip	Four 2"	(44 gm)	5	10	219
Chocolate chip, typical deli	One 3¼"	(58 gm)	6	13	289
Chocolate chip, giant size	One 5¼"	(128 gm)	14	30	637
BAR COOKIES					
Brownies:					
Jamocha Squares	2" x 2"	(28 gm)	<1	4	103
Butterscotch Brownies	2" x 2½"	(39 gm)	<1	5	133
Brownies	2½" x 2½"	(41 gm)	1	5	133
Cocoa Cake, unfrosted	3" x 3"	(50 gm)	1	5	205
Brownies from mix, unfrosted (with oil, no nuts, egg whites)	3" x 3"	(76 gm)	1	8	294
Brownies from scratch, unfrosted (with shortening, egg whites, chocolate, nuts)	3" x 3"	(124 gm)	8	30	519
Brownies, typical, unfrosted (with shortening, chocolate, nuts, whole eggs)	3" x 3"	(124 gm)	15	33	543
Brownies, typical, frosted	3" x 3"	(169 gm)	20	42	721
Chocolate Banana Bars	2" x 2¼"	(35 gm)	tr.	1	86
Apricot Meringue Bars	2" x 2"	(26 gm)	<1	3	91
Northwest Harvest Bars	2¼" x 2¼"	(42 gm)	<1	3	102
Molasses Orange Bars	2" x 2"	(58 gm)	<1	4	123

PB & J Bars	1½" x 2¼"	(24 gm)	<1	4	106
Rice Krispie bar, no chocolate	3" x 3"	(21 gm)	<1	4	98
Rice Krispie bar, with chocolate	3" x 3"	(50 gm)	5	11	228
Date bar, typical	2" x 2"	(59 gm)	3	6	188
Pumpkin bar, typical	2" x 2"	(47 gm)	5	8	164
Lemon bar, typical	2" x 2"	(37 gm)	6	6	140
Walnut Squares	1½" x 1½"	(14 gm)	tr.	1	40
Baklava	2" x 2"	(78 gm)	8	29	428

OTHER LUNCH FOODS

Fruits, most varieties:	1 medium piece, 1 cup melon or berries, ½ cup grapes, ½ cup canned fruit, ½ cup juice, ¼ cup dried	(100 gm)	tr.	tr.	60
Vegetables (carrots, celery, green beans, tomatoes, broccoli, cauliflower, etc.) cooked	½ cup	(93 gm)	tr.	tr.	25
raw	1 cup	(123 gm)	tr.	tr.	25
Vegetables (peas, corn, potatoes, winter squash, hominy, etc.)	½ cup	(80 gm)	tr.	tr.	65
Leafy vegetables (lettuce, spinach, etc.), raw	1 cup	(55 gm)	tr.	tr.	10

The abbreviation *tr.* stands for trace (less than 0.5); the symbol <1 stands for less than one (0.5 to 0.9). Recipes in **bold italics** can be found in Part III.

OTHER LUNCH FOODS *(continued)*

	SERVING SIZE		CSI	FAT (GM)	CALORIES
Beans, no fat added (navy, pinto, kidney, black, etc.)	½ cup	(90 gm)	tr.	1	106
Lentils, split peas, no fat added	½ cup	(100 gm)	tr.	1	115
Garbanzo (chick peas), black-eyed peas	½ cup	(124 gm)	tr.	3	212

MILK (SELECT CSIs OF 2 OR LOWER PER CUP)

Milk, skim or powdered nonfat	1 cup	(245 gm)	<1	tr.	85
Buttermilk, 1% fat	1 cup	(245 gm)	2	2	98
Milk, 1% fat	1 cup	(244 gm)	2	3	102
Milk, 2% fat	1 cup	(244 gm)	4	5	122
Milk, chocolate, 2% fat	1 cup	(250 gm)	5	7	194
Milk, whole	1 cup	(244 gm)	7	8	149

YOGURT (SELECT CSIs OF 3 OR LOWER PER CUP)

Plain:

Nonfat	1 cup	(227 gm)	<1	tr.	127
Low-fat	1 cup	(227 gm)	3	4	143
Whole Milk	1 cup	(227 gm)	7	8	141

All flavors:

Nonfat	1 cup	(227 gm)	<1	tr.	200
Low-fat	1 cup	(227 gm)	3	3	250
Whole milk	1 cup	(227 gm)	7	8	275

The abbreviation *tr.* stands for trace (less than 0.5); the symbol <1 stands for less than one (0.5 to 0.9). Recipes in **bold italics** can be found in Part III.

CHAPTER

8

Dinner

SAVING THE BEST FOR LAST

So now you're well on your way towards the Phase Three CSI goal for breakfast of 1 to 2 and the Phase Three CSI goal for lunch of 3 to 4. Chances are you're feeling pretty good about this—and you should. An eating style characterized by these low CSIs gets you through the day running lean and clean so that you're more likely to remain alert and performing optimally right up until evening. Your low-CSI fuel promotes high-octane energy. By making wise food choices—guided by the CSI—you're far less likely to suffer those mid-morning slumps and after-lunch blahs that affect so many who consume typical high-CSI breakfasts and lunches.

And now for dinner. Because dinner is typically the big meal of the day, we have left most of your daily CSI allotment for dinner. As shown in Table 20, this means women and children have a *maximum* CSI for dinner of 20 in Phase One, 18 in Phase Two, and 11 in Phase Three. For men and teens, the *maximum* dinner CSI is 24½ in Phase One, 22 in Phase Two, and 15½ in Phase Three. Note that these dinner CSIs *include dessert*. (See Chapter 9 later in Part II for more information on desserts and their individual CSIs.)

At dinner, more than ever, it's important to increase your intake of complex carbohydrates, to replace the fats you're cutting out of your daily fare. Review Chapter 5 for guidelines on how (and by how much) to increase your consumption of whole grains, potatoes, breads, pastas, beans and other legumes, vegetables, and

143

TABLE 20
THE CHOLESTEROL–SATURATED FAT INDEX (CSI) DAILY GOALS*

	BREAKFAST	LUNCH	**DINNER**	SNACKS	TOTAL
Women/Children	(2,000 Calories)				
CSI American Diet	5	12	**28**	6	51
CSI Phase One	4	9	**20**	4	37
CSI Phase Two	2	5	**18**	3	28
CSI Phase Three	1	3	**11**	2	17
Men/Teens	(2,800 Calories)				
CSI American Diet	8	18	**35**	8	69
CSI Phase One	5½	12½	**24½**	5½	48
CSI Phase Two	3	7	**22**	4	36
CSI Phase Three	1½	4	**15½**	3	24

* This is only one of many possible distributions.

fruit. For dinner, this means working towards eating 1½ cups (women/children) to 2 cups (men/teens) of grains, potatoes, and pasta, along with bread, while also putting a few beans (about ⅓ cup per person) on your green salads, in your soups, or in your casseroles. Always have vegetables for dinner—one is good, two are better. Fruit makes a good dessert whether it is served as is or used in one of our recipes. Our fruit desserts, by the way, also provide a lot of fiber.

Be reminded that when we recommend increasing intake of these "carbo" foods, we are focusing on their *low-fat versions*. As noted in a preceding chapter, many complex carbohydrate dishes are "corrupted" by the addition of excess fats. So when we urge you to eat more pasta, for example, we are *not* advising you to simply up your intake of *typical* pasta dishes, the type that come smothered in cheeses, creamy sauces, and other fats. Follow the recommendations we've made earlier in this book to ensure the "purity" of your pasta and other complex "carbos." Table 21 demonstrates the considerable CSI chasm that can exist between cleaned-up, "fat-modified" carbohydrates and the fat-polluted versions.

More often than not, when people go to a lower-CSI eating style, they are forced to eat plain pasta and plain potatoes. This is because there have been almost no fat-modified recipes or food products to choose from. And this is still by far the most limiting factor in lower-CSI eating—too few low-CSI "carbo" choices. We think you'll be pleased to find a number of very tasty choices listed in our CSI tables. The recipes can be found in Part III of this book. Additional recipes for these foods can be found in *The New American Diet* (our earlier book).

Now let's turn to a tasty—and educational—way to get your complex carbohydrates at dinner.

Let Your Dinner CSIs "Travel"

When it comes to dinner, one of the best ways to keep your palate pleased and your paunch puny (or nonexistent) is to try low-CSI *ethnic* foods. We invite you to experience the cuisines of many exciting parts of the world. This is one "travel" experience you will find broadening—but not in the physical sense. The cuisines we're talking about are notably low in saturated fat and cholesterol, yet exciting in taste and variety. We have included many selections from these cuisines in the cookbook section, and you'll find the CSIs of many of these foods and mixed dishes in Table 23 at the end of this chapter. We concentrate especially on Mexican, Oriental, Middle Eastern, and Mediterranean dishes. These are all rich in complex carbohydrates and low in fat, when properly prepared. Let's look at each, in turn.

Mexican Cuisine: If your only experience with Mexican dishes relates to the Americanized versions, you may be wondering why we've included Mexican food at all. "North of the border" versions of Mexican dishes are typically laden with cheese, sour cream, meat, eggs, and fat from the deep fryer. This is *not* what the Mexicans have traditionally eaten, except infrequently on feast days and the like. The *real* Mexican cuisine is a low-CSI way of eating, utilizing tomatoes, beans, corn, chiles, squash, vanilla, tropical fruits, and avocados long harvested by the native Indians of Mexico and the rice, wheat, chicken, and dairy products later added by the Spanish who settled in Mexico in the 1500s. Mexican

TABLE 21
THE CHOLESTEROL–SATURATED FAT INDEX (CSI) AND FAT AND CALORIE CONTENT OF MODIFIED AND TYPICAL RECIPES FOR COMPLEX CARBOHYDRATE DISHES

COMPLEX CARBOHYDRATE 1 CUP SERVING	CSI	TOTAL FAT		CALORIES
		Grams	Teaspoons	
Macaroni or Pasta Salad				
Four-Star Pasta Salad	<1	3	½	154
Typical	7	36	7	510
Potato Salad				
Potato Salad	1	4	1	206
Typical	10	26	5	392
French Fries				
Skinny "French Fries"	<1	4	1	134
Typical	5	17	3½	392

Recipes in **bold italics** can be found in Part III.
The symbol <1 stands for less than one (0.5 to 0.9).

cuisine, at its best, is among the most healthful, tasty, colorful, and varied fare in the world.

It is easy to embrace the basics of Mexican cooking: corn, beans, chiles, and fruit. All are low in fat, calories, and cholesterol, high in fiber, easy to prepare, and good for obtaining needed vitamins and minerals. Some of the Mexican dishes you'll find recipes for in Part III are *Acapulco Enchiladas* and *Creamy Enchiladas* (both with CSIs of 3 per enchilada, compared with 12 for a typical cheese enchilada), *Your Basic Bean Burrito* (CSI of 2 compared with a CSI of 9 for the same-sized serving of a typical Americanized beef burrito), *Chile Relleno Casserole* (CSI of 2 versus 19 for one serving of the standard Americanized version), and *Halibut Mexicana* (CSI of 7 for 6 ounces of fish).

You'll be happy to learn, too, that with Mexican cooking growing in popularity in the United States, you can often find even the more exotic ingredients called for in some Mexican dishes in ordinary grocery stores and supermarkets.

Asian Cuisine: We've long been attracted to Asian cooking because of its abundant and imaginative use of vegetables, its sparing use of fats (with meat used as a condiment rather than as a main attraction), and its intriguing and delicious blends of spices. Once again, however, we must warn you that the kind of food that is served in many Chinese restaurants in our country is not typical of what the Chinese themselves have traditionally eaten. Many of these restaurant dishes are fattened up, over-salted, and/or sweetened to cater to American palates. We think that, if you'll try some of

our Oriental dishes, such as *Spicy Chicken with Peppers* (CSI of 5 for 2 pieces), *Beef-Tomato Chow Yuk* (CSI of 3 per 1½ cups), *Pinto Bean Chow Mein* (CSI nearly 0 per cup), *Seafood Teriyaki and Kabobs* (CSI of 6 for 6 ounces of fish), and *Cashew Chicken* (CSI 4 per 1¾ cups), you'll find that the low-CSI versions can be just as tasty—or even more so—than the high-CSI varieties.

Middle Eastern and Mediterranean Cuisines: These are remarkable cuisines that feature such wonderfully varied and zesty foods and spices as fish, figs, grains, lentils, olives, fruits, garbanzo beans, vegetables, fermented dairy products (yogurt), garlic, onions, mint, cumin, thyme, leeks, and pasta. Especially fish and pasta. These are the cuisines of Spain, Southern France, Italy, Greece, Morocco, Northern Africa and Lebanon, and other countries in the Middle East.

Examples of these cuisines that you'll find in our cookbook section include our *Salad Athene* (CSI of 1 per cup), *Pizza Rice Casserole* (CSI of 3 per cup), *Chicken Cacciatore* (CSI of 4 per breast, half the CSI of 8 for typical chicken cacciatore), *Parmesan Yogurt Chicken* (CSI of 7 for 2 pieces versus 18 for the usual version), *Beef and Bean Ragout* (CSI of 2 per cup), *Cheese-Stuffed Manicotti* (CSI of 2 per manicotti versus 11 for the high-fat Americanized version), *Easy Oven Lasagna* (CSI of 3 per three-inch-square piece), *Spicy Cheese Pizza* (CSI of 5 for ¼ of fourteen-inch pizza), *Salmon Mousse* (CSI of 3 per ½ cup), *Bouillabaisse* (CSI of 3 per 1½ cups), *Fish à la Mistral* (CSI of 6 per ¼ recipe), *Fish Fillets with*

Walnuts (CSI of 7 per ¼ recipe), and *Moroccan Salad* (CSI of 1 per cup). *Garlic Chicken with Balsamic Vinegar* (CSI of 5 for 1 breast) and *Pasta with Fresh Tomato Sauce* (CSI of 2 per serving) make for a meal straight from Florence, Italy.

American Cuisine: You are probably very surprised that we would include a section on American cuisine. Don't be, because, with a little modification, many of our "favorites" can fit a lower-CSI way of eating. Chili con carne without beans (CSI of 11 per cup), for example, can be converted to *Rick's Chili* (CSI of 1 per cup) or our new, delicious *Black Bean Chili* (CSI of 1 per cup). The all-American meat loaf, at a CSI of 17 per slice, can be made with 10-percent-fat ground beef and egg white and be reborn with a CSI of 4 per slice. Our new *Old-Fashioned Meat Loaf* recipe is just like Mother's! And the typical hamburger (CSI of 25) can be converted to one of our *Skinny Burgers* (CSI of 8) or *Very Skinny Burgers* (CSI of 5). We don't have to give up fried chicken either—just trade in the grease-soaked version (CSI of 11 per 2 pieces) for our *Portland Fried Chicken* (CSI of 5 per 2 pieces). We hope you can be talked into trading in fried fish (CSI of 14 per 8 ounces) for skinny fried fish, such as our *Skinny Sole* (CSI of 7 for 7 ounces). Tuna noodle casserole (CSI of 10 per 2 cups) can have a CSI of 2 per 2 cups— when it's our *Tuna Noodle Casserole*. We know you'll want to try our *Skinny "French Fries"* or our *Skinny Hash Browns* (CSI of <1 per cup), instead of typical French fries or hash browns at CSIs of 5 per cup. Scalloped potatoes (CSI of 4 per cup) can be made with a CSI of <1 per cup—*Scalloped*

Potatoes. Those all-American baked beans (CSI of 5 per cup) can be made with a CSI of trace per cup—*Classic Baked Beans* or *Rancher's Beans.* Candied yams (CSI of 6 per serving) need not be eliminated because our *Holiday Yams* have a CSI of trace per serving!

SAMPLE LOW-CSI DINNERS

Table 22 provides you with twenty-one low-CSI dinners corresponding to the three CSI phases. These will give you a starting place to implement what you've learned in this chapter and will no doubt provide you with many menu ideas of your own. These particular dinner choices are a bit lower in CSI than they have to be, demonstrating that even the leanest of CSIs can still yield tasty and varied fare. Let's take a close look at Phase One, Phase Two, and Phase Three dinners to see just how they differ.

Phase One dinners: In the week of Phase One dinners, lean red meat (10–20 percent fat) is served four times (instead of typical red meat of 25–30 percent fat). Poultry is served two times—chicken once and turkey once. One dinner is meatless (broccoli quiche). In the meat category, 6-ounce serving sizes are maximum for 2,000 Calories (women/children), 8-ounce serving sizes for 2,800 Calories (men/teens). Regular salad dressings with low CSIs are suggested (Russian and Italian).

TABLE 22
CSI PHASE ONE, PHASE TWO, AND PHASE THREE WEEK OF DINNERS

Day 1	Day 2	Day 3	Day 4	Day 5	Day 6	Day 7
CSI Phase One Dinner Plans						
Portland Fried Chicken, 3 pieces Corn on the cob, 1 piece Soft margarine, 2 tsp. Tomato, sliced Potato salad, ½ cup Gelatin fruit dessert, 1 cup	Broccoli quiche, ⅙ of 9″ pie with no egg yolk and typical crust *Sunshine Spinach Salad*, 2 cups French bread, 2 pieces (4″ diameter) Soft margarine, 2 tsp.	Baked ham, 3 oz. *Scalloped Potatoes*, 1 serving Steamed broccoli, ¾ cup with Soft margarine, 1 tsp.	Spaghetti with *Marinara Sauce*, 1½ cups and Ground beef (15% fat), 4 oz. cooked Green salad, 1 cup Italian dressing, 2 Tbsp. French bread, 1 piece (4″ diameter) Soft margarine, 2 tsp. Rainbow sherbet, ¾ cup	Special Dinner: **Stuffed Flank Steak Florentine**, 1 serving Fluffy white rice, ¾ cup Steamed broccoli, ½ cup, with Soft margarine, 1 tsp. *Caraway Dinner Roll* Soft margarine, 1 tsp. *All Season Shortcake* with Strawberries and Yogurt, 1 serving	Roast Turkey (no skin), 6 oz. Mashed potatoes, 1 cup *Turkey Gravy*, ⅓ cup French-cut green beans, ¾ cup, with Slivered almonds, 1 Tbsp. Homemade biscuits, 2 Strawberry jam, 2 tsp. *Apple Loaf Cake*, 1 serving	Lasagna, 3″ x 3″ (made with 20% fat ground beef, mozzarella and cottage cheeses) Green salad, 1 cup Russian salad dressing, 2 Tbsp. Sourdough roll, 1 large, with Soft margarine, 2 tsp. *Fruit Salad Alaska*, 1 serving
CSI Phase Two Dinner Plans						
Chicken Cacciatore, 1 breast Steamed rice, ¾ cup *Stir-Fried Mushrooms and Broccoli*, 1 serving Dinner roll, 1 Soft margarine, 2 tsp. Fortune cookies, 2 1% milk, ½ cup	*Marinated Mushrooms*, 1 serving Spaghetti with Red clam sauce, 1½ cups Parmesan cheese, 2 Tbsp. *Ratatouille Provençale*, 1 serving *Whole Wheat French Bread*, four (2″-diameter) pieces Soft margarine, 2 tsp. Cherry cobbler, ½ cup	*Baked Corn Chips*, ½ cup Guacamole, ¼ cup *Acapulco Bean Casserole*, 2 cups Green salad, 1 cup Low-cal French dressing, 2 Tbsp. Daiquiri ice, ½ cup	*Beef Stroganoff*, 1 cup Noodles (eggless), 1½ cups Spinach salad, 1 cup Low-cal Italian dressing, 2 Tbsp. Steamed broccoli, ¾ cup Wheatberry roll, 1 Soft margarine, 2 tsp.	*Pepper Steak*, 1 serving Brown rice, 1 cup Green salad, 1 cup with *Red French Salad Dressing*, 2 Tbsp. Whole wheat dinner rolls, 2 Soft margarine, 2 tsp. *Cocoa Cake*, 1 serving	Barbecued chicken, no skin, 2 pieces *Potato Puff*, 1 serving *Tomatoes "Provençale,"* 1 serving Baked winter squash, ½, with Brown sugar, 1 tsp. *Poppyseed Cake*, 1 serving	*Popeye's Spinach Dip*, ½ cup with Vegetables: Radishes, Green pepper, Cauliflower, ¼ cup each *Bouillabaisse*, 2 cups Green salad, 1 cup, with *Hearty Ranch Salad Dressing*, 2 Tbsp. Hard roll, 1 *Apple Crisp*, 1 serving with Plain nonfat yogurt, 2 Tbsp.
CSI Phase Three Dinner Plans						
Cashew Chicken, 1¾ cups Steamed rice, 1½ cups Green salad, 1 cup, with *Red French Salad Dressing*, 2 Tbsp. Fresh sliced pineapple, 1¼ cups *Hot Fudge Pudding Cake*, 1 serving	*Turkey-Vegetable Chowder*, 2 cups Baked potato Soft margarine, 2 tsp. *Carrot Raisin Salad*, ¾ cup Whole wheat dinner rolls, 2	Charcoal-grilled halibut, 6 oz., with margarine, 1 tsp. *Four-Star Pasta Salad*, 1 cup Whole wheat sourdough rolls, 2 *Apricot Meringue Bars*, 2	*Pizza Rice Casserole*, 1 serving Green peas, ⅔ cup Baked squash, ½ cup *Whole Wheat French Bread*, 4 pieces (2″ diameter) Fresh peach	*Parmesan Yogurt Chicken*, 1 serving Fettuccine, 1½ cups Steamed broccoli, 1 cup Whole wheat dinner rolls, 2 Chocolate frozen yogurt (low-fat), ⅔ cup	*Fish Almondine with Dilly Sauce*, 6 oz. cooked fish Baked potato Soft margarine, 2 tsp. *Stuffed Zucchini Boats*, 1 serving *Waldorf Salad*, 1 serving *Caraway Dinner Rolls*, 2 *Pinto Fiesta Cake*, 1 serving	Spaghetti with *Marinara Sauce*, 1½ cups, and Parmesan cheese, 2 Tbsp. Green salad, 1 cup, with *Western Salad Dressing*, 2 Tbsp. Steamed green beans, ½ cup *Whole Wheat French Bread*, 4 pieces (2″ diameter) Wine or sparkling grape juice, 6 oz.

Recipes in **bold italics** can be found in Part III. The food amounts shown are for women and children; men and teens need one-third more.

Potatoes, rice, or pasta are included in six of the seven dinners, and bread is served five times. Margarine is served on the bread. Vegetables are included in all seven dinners and fruit in four of the dinners in low-fat desserts. There are five low-fat desserts in the week of Phase One dinners.

Phase Two dinners: Red meat is served three times in the week of Phase Two dinners, poultry two times, and fish two times—with the maximum serving size of 4 ounces for 2,000 Calories (women/children) and 6 ounces for 2,800 Calories (men/teens). Pasta, rice, potatoes, or tortillas are included in six of the dinners. Bread is served five times, with margarine offered as the spread. Vegetables are served in all seven of the dinners. Low-CSI salad dressings are used. Fruit is included in two of the desserts. Low-fat desserts are served in six of the dinners.

Phase Three dinners: In Phase Three dinners, fish is served two times, poultry three times, red meat one time, and one dinner is meatless. The maximum serving size for meat is 3 ounces for 2,000 Calories (women/children) and 4 ounces for 2,800 Calories (men/teens). Pasta, rice, or potatoes are served in all seven dinners (1½-cup servings for 2,000 Calories and 2-cup servings for 2,800 Calories). Bread—without spread—is offered in six dinners, and the dinner without bread is a Chinese meal with lots of rice. Only low-fat salad dressings are used. Vegetables are included in all seven dinners and fruit is included in three dinners and in one dessert. Low-fat desserts are served in four dinners.

Quick dinners: Let's be realistic. Some meals need to be prepared in a hurry. Many evenings the cook doesn't have much time to spend in the kitchen, or the family needs to have a quick meal. Here are some suggestions for "quick-and-easy" main dishes (you can easily add a green salad and bread, and cut up some fresh fruit to complete the meal): Fresh pasta (the kind with no egg yolk) with bottled marinara sauce, *Turkey Lettuce Stir-Fry* over leftover rice (heats well in the microwave oven) or quick-cook rice, *Bean Sprout Tuna Chow Mein* served over leftover spaghetti, *Quick-and-Easy Pan Bread Pizza* using a prepared pizza sauce, *Baked Herbed Fish* with corn on the cob, *Skinny Sole* with *Rancher's Beans*, Hearty Chicken Soup (a canned soup made by Progresso) with dumplings, or baked potatoes (in microwave—can be finished off in the oven to crisp the skin) and light canned chili with beans over the top. The trick to making these ideas a reality is to have the ingredients *on hand* so you only have to open the cupboard, set the pan on the stove, and produce another low-CSI dinner—while avoiding another trip to the fast-food establishment. The number of frozen dinners is ever-increasing. Select entrées that contain 10 grams or less fat per serving.

DINNER CSIs

Table 23 provides the CSIs for individual dinner foods and dishes.

TABLE 23
THE CSIs OF DINNER CHOICES*

MAIN ENTRÉES: ASIAN DISHES
(SELECT CSIs OF 9 OR LOWER PER SERVING)

	SERVING SIZE		CSI	FAT (GM)	CALORIES
Beef-Tomato Chow Yuk	1½ cups	(270 gm)	3	7	211
Beef Broccoli Oriental	¼ recipe	(230 gm)	7	11	251
CHOW MEIN DISHES					
Pinto Bean Chow Mein	1 cup	(156 gm)	tr.	2	96
Bean Sprout Tuna Chow Mein	1 cup	(134 gm)	1	3	91
Chicken chow mein, typical	1 cup	(69 gm)	4	9	224
Pork chow mein, typical	1 cup	(69 gm)	7	15	270
Stir-Fried Mushrooms and Broccoli	⅛ recipe	(101 gm)	<1	3	69
"Fire" on Rice	1 cup	(200 gm)	2	11	176
Turkey Lettuce Stir-Fry	¼ recipe	(185 gm)	2	5	147
Cashew Chicken	1¾ cups	(288 gm)	4	10	242
Spicy Chicken with Peppers	⅙ recipe (2 pieces)	(245 gm)	5	8	221
Zesty Stir-Fried Chicken	¼ recipe	(315 gm)	5	9	266
Thai Barbecued Chicken	⅙ recipe	(133 gm)	5	5	191
Seafood Teriyaki and Kabobs	¼ recipe	(183 gm)	6	3	258
Wonderful Oriental Steamed Fish	¼ recipe	(326 gm)	7	4	268
Peppers and Prawns	¼ recipe	(200 gm)	9	5	174

* The dessert CSI tables are in Chapter 9.

Egg foo Yong	1 serving	(78 gm)	10	12	131
Tempura	6 prawns	(124 gm)	14	14	272
Fried rice	1 cup	(260 gm)	18	14	338
Chinese Noodles	2¼ cups	(338 gm)	tr.	3	192
Top Raamen	1 cup	(227 gm)	2	8	161

MAIN ENTRÉES: BEEF AND PORK DISHES
(SELECT CSIs OF 9 OF LOWER PER SERVING)

Beef Stroganoff	1 cup	(185 gm)	6	10	242
Beef stroganoff, typical	1 cup	(242 gm)	27	44	571
Beef and Bean Ragout	1 cup	(243 gm)	2	3	168
Bean Hot Dish	1 cup	(186 gm)	2	3	231
Stay-Abed Stew	1 cup	(190 gm)	2	2	121
Beef vegetable stew	1 cup	(245 gm)	8	14	246
Cabbage Roll with rice and tofu	1 roll	(130 gm)	tr.	<1	80
Cabbage roll with rice and cheese	1 roll	(87 gm)	3	8	117
Cabbage roll with ground beef and rice	1 roll	(139 gm)	5	9	176
Black Bean Chili	1 cup	(244 gm)	<1	4	277
Rick's Chili	1 cup	(215 gm)	<1	3	126
Chicken chili with beans	1 cup	(213 gm)	1	4	190
Rose Bowl Chili	1 cup	(267 gm)	2	5	213
Chili con carne with beans	1 cup	(255 gm)	8	14	282

The abbreviation *tr.* stands for trace (less than 0.5); the symbol <1 stands for less than one (0.5 to 0.9). Recipes in **bold italics** can be found in Part III.

151

TABLE 23 *(continued)*

	SERVING SIZE		CSI	FAT (GM)	CALORIES
Chili con carne without beans	1 cup	(255 gm)	11	18	282
Pizza Rice Casserole	1 cup	(144 gm)	3	3	137
Hamburger Helper with ground beef	1 cup	(231 gm)	11	18	356
Hamburger rice casserole	1 cup	(240 gm)	12	24	385
Meat loaf, 10% fat ground beef, egg white (smaller piece)	1 thin slice (2½" x 5" x ¾")	(101 gm)	3	4	126
Old-Fashioned Meat Loaf	⅙ recipe	(130 gm)	4	6	195
Meat loaf, 10% fat ground beef, egg white (larger piece)	1 slice (2½" x 5" x 1½")	(202 gm)	7	7	253
Meat loaf, typical	1 slice (2½" x 5" x 1½")	(199 gm)	17	25	391
Pepper Steak	¼ recipe	(199 gm)	5	7	217
Juicy Flank Steak	⅙ recipe	(76 gm)	6	8	188
Stuffed Flank Steak Florentine	⅛ recipe (3 oz. cooked meat)	(243 gm)	8	10	281
HAMBURGERS					
Very Skinny Burgers	One	(156 gm)	5	10	288
Skinny Burgers	One	(212 gm)	8	15	375
"Hamburger" (typical, at home): 5 oz. (cooked) ground beef (30% fat), 1 Tbsp. ketchup, 3 slices dill pickle, 1 Tbsp. mayonnaise, lettuce, tomato, onion, bun	One	(236 gm)	25	50	763
Quarter Pounder	One	(160 gm)	13	24	427
Quarter Pounder, cheese	One	(186 gm)	18	32	525
Pork Chops Dijon	⅙ recipe	(112 gm)	7	10	199

MAIN ENTRÉES: CHICKEN AND TURKEY DISHES
(SELECT CSIs OF 9 OR LOWER PER SERVING)

Chicken Cacciatore	1 breast	(228 gm)	4	6	222
Chicken cacciatore, typical	1 breast	(222 gm)	8	16	298
Carmen's Curry	1/6 recipe	(433 gm)	5	6	293
Curried Chicken Quickie	1/6 recipe	(269 gm)	3	4	415
Chicken rice casserole	1/6 recipe (1 cup)	(242 gm)	10	16	311
Chicken Parmesan	1/4 recipe (1 piece)	(100 gm)	6	6	205
Parmesan Yogurt Chicken	1/6 recipe (2 pieces)	(155 gm)	7	10	235
Parmesan chicken	1/6 recipe (2 pieces)	(222 gm)	18	47	606
Cashew Chicken	1/4 recipe	(288 gm)	4	10	242
Chicken in Pastry	1/4 recipe	(161 gm)	5	10	314
Zesty Stir-Fried Chicken	1/4 recipe	(315 gm)	5	9	266
Spicy Chicken with Peppers	1/6 recipe (2 pieces)	(245 gm)	5	8	221
Garlic Chicken with Balsamic Vinegar	1/4 recipe (1 piece)	(209 gm)	5	7	220
Chicken with Apricot-Wine Glaze	1/6 recipe (1 piece)	(166 gm)	5	5	270
Chicken Paprika	1/6 recipe (1 piece)	(188 gm)	5	6	214
Chicken Broccoli Roll-Ups	1/4 recipe	(221 gm)	6	5	195

The abbreviation *tr.* stands for trace (less than 0.5); the symbol <1 stands for less than one (0.5 to 0.9). Recipes in **bold italics** can be found in Part III.

MAIN ENTRÉES: CHICKEN AND TURKEY DISHES (continued)

	SERVING SIZE		CSI	FAT (GM)	CALORIES
Oven-Fried Chicken	2 pieces	(139 gm)	5	6	173
Portland Fried Chicken	2 pieces	(139 gm)	5	5	187
Chicken McNuggets	8 pieces	(146 gm)	11	27	433
Chicken, fried, typical	2 pieces	(177 gm)	11	17	335
Chicken, Kentucky Fried	2 pieces	(232 gm)	11	23	431
Curried Chicken and Peanut Salad	1⅓ cups	(204 gm)	3	8	198
Chicken Salad with Yogurt-Chive Dressing	1 cup	(314 gm)	5	5	252
Chicken salad, with mayonnaise	1 cup	(209 gm)	17	64	705
Thai Barbecued Chicken	2 pieces	(133 gm)	5	5	191
Barbecued chicken (no skin)	2 pieces	(147 gm)	6	7	230
Barbecued chicken (with skin)	2 pieces	(176 gm)	9	16	334
Turkey-Vegetable Chowder	2 cups	(418 gm)	3	7	280
Mulligatawny Stew	1 cup	(244 gm)	3	5	174
Rose Bowl Chili	1 cup	(267 gm)	2	5	213
Sesame Linguini with Chicken	1½ cups	(256 gm)	2	5	311
Turkey Tetrazzini	⅙ recipe	(353 gm)	4	8	422
Poppyseed and Turkey Casserole	¼ recipe	(302 gm)	8	9	344
Chicken Fajitas with Lime	One	(191 gm)	4	9	297
Chicken Fajitas Spicy-Style	One	(253 gm)	4	8	290
Chicken Marbella	⅙ recipe	(218 gm)	5	9	289

MAIN ENTRÉES: FISH AND SHELLFISH DISHES
(SELECT CSIs OF 9 OR LOWER PER SERVING)

Poached	6 ounces	(170 gm)	5	2	141
Baked:					
Baked Herbed Fish	7 ounces	(205 gm)	5	5	189
Baked Salmon (3 ounces cooked)	3 ounces	(86 gm)	7	11	185
Baked fish with butter	7 ounces	(193 gm)	14	13	246
Fish sticks, commercial	Six	(227 gm)	14	29	405
Broiled or charcoal grilled: no fat added	6 ounces	(170 gm)	5	2	141
Broiled or charcoal grilled: with butter added	6½ ounces	(184 gm)	14	13	241
Skinny Sole	7 ounces	(202 gm)	7	11	303
Panfried	8 ounces	(229 gm)	14	20	420
Deep-fried (batter coated)	11 ounces	(320 gm)	21	52	725
Fish Almondine with Dilly Sauce (6 ounces cooked fish)	9 ounces	(263 gm)	7	8	248
Fish almondine with dilly sauce (6 ounces cooked fish), typical	10½ ounces	(299 gm)	20	44	566
Fancy Baked Scallops	¼ recipe	(280 gm)	5	8	226
Baked Scallops with Feta Cheese	¼ recipe	(320 gm)	15	24	453
Scallops in Creamy Sauce (3 ounces cooked scallops)	6 ounces	(181 gm)	4	6	218
Coquilles St. Jacques (3 ounces cooked scallops)	9 ounces	(252 gm)	34	41	528

The abbreviation tr. stands for trace (less than 0.5); the symbol <1 stands for less than one (0.5 to 0.9). Recipes in **bold italics** can be found in Part III.

155

MAIN ENTRÉES: FISH AND SHELLFISH DISHES (continued)

	SERVING SIZE		CSI	FAT (GM)	CALORIES
Tuna Noodle Casserole	2 cups	(344 gm)	2	4	292
Tuna noodle casserole, typical	2 cups	(480 gm)	10	30	642
Salmon Loaf	One ¾" slice	(72 gm)	1	4	87
Salmon loaf, typical	One ½" slice	(115 gm)	8	11	212
Salmon Mousse	½ cup	(94 gm)	3	7	140
Salmon mousse, typical	½ cup	(91 gm)	6	19	218
Fish and Leek Chowder	1 cup	(240 gm)	2	2	142
Bouillabaisse	1½ cups	(285 gm)	3	3	123
Northwest Gumbo	2½ cups	(635 gm)	6	5	418
Cioppino	2¼ cups	(529 gm)	8	7	299
Seafood Pilaf	1 cup	(240 gm)	4	3	209
Seafood Strudel	⅙ recipe	(158 gm)	4	6	232
Peppered Salmon Steak	¼ recipe	(135 gm)	5	10	251
Sole with Spring Vegetables	¼ recipe	(241 gm)	5	3	184
Fish à la Mistral	¼ recipe	(324 gm)	6	5	203
Fish Fillets with Walnuts	¼ recipe	(252 gm)	7	11	246
Halibut Mexicana	¼ recipe	(293 gm)	7	6	259
Halibut and Vegetables	¼ recipe	(259 gm)	7	10	289
Lively Lemon Roll-ups	⅙ recipe	(362 gm)	7	6	281
Wonderful Oriental Steamed Fish	¼ recipe	(326 gm)	7	4	268
Oysters Sauté	½ recipe	(229 gm)	7	7	173
Peppers and Prawns	¼ recipe	(200 gm)	9	5	174
Oysters in Crusty French Bread	½ recipe	(318 gm)	9	10	527

156

MAIN ENTRÉES: INDIAN DISHES
(SELECT CSIs OF 9 OR LOWER PER SERVING)

Curried Chicken Quickie	⅙ recipe	(269 gm)	3	4	415
Chicken rice casserole	⅙ recipe (1 cup)	(242 gm)	10	16	311
Carmen's Curry	⅙ recipe	(433 gm)	5	6	293
Vegetable Pulav	¼ recipe	(349 gm)	1	6	389
Pulihora (tamarind rice)	1 cup	(142 gm)	<1	5	264
Spicy Lentils	1 cup	(201 gm)	<1	4	137

MAIN ENTRÉES: MEXICAN DISHES
(SELECT CSIs OF 9 OR LOWER PER SERVING)

ENCHILADAS

Acapulco Enchilada	One 6"	(177 gm)	3	5	193
Creamy Enchilada	One 6"	(196 gm)	3	4	179
No-Meat enchilada	One 6"	(131 gm)	4	7	202
Chicken enchilada	One 6"	114 (gm)	7	10	197
Beef enchilada	One 6"	(114 gm)	9	15	234
Cheese enchilada	One 6"	(114 gm)	12	17	256

BURRITOS (NOT DEEP-FRIED)

Burritos with Black Beans	One	(217 gm)	2	4	242
Your Basic Bean Burrito	One 8"	(202 gm)	2	5	269
Baked Burrito Squares	One	(149 gm)	4	8	298
Bean burrito	One 8"	(161 gm)	7	16	384
Beef burrito	One 8"	(125 gm)	9	16	353

The abbreviation *tr.* stands for trace (less than 0.5); the symbol <1 stands for less than one (0.5 to 0.9). Recipes in *bold italics* can be found in Part III.

157

MAIN ENTRÉES: MEXICAN DISHES (*continued*)

	SERVING SIZE		CSI	FAT (GM)	CALORIES
CHILE RELLENOS					
Chile Relleno Casserole	One chile	(152 gm)	2	4	155
Chile relleno	One chile	(110 gm)	19	21	267
SALADS					
Taco Salad	2 cups	(261 gm)	4	8	252
Taco salad, typical	2 cups	(212 gm)	15	25	336
CASSEROLES					
Tamale Pie	1 cup	(276 gm)	3	4	205
Acapulco Bean Casserole	1 cup	(201 gm)	5	9	236
Tamale pie, typical	1 cup	(286 gm)	16	28	441
SIDE DISHES					
Black Beans with 1,000 Uses	1 cup	(212 gm)	tr.	tr.	126
Refried Beans	1 cup	(174 gm)	1	6	225
Refried beans (canned)	1 cup	(241 gm)	1	4	248
Refried beans, typical	1 cup	(243 gm)	12	28	485
FISH					
Halibut Mexicana	6 oz. fish	(293 gm)	7	6	259
FAJITAS					
Chicken Fajitas with Lime	One	(191 gm)	4	9	297
Chicken Fajitas Spicy-Style	One	(253 gm)	4	8	290

MAIN ENTRÉES: PASTA DISHES
(SPAGHETTI, MACARONI, NOODLES)
(SELECT CSIs OF 9 OR LOWER PER SERVING)

GOULASH TYPE

Garbanzo Goulash	1 cup	(186 gm)	tr.	3	208
Texas Hash	1 cup	(240 gm)	1	3	170
Beef & macaroni casserole	1 cup	(240 gm)	9	19	328

LASAGNA

Bean Lasagna	3" x 3"	(224 gm)	3	5	220
Easy Oven Lasagna	3" x 3"	(321 gm)	3	6	185
Spinach Lasagna	3" x 3"	(245 gm)	3	6	223
Lasagna Primavera	3" x 3"	(221 gm)	4	7	240
Lasagna with meat sauce	3" x 3"	(235 gm)	14	19	390

MACARONI & CHEESE

Macaroni Bake	1 cup	(219 gm)	2	5	246
From packaged mix	1 cup	(209 gm)	6	18	401
Homemade (2% milk)	1 cup	(200 gm)	12	19	336

RAVIOLIS

Homemade Ravioli (Chicken)	6 large, 12 small	(490 gm)	2	10	366
Ravioli, cheese (canned)	1 cup	(223 gm)	4	5	229
Ravioli, meat (canned)	1 cup	(223 gm)	5	7	240
Ravioli, cheese (homemade), with to-mato sauce	6 large, 12 small	(131 gm)	10	11	216

The abbreviation *tr.* stands for trace (less than 0.5); the symbol <1 stands for less than one (0.5 to 0.9). Recipes in **bold italics** can be found in Part III.

MAIN ENTRÉES: PASTA DISHES

	SERVING SIZE		CSI	FAT (GM)	CALORIES
Ravioli, meat (homemade), with tomato sauce	6 large, 12 small	(149 gm)	13	20	302
SALADS					
Montana Pasta Salad	1 cup	(196 gm)	<1	4	169
Four-Star Pasta Salad	1 cup	(137 gm)	<1	3	154
Macaroni (with mayonnaise)	1 cup	(184 gm)	7	36	510
STUFFED					
Cheese-Stuffed Manicotti	1 piece	(178 gm)	2	4	135
Manicotti with cheddar cheese	1 piece	(173 gm)	11	10	220
SPAGHETTI					
Spaghetti with *Marinara Sauce*	1½ cups	(302 gm)	tr.	3	251
Spaghetti with *Beef-Mushroom Spaghetti Sauce*	1½ cups	(235 gm)	1	2	267
Spaghetti with *Turkey-Mushroom Spaghetti Sauce*	1½ cups	(250 gm)	1	2	266
Spaghetti with *Light Mushroom Sauce*	1½ cups	(242 gm)	1	3	262

160

Spaghetti with **Clam Sauce**	1½ cups	(210 gm)	4	6	303
Spaghetti with meat sauce	1½ cups	(259 gm)	6	11	356
TUNA DISHES					
Tuna Noodle Casserole	1 cup	(172 gm)	1	2	146
Tuna noodle casserole, typical	1 cup	(240 gm)	5	15	321
OTHER DISHES					
Fettuccine, at Last!	¼ recipe	(205 gm)	2	5	358
Fettuccine Alfredo	¼ recipe	(234 gm)	31	39	573
Sesame Linguini with Chicken	1½ cups	(256 gm)	2	5	311
Baked Spaghetti Pie	⅙ recipe	(160 gm)	2	3	213
Savory Eggplant Pasta Sauce	1 cup	(250 gm)	1	3	131
Pasta with Fresh Tomato Sauce	⅙ recipe	(362 gm)	2	6	397
Turkey Tetrazzini	⅙ recipe	(353 gm)	4	8	422
Poppyseed and Turkey Casserole	¼ recipe	(302 gm)	8	9	344
Calico Pasta	1 cup	(192 gm)	tr.	3	142

The abbreviation *tr.* stands for trace (less than 0.5); the symbol <1 stands for less than one (0.5 to 0.9). Recipes in **bold italics** can be found in Part III.

MAIN ENTRÉES: PIZZAS
(SELECT CSIs OF 9 OR LOWER PER SERVING)

	SERVING SIZE	CSI	FAT (GM)	CALORIES
THIN CRUST PIZZA				
Spicy Cheese Pizza	¼ of 14" pizza (357 gm)	5	9	390
Green pepper-mushroom-onion	¼ of 14" pizza (292 gm)	9	14	419
Canadian bacon	¼ of 14" pizza (229 gm)	10	16	446
Pepperoni	¼ of 14" pizza (229 gm)	13	23	509
Cheese	¼ of 14" pizza (257 gm)	16	24	552
Combination	¼ of 14" pizza (279 gm)	20	38	676
THICK CRUST PIZZA				
Spicy Cheese Pizza	¼ of 14" pizza (417 gm)	4	7	565
Green pepper-mushroom-onion	¼ of 14" pizza (360 gm)	6	9	574
Canadian bacon	¼ of 14" pizza (334 gm)	7	12	611
Pepperoni	¼ of 14" pizza (334 gm)	10	19	674
Cheese	¼ of 14" pizza (343 gm)	11	16	664
Combination	¼ of 14" pizza (384 gm)	17	33	842
Quick-and-Easy Pan Bread Pizza	⅙ of recipe (251 gm)	2	11	339
Pita Pizza	1 pizza (149 gm)	3	5	255
Baguette with Vegetable Filling	½ of recipe (354 gm)	2	10	500
Vegetable Calzone	¼ of recipe (301 gm)	5	11	437

162

MAIN ENTRÉES: QUICHES
(SELECT CSIs OF 9 OR LOWER PER SERVING)

Broccoli Quiche				
Broccoli Quiche	⅙ of 9" quiche	(229 gm)	2	6	189
Broccoli quiche—no egg yolk, 2% fat milk, typical crust	⅙ of 9" quiche	(209 gm)	9	21	327
Broccoli quiche, typical	⅙ of 9" quiche	(209 gm)	30	38	480
Zucchini Pie	3" x 4½"	(145 gm)	5	7	188
Zucchini casserole	3" x 4½"	(330 gm)	17	14	210

SALADS
(SELECT CSIs OF 3 OR LOWER PER SERVING)

GREEN SALADS

Green salad (1 cup, 55 gm) with: low-calorie blue cheese dressing	2 tablespoons	(31 gm)	1	2	30
Blue cheese dressing	2 tablespoons	(30 gm)	3	16	147
Blue cheese dressing	¼ cup	(59 gm)	6	32	287
Green salad (1 cup, 55 gm) with: low-calorie French dressing	2 tablespoons	(33 gm)	tr.	2	51
Red French Dressing	2 tablespoons	(31 gm)	<1	5	87
Russian Salad Dressing	2 tablespoons	(30 gm)	<1	4	57
French dressing	2 tablespoons	(32 gm)	3	13	140
French dressing	¼ cup	(63 gm)	6	25	274

The abbreviation *tr.* stands for trace (less than 0.5); the symbol <1 stands for less than one (0.5 to 0.9). Recipes in ***bold italics*** can be found in Part III.

SALADS *(continued)*

	SERVING SIZE		CSI	FAT (GM)	CALORIES
Green salad (1 cup, 55 gm) with: low-calorie Italian dressing	2 tablespoons	(30 gm)	1	3	39
Italian dressing	2 tablespoons	(30 gm)	1	8	97
Italian dressing	¼ cup	(59 gm)	2	16	187
Green salad (1 cup, 55 gm) with: 3 Tbsp. vinegar + 1 Tbsp. olive oil	¼ cup	(59 gm)	2	14	129
2 Tbsp. vinegar + 2 Tbsp. olive oil	¼ cup	(57 gm)	4	27	250
Green salad (1 cup, 55 gm) with: *Western Salad Dressing*	2 tablespoons	(29 gm)	tr.	1	31
Ranch dressing (typical restaurant)	2 tablespoons	(30 gm)	2	11	114
Green salad (1 cup, 55 gm) with: *Thousand Island Salad Dressing*	2 tablespoons	(28 gm)	tr.	1	37
low-calorie Thousand Island dressing	2 tablespoons	(31 gm)	1	3	56
Thousand Island dressing	2 tablespoons	(30 gm)	2	10	127
Thousand Island dressing	¼ cup	(59 gm)	4	20	247
Sunshine Spinach Salad	1 cup	(105 gm)	tr.	2	51
Snowbird Salad	1 cup	(120 gm)	<1	5	58
Vinaigrette Salad Dressing with Greens	1 cup	(61 gm)	tr.	2	31
Caesar salad	1 cup	(87 gm)	6	20	207
CHEF-TYPE SALADS					
Crab Louis without egg, with ¼ cup *Thousand Island Salad Dressing*	1 salad	(389 gm)	7	7	232
Crab Louis without egg, with ½ cup low-calorie Thousand Island salad dressing	1 salad	(455 gm)	8	18	348
Crab Louis with egg, ½ cup low-calorie Thousand Island salad dressing	1 salad	(505 gm)	20	24	427

Food	Amount	Weight			
Crab Louis with egg, ½ cup Thousand Island salad dressing	1 salad	(501 gm)	26	51	714
Shrimp Louis without egg, with ¼ cup *Thousand Island Salad Dressing*	1 salad	(389 gm)	8	7	232
Shrimp Louis without egg, with ½ cup low-calorie Thousand Island salad dressing	1 salad	(455 gm)	10	17	364
Shrimp Louis with egg, ½ cup low-calorie Thousand Island salad dressing	1 salad	(505 gm)	22	23	443
Shrimp Louis with egg, ½ cup Thousand Island salad dressing	1 salad	(501 gm)	28	50	730
Chef's salad without egg, with Cheddar cheese, ham, turkey, ½ cup low-calorie Thousand Island dressing	1 salad	(466 gm)	19	34	545
Chef's salad with egg, with Cheddar cheese, ham, turkey, ½ cup low-calorie Thousand Island salad dressing	1 salad	(516 gm)	31	40	624
Chef's salad with egg, with Cheddar cheese, ham, turkey, ½ cup Thousand Island salad dressing (typical restaurant)	1 salad	(512 gm)	40	67	910
MISCELLANEOUS SALADS					
Confetti Appleslaw	1 cup	(105 gm)	tr.	1	55
Orange Yogurt Fruit Slaw	1 cup	(144 gm)	tr.	2	96
Sesame Slaw	1 cup	(114 gm)	tr.	3	91
Sesame slaw, typical	1 cup	(145 gm)	4	30	331
Cole slaw with salad dressing	1 cup	(120 gm)	4	19	201
Cole slaw with mayonnaise	1 cup	(120 gm)	6	29	282

The abbreviation *tr.* stands for trace (less than 0.5); the symbol <1 stands for less than one (0.5 to 0.9). Recipes in **bold italics** can be found in Part III.

SALADS *(continued)*

		SERVING SIZE		CSI	FAT (GM)	CALORIES
Potato Salad	1 cup	(255 gm)		1	4	206
German potato salad	1 cup	(188 gm)		2	5	163
Potato salad, typical	1 cup	(240 gm)		10	26	392
California Beans	1 cup	(155 gm)		tr.	2	126
Summer Bean Salad	1 cup	(178 gm)		<1	4	199
Spicy Black Bean Salad	1 cup	(170 gm)		<1	4	228
Chili Bean Salad	1 cup	(221 gm)		<1	5	255
Three-bean salad	1 cup	(167 gm)		4	23	287
Curried Chicken with Peanut Salad	1 cup	(123 gm)		2	5	119
Chicken Salad with Yogurt-Chive Dressing	1 cup	(172 gm)		3	3	169
Simply Wonderful Turkey Salad	1 cup	(171 gm)		1	4	156
Chicken salad with mayonnaise	1 cup	(209 gm)		17	64	705
Orange Bulgur Salad	1 cup	(397 gm)		tr.	1	252
Tabouli	1 cup	(220 gm)		1	8	178
Tabouli, typical	1 cup	(219 gm)		3	19	269
Carrot Raisin Salad	1 cup	(136 gm)		<1	2	166
Carrot raisin salad, typical	1 cup	(108 gm)		6	9	152
Waldorf Salad	1 cup	(147 gm)		2	10	196
Waldorf salad, typical	1 cup	(155 gm)		6	36	382
Greek Salad	1 cup	(114 gm)		<1	3	55
Aspic with mayonnaise, crab, asparagus	1 cup	(209 gm)		3	12	162
Absolutely Delicious Molded Salad	1/15 recipe	(185 gm)		tr.	tr.	150

166

	Serving	(weight)			
Holiday Wreath Salad	1 cup	(262 gm)	2	5	274
Fruit salad with marshmallows and whipped cream	1 cup	(152 gm)	7	9	180
Crunchy Vegetable Salad	1 cup	(191 gm)	1	5	136
Crunchy vegetable salad, typical	1 cup	(257 gm)	13	47	561
Cheese and pea salad	1 cup	(187 gm)	15	13	247
Moroccan Salad	1 cup	(163 gm)	<1	4	229
Montana Pasta Salad	1 cup	(196 gm)	<1	4	169
Four-Star Pasta Salad	1 cup	(137 gm)	<1	3	154
Alphabet Seafood Salad	1 cup	(181 gm)	2	3	242
Macaroni (with mayonnaise)	1 cup	(184 gm)	7	36	510
Salad Athene	1 cup	(69 gm)	1	4	103
Salad Athene, typical	1 cup	(137 gm)	3	14	195
Crunchy Confetti Salad	1 cup	(186 gm)	<1	6	170
Curried Rice and Artichoke Salad	1 cup	(250 gm)	<1	3	206
Fruit and Rice Salad	1 cup	(155 gm)	tr.	3	169
Lemony Beets	⅙ recipe	(58 gm)	<1	5	66
Green Bean, Mushroom, and Tomato Salad	⅛ recipe	(109 gm)	1	4	67

The abbreviation *tr.* stands for trace (less than 0.5); the symbol <1 stands for less than one (0.5 to 0.9). Recipes in **bold italics** can be found in Part III.

SAUCES AND GRAVIES
(SELECT CSIs OF 2 OR LOWER PER SERVING)

	SERVING SIZE		CSI	FAT (GM)	CALORIES
Basic White Sauce (made with skim milk)	¼ cup	(59 gm)	<1	3	47
White sauce (made with whole milk)	¼ cup	(63 gm)	3	8	101
Cheese sauce, low-fat	¼ cup	(53 gm)	1	3	51
Cheese sauce	¼ cup	(63 gm)	6	11	133
Mock Hollandaise Sauce	¼ cup	(67 gm)	2	7	90
Hollandaise, canned or from a mix	¼ cup	(64 gm)	13	17	176
Hollandaise or Bearnaise, homemade	¼ cup	(65 gm)	16	27	250
Turkey Gravy	¼ cup	(68 gm)	tr.	2	32
Turkey gravy	¼ cup	(65 gm)	1	2	28
Au jus	¼ cup	(63 gm)	tr.	tr.	10
Cream gravy for chicken made with skim milk	¼ cup	(60 gm)	<1	2	39
Cream gravy for chicken made with whole milk	¼ cup	(60 gm)	2	4	55
Tartar Sauce	¼ cup	(47 gm)	<1	<1	40
Tartar sauce, typical	¼ cup	(58 gm)	6	33	305
Cranberry sauce	¼ cup	(68 gm)	0	tr.	103
Baked Cranberry-Nut Relish	¼ cup	(70 gm)	tr.	2	152
Sweet & sour sauce	¼ cup	(78 gm)	0	0	73
Barbecue sauce (bottled)	¼ cup	(63 gm)	tr.	2	70
Marinara Sauce	¼ cup	(86 gm)	tr.	1	29

168

Italian sauce (meatless)	¼ cup (60 gm)	tr.	2	42
Italian sauce (with meat)	¼ cup (64 gm)	3	5	82
Onion Chutney	¼ cup (53 gm)	tr.	tr.	112
Homemade Enchilada Sauce	¼ cup (62 gm)	tr.	tr.	14
Cucumber-Dilly Sauce	¼ cup (60 gm)	tr.	<1	30
Cucumber-dilly sauce, typical	¼ cup (60 gm)	3	6	64

POTATO DISHES
(SELECT CSIs OF 2 OR LOWER PER SERVING)

Baked potato, plain	1 potato/1 cup (156 gm)	<1	<1	170
Potato Puff	1 potato (215 gm)	1	2	142
Super Stuffed Potato	½ potato (131 gm)	1	3	113
Cheese-stuffed baked potato	1 potato (188 gm)	4	10	236
Plank Potatoes	¼ recipe (187 gm)	<1	4	231
Skinny "French Fries"	1 cup (163 gm)	<1	4	134
French fries	1 cup (137 gm)	5	17	392
Skinny Hash Browns	1 cup (155 gm)	<1	5	174
Hash browns	1 cup (155 gm)	5	17	375
Homemade Tatertots	1 cup (93 gm)	2	7	192
Tatertots	1 cup (104 gm)	5	11	222

The abbreviation *tr.* stands for trace (less than 0.5); the symbol <1 stands for less than one (0.5 to 0.9). Recipes in **bold italics** can be found in Part III.

POTATO DISHES (continued)

	SERVING SIZE		CSI	FAT (GM)	CALORIES
Mashed Potatoes	1 cup	(180 gm)	tr.	tr.	111
Mashed potatoes, typical	1 cup	(210 gm)	2	9	241
Potato Salad	1 cup	(255 gm)	1	4	206
German potato salad	1 cup	(188 gm)	2	5	163
Potato salad, typical	1 cup	(240 gm)	10	26	392
Scalloped Potatoes	1 cup	(314 gm)	<1	2	219
Scalloped potatoes made with skim milk	1 cup	(245 gm)	1	6	232
Scalloped potatoes made with whole milk	1 cup	(245 gm)	4	9	259
Au gratin potatoes, homemade	1 cup	(245 gm)	15	19	322
Holiday Yams	1 potato	(198 gm)	tr.	2	287
Candied sweet potatoes	1 potato	(206 gm)	6	8	338
Spuds and Onions	1 cup	(146 gm)	tr.	2	185
Italian Potatoes	¼ recipe	(161 gm)	<1	4	200

VEGETABLE AND GRAIN DISHES
(SELECT CSIs OF 2 OR LOWER PER SERVING)

Corn Bake	1 cup	(154 gm)	tr.	<1	118
Onion Squares	3" x 3"	(93 gm)	1	5	140
Corn pudding	1 cup	(255 gm)	13	14	280
Calico Pasta	1 cup	(192 gm)	tr.	3	142
Bulgur Pilaf	1 cup	(218 gm)	tr.	3	209

Recipe	Serving	Weight			
Spicy Peanut Noodles	1 cup	(148 gm)	<1	4	223
Mushroom Barley Pilaf	1 cup	(217 gm)	<1	3	262
Rice pilaf	1 cup	(220 gm)	4	16	365
Barley pilaf	1 cup	(238 gm)	8	13	290
Spanish Rice	1 cup	(219 gm)	tr.	3	149
Spanish rice, typical	1 cup	(245 gm)	<1	3	195
Lemon Rice	1 cup	(167 gm)	tr.	<1	221
Pine Needle Rice	1 cup	(245 gm)	<1	5	318
Gourmet Curried Rice	¼ recipe	(139 gm)	1	4	212
Spinach and Rice Casserole	3" x 4½"	(191 gm)	2	4	174
Broccoli with Rice	1 cup	(182 gm)	2	5	157
Green Rice	1 cup	(130 gm)	3	5	169
Green rice, typical	1 cup	(200 gm)	15	16	299
Eggplant Parmesan	1 cup	(290 gm)	2	6	124
Eggplant Parmesan, typical	1 cup	(209 gm)	10	24	344
Rancher's Beans	1 cup	(238 gm)	tr.	<1	342
Classic Baked Beans	1 cup	(190 gm)	tr.	2	230
Baked beans with ham	1 cup	(256 gm)	5	12	384
Tomatoes "Provençale"	1 tomato	(197 gm)	tr.	3	73
Ratatouille Provençale	⅛ recipe	(237 gm)	<1	2	72
Stuffed Zucchini Boats	1 boat	(168 gm)	1	4	66
Fettuccine, at Last!	¼ recipe	(205 gm)	2	5	358

The abbreviation tr. stands for trace (less than 0.5); the symbol <1 stands for less than one (0.5 to 0.9). Recipes in **bold italics** can be found in Part III.

171

VEGETABLE AND GRAIN DISHES *(continued)*

	SERVING SIZE		CSI	FAT (GM)	CALORIES
Fettuccine Alfredo	¼ recipe	(234 gm)	31	39	573
Vegetable Pulav	2 cups	(349 gm)	1	6	389
Pulihora (Tamarind Rice)	1 cup	(142 gm)	<1	5	264
Spicy Lentils	1 cup	(201 gm)	<1	4	137
Oriental Broccoli	1 cup	(105 gm)	tr.	2	70
Easy Acorn Squash	¼ recipe	(275 gm)	tr.	2	101
Grilled Zucchini	¼ recipe	(200 gm)	tr.	1	32
Lemony Beets	⅙ recipe	(58 gm)	<1	5	66
Acorn Squash with Roasted Onions	⅛ recipe	(315 gm)	<1	3	135
Stir-Fried Mushrooms and Broccoli	⅛ recipe	(101 gm)	<1	3	69
Cheesy Cauliflower	¼ recipe	(167 gm)	2	3	76
Zucchini Puff	¼ recipe	(76 gm)	3	4	93

BREADS
(SELECT CSIs OF 1 OR LOWER PER SERVING)

YEAST BREADS					
White	1 slice	(25 gm)	tr.	<1	68
Whole wheat	1 slice	(29 gm)	tr.	<1	70
Raisin	1 slice	(23 gm)	tr.	<1	61
Rye	1 slice	(29 gm)	tr.	tr.	70

Food	Serving	Weight			
Pumpernickel	1 slice	(25 gm)	tr.	tr.	62
English muffin	One	(57 gm)	tr.	1	135
Whole Wheat French Bread	⅕ loaf	(38 gm)	tr.	<1	125
Grape-nut Bread	1 slice or roll	(42 gm)	tr.	1	99
French, Italian, sourdough	4¼" x 2¾" x 1"	(30 gm)	tr.	tr.	83
Pita or pocket	One	(64 gm)	tr.	<1	180
Boston brown	1 slice	(48 gm)	tr.	<1	101
Cinnamon swirl	1 slice	(22 gm)	tr.	<1	59
Egg	1 slice	(33 gm)	2	2	89
Cheese	1 slice	(29 gm)	2	3	87
Challah	1 slice	(33 gm)	2	2	89
Focaccia	⅛ loaf	(60 gm)	1	5	190
Boboli	⅛ loaf	(60 gm)	2	8	183
YEAST ROLLS					
Hard	1 small	(25 gm)	tr.	<1	77
Kaiser	One	(50 gm)	tr.	2	153
Caraway Dinner Roll	One	(48 gm)	tr.	<1	108
Pan or dinner-type	One	(28 gm)	<1	2	83
Poor boy or submarine	3" x 11½"	(135 gm)	1	4	385
Crescent	One	(28 gm)	3	6	101
Croissant	One	(55 gm)	9	12	167

The abbreviation *tr.* stands for trace (less than 0.5); the symbol <1 stands for less than one (0.5 to 0.9). Recipes in **bold italics** can be found in Part III.

BISCUITS	SERVING SIZE	CSI	FAT (GM)	CALORIES
Old-style Wheat Biscuit	One (34 gm)	<1	4	86
Canned	One ½" (21 gm)	<1	3	68
Baking powder	One½ 2" (28 gm)	2	5	118
Scone	One½ 4" (56 gm)	6	12	294

OTHER DINNER FOODS

	SERVING SIZE	CSI	FAT (GM)	CALORIES
Fruits, most varieties:	1 medium piece, (100 gm) 1 cup melon or berries, ½ cup grapes, ½ cup canned fruit, ½ cup juice, ¼ cup dried	tr.	tr.	60
Vegetables (carrots, celery, green beans, tomatoes, broccoli, cauliflower, etc.) cooked	½ cup (93 gm)	tr.	tr.	25
raw	1 cup (123 gm)	tr.	tr.	25
Vegetables (peas, corn, potatoes, winter squash, hominy, etc.)	½ cup (80 gm)	tr.	tr.	65
Leafy vegetables (lettuce, spinach, etc.), raw	1 cup (55 gm)	tr.	tr.	10

174

MILK (SELECT CSIs OF 2 OR LOWER PER CUP)

		<1	tr.	85
Milk, skim or powdered nonfat	1 cup	(245 gm)	tr.	85
Buttermilk, 1% fat	1 cup	(245 gm)	2	98
Milk, 1% fat	1 cup	(244 gm)	2	102
Milk, 2% fat	1 cup	(244 gm)	4	122
Milk, chocolate, 2% fat	1 cup	(250 gm)	5	194
Milk, whole	1 cup	(244 gm)	7	149

MARGARINE AND BUTTER (SELECT CSIs OF 0.7 OR LOWER PER TEASPOON)

Margarine, diet (40% fat, not recommended for baking)	1 teaspoon	(5 gm)	0.3	17
Margarine, table spread (60% fat, Country Crock)	1 teaspoon	(5 gm)	0.5	27
Margarine, liquid (squeeze type)	1 teaspoon	(5 gm)	0.7	35
Margarine, tub or soft stick (Saffola, Mazola, Fleischmann's)	1 teaspoon	(5 gm)	0.7	35
Margarine, hard stick (inexpensive store brands)	1 teaspoon	(5 gm)	0.8	35
Butter	1 teaspoon	(5 gm)	3.1	36

The abbreviation *tr.* stands for trace (less than 0.5); the symbol <1 stands for less than one (0.5 to 0.9). Recipes in ***bold italics*** can be found in Part III.

175

CHAPTER

9

Desserts

THE PRECIOUS CSIs

We all love desserts—so much so that we can't seem to make changes as easily here as we do in other areas. Even though we are eating leaner meats, lower-fat dairy products, and more grains and beans, many of us are still eating too many sugar-coated fats, which is what most desserts are. One reason, in our opinion, is the erroneous, widely held belief that, when it comes to dessert, there is no middle ground—either you indulge freely in them or you abstain, settling for fresh fruit instead. The good news in this chapter is that *some* sweet desserts containing a little fat *do* fit into a lower-CSI eating style. Rating desserts by their CSIs, we've found, is a most effective way of putting the sweet/fat stuff in proper perspective. This chapter will show you how to use these very precious CSIs.

Desserts can be modified so that they have *less* fat and sugar and *fewer* calories, but, let's not kid ourselves, they will *still* pose serious problems if we consume typical, large serving sizes several times a day. If *you* have developed the dessert habit to the extent that you've got to have it with *both* lunch and dinner, then the obvious way to start is to cut back on dessert at *one* of these meals. Once you're down to one dessert a day, start whittling away at that by having *smaller* portions. And note, as you pursue your CSI goals, the dinner CSI goals discussed in the preceding chapter *include* dessert.

If you'll look at Table 25 at the end of the chapter, you'll see that single servings of most typical desserts deliver downright scary CSIs and a heavy load of calories.

176

Some examples: German chocolate cake with frosting (CSI 17, 472 Calories for a 3" x 3" x 2" piece), cheesecake (CSI 22, 355 Calories for 1/12 of 10"), strawberry shortcake (CSI 19, 616 Calories for 1/6 of 8"), typical deli chocolate chip cookie (CSI 6, 289 Calories for one 3¼"), typical frosted brownie (CSI 20, 721 Calories for 3" x 3"), gourmet ice cream (CSI 30, 580 Calories for 1 cup), coconut cream pie (CSI 25, 455 Calories for 1/6 of 9"), chocolate mousse (CSI 33, 380 Calories for 1 cup). To help put these CSIs in perspective, the Phase Three CSI *daily* goal is 17 for women/children and 24 for men/teens.

Remember, the above numbers are for *single* servings. Double those figures if you go back for seconds. Remember the last time you couldn't stop at just one brownie or even two and ended up eating three? That "little" indulgence might take only a minute or two, but would total more than 2,100 Calories and a CSI of 60!

Review Chapters 3 and 4 in Part II for guidelines on how to handle chocolate, ice cream, and other dairy desserts. As noted in those chapters, there *are* delicious alternatives to ice cream and chocolate, including cocoa powder, carob, low-fat or nonfat frozen yogurt, sherbets, and sorbets. Table 25 in this chapter will show you the CSI differences among these choices used in desserts—and they are often dramatic. (In the following chapter, which deals with snack foods, you'll find the CSIs of candy bars and the like.)

The fat is the big item we have to watch out for in desserts. But we also need to pay attention to the sugar. Sugar itself has a zero CSI but it's one of the concentrated sources of calories. You may be shocked to learn that Americans get fully 20 percent of their total calories from sugar. The typical American eats about *100 pounds* of sugar each year! A good general goal is to try to cut sugar consumption *in half*. You can start doing this not only by cutting back on desserts and using sugar-modified desserts, but also by reducing the amount of sugar you add to foods at the table and in your cooking. If you make these sugar reductions in your cooking gradual, no one in your family will even notice.

Most Americans consume 20 to 30 teaspoons of sugar daily, some directly in prepared foods, pop, and candy. This should be reduced gradually to no more than 14 teaspoons per day for men and teens and to no more than 10 teaspoons daily for women and children. That's sugar from *all* sources, including sugar "hidden" in prepared foods. *Read labels.* The ingredients are listed in order of amounts (most to least). The higher up on a label's list of ingredients sugar is mentioned, the more of it there is in the product. And sugar is sugar no matter what form it comes in—sucrose, glucose, fructose, etc. Sugar is a prominent ingredient in many foods you might not suspect, including many cereals, salad dressings, frozen pizza, wieners, lunch meats, ketchup, crackers, spaghetti sauce, etc. Some prepared mixes used for coating meat and chicken are, for example, 65 percent sugar. A 12-ounce can of soda pop contains a staggering 7 or 8 teaspoons of sugar. When you reduce your sugar intake from pop and prepared foods, you'll be able to have more in those precious desserts.

We think the proper use of sugar is to sweeten our sour fruits and our grains (quick breads, cakes, cookies). Therefore, you'll find sugar used in these desserts—but we have reduced the amount typically used. Take, for example, our *Berry Pavlova*—the recipe for the meringue originally called for ¾ cup sugar and we reduced it to ½ cup, a savings of 240 Calories. And the meringue tastes great!

Beware Bigger—But Not Better—Desserts

A worrisome trend we've noted is the runaway dessert—the old standard, bad enough to begin with, expanded to Godzilla-like proportions. We're now confronted with "giant" chocolate chip cookies, "super" muffins, "jumbo" soft drinks,

and so on. In the new never-never land of amplified desserts, some sweets have grown to three times their original sizes. No wonder people are growing larger, too! There are gargantuan cookies out there now that can, *individually*, deliver nearly 640 Calories.

In Table 24 you can see for yourself that typical, larger servings pack big CSIs *and* provide lots of calories. Take a favorite carrot cake—a typical piece (3 inches by 3¼ inches) has a CSI of 14 and contains 662 Calories. If you simply cut this serving size in half and eat a 2-inch-by-2¼-inch piece, the CSI is 7 and there are 331 Calories—better but still too high for lower-CSI eating. But you can have your cake and eat it too if you use our fat-modified carrot cake (*Party Carrot Cake*). A larger serving size (3 inches by 3¼ inches), has a CSI of only

TABLE 24
THE CHOLESTEROL–SATURATED FAT INDEX (CSI) OF SMALLER AND LARGER SERVINGS OF TWO TYPICAL AND FAT-MODIFIED CAKES

CAKE	SERVING SIZE	CSI	CALORIES
Carrot cake, frosted:			
Carrot cake, fat-modified*	Smaller (2″ x 2¼″)	2	224
Carrot cake, fat-modified*	Larger (3″ x 3¼″)	3	449
Carrot cake, typical	Smaller (2″ x 2¼″)	7	331
Carrot cake, typical	Larger (3″ x 3¼″)	14	662
Apple Cake, unfrosted:			
Apple Cake, fat-modified†	Smaller (1/24 of cake)	<1	179
Apple cake, fat-modified†	Larger (1/12 of cake)	2	359
Apple cake, typical	Smaller (1/24 of cake)	3	229
Apple cake, typical	Larger (1/12 of cake)	6	457

* *Party Carrot Cake* (recipe can be found in Part III)

† *Apple Loaf Cake* (recipe can be found in Part III)

The symbol <1 stands for less than one (0.5 to 0.9).

3 and contains 449 Calories. Better yet, select the smaller serving size (2 inches by 2¼ inches), with a CSI of 2 and 224 Calories. This will fit nicely into a low-CSI eating pattern while helping keep your waistline fit, too. You'll find the same scenario for apple cake. Our fat-modified version, *Apple Loaf Cake*, cuts the CSI in half and saves calories. The "rule of thumb" for desserts is to use fat-modified (and sugar-modified in most cases) recipes and cut the serving size in half. Smaller servings of fat-modified recipes fit the criteria for low-CSI eating.

Other cakes that have CSIs of 1 or lower per serving are: *Pinto Fiesta Cake, Angel Quickie, Hot Fudge Pudding Cake, Chocolate Zucchini Cake, Poppyseed Cake, Cocoa Cake, Depression Cake, All-Season Short-cake*, and *Baba au Rhum*.

For the Cookie Monster

There is at least one cookie monster in every house. One quick look at our list of cookies and bars could send you into the depths of a depression. If it does—take a second look! There are at least seven kinds of cookies you can make that have very low CSIs—almost 0 to 1 per serving: *Forgotten Kisses, Lebkuchen, Gingies, Carob, Crispy Spice, Oatmeal*, and *Lace Cookies*. There are 6 kinds of cookies you can buy that have CSIs of 3 or lower per serving (gingersnaps, animal and graham crackers, vanilla wafers, fortune cookies, and fig or fruit bars). On a recent raft trip on the Salmon River in Idaho we caught the guides serving the chocolate chip cookies and hiding the "cinnamon-apple newtons" under the table to eat themselves.

There's also good news for brownie addicts. You can make low-CSI brownies using a mix and making them with oil and egg whites while leaving off the nuts and frosting (CSI of 1 per brownie). The fat and calories are still up there though: 8 grams of fat (1½ teaspoons) and 294 Calories for each brownie. For the best brownie choices, try our recipes for *Brownies* (CSI of 1 per serving with 5 grams fat and 133 Calories), *Jamocha Squares* (CSI of less than 1 per serving with 4 grams fat and 103 Calories per serving), and *Cocoa Cake*, unfrosted (CSI of 1 per serving with 5 grams fat and 205 Calories).

Other low-CSI (less than 1 per serving) bars you may want to try are: *Chocolate Banana Bars, Apricot Meringue Bars, Northwest Harvest Bars, Molasses Orange Bars*, Rice Krispie bar, and *Walnut Squares*.

Fruit—The Perfect Dessert

You don't need this book to know that fruit, by itself, is a great dessert. However, you may not fully appreciate the tastiness and nutrient value of dessert recipes that are predominantly fruit. The CSIs are 1 or less per serving, the fat varies from almost 0 to 4 grams per serving, and calories are low compared to typical desserts—125 to 244 Calories per serving. (Since the calories are not zero, we can't eat these delicious fruit desserts with abandon—we'll gain weight.) The biggest surprise is that they all contain appreciable amounts of fiber—2 to 6 grams per serving. Try our *Baked Apples*, which can be microwaved very quickly. Warm cinnamon applesauce is a great treat—and quick to prepare.

Ice Cream and Other Frozen Desserts

We discussed these desserts in great detail, earlier in Chapter 3. The table of frozen desserts is repeated at the end of this chapter in Table 25 for easy referral. Although frozen yogurt has already been discussed, its use as a dessert bears emphasis. The quality of frozen yogurt has steadily improved over the years and is now widely available. Discover for yourself how delicious *and* nutritious *nonfat* frozen yogurt is; it comes in many different flavors, including chocolate. The nonfat vanilla flavor makes an excellent topping for fruit desserts. In addition to having a CSI of almost zero and being relatively low in calories, nonfat frozen yogurt also contains natural vegetable gums, substances that may have a very mild blood-cholesterol-lowering effect. Nonfat frozen yogurts are proving as popular with children and teens as with adults. Remember to select CSIs of 3 or lower per cup.

Pies and Cobblers

Pie crust is a *big* problem. We can get the CSI low (2 per ⅙ of 9″ crust) by making an oil crust and using a single layer—but the fat (12 grams) and calories (184) for this wedge are still high. We recommend you save pies for very special occasions, such as for the once-a-year blackberry treat—put the filling in a deep dish and cover with a single oil crust. If you want a topper, select nonfat vanilla frozen yogurt. For everyday desserts, try cobblers and crisps with CSIs of 1 or lower per serving, such as our *Apple Crisp*, *Berry Cobbler*, or *Upside-Down Peach Cobbler*.

Beware of the commercial graham cracker crust (CSI of 6 per ⅙ of 9″). It is *not* better than commercial pie crust (CSI of 5) or homemade pie crust (CSI of 2 to 8) for the same size. Instead try our *Graham Cracker Crust* recipe (CSI of 1 per ⅙ of 9″) and fill it with pumpkin pie filling (*Pumpkin Pie*) or a berry yogurt filling (*Berry Yogurt Pie*). Note that the *very lowest*–CSI crust or shell that can hold your favorite pie filling is a meringue shell, which has a CSI of 0 no matter what the size. The bad news is that the calories are not 0, but they are much lower than other crusts or shells. Give the meringue shell a try.

Puddings

People in the United States love pudding. You'll be happy to learn that simply using *skim* milk in your favorite pudding mix gives a dessert or snack with a CSI of less than 1 per cup. Our *Chocolate Pudding* and *Pumpkin Bread Pudding* recipes are very tasty (CSIs of less than 1 per cup). Gelatins made from mixes (Jell-O) or using unflavored gelatin and fruit juice have CSIs of 0. But beware of soufflés, custards, mousses, and Bavarian creams—all of these desserts soar into the CSI stratosphere: 22 to 37 per cup.

Dessert Sauces

If you like sauces on your desserts, try nonfat or low-fat vanilla yogurt or our *Yogurt Dessert Sauce* (CSIs of less than 1 per ¼ cup). They are great on warm crisp and cobbler desserts and make a good substitute for custard sauce (CSI of 9 per ¼ cup). Use caramel- or butterscotch-flavored sauces or chocolate syrup with CSIs of less than 1 per ¼ cup, instead of the richer versions with CSIs of 2 to 7 per ¼ cup.

Lower-CSI Desserts Choices

Referring back to the sample dinners in Chapter 8, note that desserts were included in most of the dinners for each of the three phases. The CSIs for all of the desserts ranged from almost 0 to 2 per serving. In order for desserts to fit into the low-CSI way of eating, they *must* be served with low-CSI meals. We find that desserts fit best with lower-calorie dinners, such as with Spaghetti with *Marinara Sauce*, or one of our fish dinners, such as *Halibut Mexicana*. Lower-fat desserts with CSIs greater than 2 per serving, or typical desserts with much higher CSIs, do *not* fit into everyday lower-CSI eating. To put it bluntly, they are special-occasion foods—which means no more than once a month.

CSIs OF DESSERTS

Table 25 provides the CSIs for individuals desserts.

TABLE 25
THE CSIs OF DESSERT CHOICES

DESSERTS: CAKES
(SELECT CSIs OF 5 OR LOWER PER SERVINGS)

	SERVING SIZE		CSI	FAT (GM)	CALORIES
CARROT CAKES, FROSTED					
Carrot-Raisin Cake with Penuche Frosting	2¼" x 2½"	(112 gm)	<1	4	271
Party Carrot Cake (smaller piece)	2" x 2¼"	(81 gm)	2	6	224
Party Carrot Cake (larger piece)	3" x 3¼"	(161 gm)	3	12	449
Carrot cake, typical	3" x 3¼"	(197 gm)	14	29	662
APPLE CAKES, UNFROSTED					
Pinto Fiesta Cake	⅟₁₆ of cake	(66 gm)	<1	5	182
Apple Loaf Cake (smaller piece)	⅟₂₄ of cake	(60 gm)	<1	6	179
Apple Loaf Cake (larger piece)	⅟₁₂ of cake	(121 gm)	2	11	359
Apple cake, typical	⅟₁₂ of cake	(122 gm)	6	23	457
CHIFFON-TYPE CAKES, UNFROSTED					
Angel food cake, plain	⅟₁₀ of cake	(72 gm)	0	0	170
Angel Quickie (chocolate angel food)	⅟₁₀ of cake	(76 gm)	<1	1	186
Chiffon	⅟₁₀ of cake	(105 gm)	9	14	336
Sponge	⅟₁₀ of cake	(98 gm)	12	4	279
PUDDING CAKES, UNFROSTED					
Hot Fudge Pudding Cake	3" x 3"	(78 gm)	1	5	259
White pudding cake, typical	3" x 3"	(88 gm)	3	9	238

Yellow, chocolate, spice, or apple-sauce pudding cake, typical	3" x 3"		7	10	254
ZUCCHINI CAKES, UNFROSTED					
Chocolate Zucchini Cake (smaller piece)	1/24 of cake	(51 gm)	<1	5	142
Chocolate Zucchini Cake (larger piece)	1/12 of cake	(101 gm)	2	10	284
Zucchini cake, typical	1/12 of cake	(85 gm)	6	9	285
POUND CAKES					
Poppyseed Cake (glazed)	5" x 3" x 1/2"	(62 gm)	1	7	180
Pound cake, typical (unglazed)	5" x 3" x 1/2"	(42 gm)	7	9	178
Chocolate, typical (unglazed)	5" x 3" x 1/2"	(53 gm)	9	13	250
JELLY ROLL CAKES					
All flavors except chocolate (jelly filling)	4" diameter, 1" thick	(71 gm)	4	1	198
Chocolate (cream filling)	4" diameter, 1" thick	(56 gm)	9	7	192
CHOCOLATE CAKES					
Cocoa Cake (unfrosted)	3" x 3" x 2"	(50 gm)	1	5	205
Cocoa Cake (Seven Minute frosting)	3" x 3" x 2"	(69 gm)	1	5	254
Cocoa Cake (Cocoa frosting)	3" x 3" x 2"	(82 gm)	2	9	331
Chocolate cake, typical (seven minute frosting)	3" x 3" x 2"	(100 gm)	5	7	271
Chocolate cake, typical (Chocolate fudge frosting)	3" x 3" x 2"	(115 gm)	8	12	346

The abbreviation *tr.* stands for trace (less than 0.5); the symbol <1 stands for less than one (0.5 to 0.9). Recipes in **bold italics** can be found in Part III.

DESSERTS: CAKES (continued)

	SERVING SIZE		CSI	FAT (GM)	CALORIES
Devil's Food, typical (Seven Minute frosting)	3" x 3" x 2"	(107 gm)	10	15	378
Devil's Food, typical (Chocolate fudge frosting)	3" x 3" x 2"	(122 gm)	13	19	453
German chocolate (frosted)	3" x 3" x 2"	(118 gm)	17	24	472
SPICE-TYPE CAKES					
Depression Cake	3" x 3" x 2"	(73 gm)	<1	4	263
Spice-cake, typical (unfrosted)	3" x 3" x 2"	(83 gm)	4	6	203
Gingerbread, typical	3" x 3" x 2"	(117 gm)	7	12	330
WHITE CAKES					
From mix with water, egg whites (Cocoa frosting)	3" x 3" x 2"	(120 gm)	3	9	319
From mix with water, egg whites (Chocolate fudge frosting)	3" x 3" x 2"	(122 gm)	5	10	317
Homemade with milk and butter (Chocolate fudge frosting)	3" x 3" x 2"	(119 gm)	8	14	380
CHEESECAKES					
"Royal" No-bake Cheesecake Mix made with skim milk	⅛	(100 gm)	3	10	270
made with whole milk	⅛	(100 gm)	4	12	280
Ricotta Cheesecake	½2 of 10"	(116 gm)	4	7	211
Crème de Menthe Cheesecake	½2 of 10"	(106 gm)	5	8	210
Cheesecake, typical	½2 of 10"	(110 gm)	22	25	355
SHORTCAKES					
All-Season Shortcake	3" x 3"	(242 gm)	1	3	292

Red-headed Shortcake	2½" x 2½"	(206 gm)	2	7	241
Strawberry Shortcake, typical	⅙ of 8"	(286 gm)	19	31	616

OTHERS

New and Improved Baked Alaska	1/10 recipe	(71 gm)	tr.	tr.	156
Baba au Rhum	1/24 of cake	(67 gm)	<1	3	190
Trifle (pound cake, fruit, jam, custard)	½ cup	(130 gm)	14	20	290
Fruitcake, typical	3" x 3" x 2"	(221 gm)	17	30	769

DESSERTS: COOKIES AND BARS
(SELECT CSIs OF 3 OR LESS PER SERVING)

HOMEMADE COOKIES

Modified:

Forgotten Kisses	3 cookies	(21 gm)	tr.	2	70
Lace Cookies	3 cookies	(14 gm)	tr.	2	60
Lebkuchen	2 cookies	(36 gm)	tr.	1	115
Gingies	1 large	(33 gm)	tr.	2	110
Carob	2 large	(41 gm)	1	8	166
Crispy Spice	3 large	(44 gm)	1	8	187
Oatmeal	2 medium	(24 gm)	1	5	124

Typical:

Oatmeal	2 cookies	(53 gm)	2	9	186

DESSERTS: COOKIES AND BARS *(continued)*

	SERVING SIZE	CSI	FAT (GM)	CALORIES
Peanut butter	2 cookies	(37 gm)	4	9	166
Sugar	2 cookies	(33 gm)	4	6	134
Chocolate chip	2 cookies	(40 gm)	6	11	186
COMMERCIAL COOKIES				
Fortune cookies	3 cookies	(23 gm)	1	2	103
Gingersnaps	Six 2"	(42 gm)	2	4	176
Animal	16 small	(43 gm)	2	4	181
Graham crackers	6 squares	(42 gm)	2	4	176
Vanilla wafers	Twelve 1½"	(45 gm)	3	4	189
Fig bars	Three 1½"	(47 gm)	3	4	197
Pecan shortbread	Three 2"	(43 gm)	4	10	204
Oatmeal	Three 3"	(41 gm)	4	10	204
Oreos	Four 2"	(44 gm)	5	10	219
Chocolate chip	Four 2"	(44 gm)	5	10	219
Chocolate chip, typical deli	One 3¼"	(58 gm)	6	13	289
Chocolate chip, giant size	One 5¼"	(128 gm)	14	30	637
BAR COOKIES				
Brownies:				
Jamocha Squares	2" x 2"	(28 gm)	<1	4	103
Butterscotch Brownies	2" x 2½"	(39 gm)	<1	5	133
Brownies	2½" x 2½"	(41 gm)	1	5	133
Cocoa Cake, unfrosted	3" x 3"	(50 gm)	1	5	205

186

Brownies from mix, unfrosted (with oil, no nuts, egg whites)	3" x 3"	(76 gm)	1	8	294
Brownies from scratch, unfrosted (with shortening, egg whites, chocolate, nuts)	3" x 3"	(124 gm)	8	30	519
Brownies, typical, unfrosted (with shortening, chocolate, nuts, whole eggs)	3" x 3"	(124 gm)	15	33	543
Brownies, typical, frosted	3" x 3"	(169 gm)	20	42	721
Chocolate Banana Bars	2" x 2¼"	(35 gm)	tr.	1	86
Apricot Meringue Bars	2" x 2"	(26 gm)	<1	3	91
Northwest Harvest Bars	2¼" x 2¼"	(42 gm)	<1	3	102
Molasses Orange Bars	2" x 2"	(58 gm)	<1	4	123
PB & J Bars	1½" x 2¼"	(24 gm)	<1	4	106
Rice Krispie bar, no chocolate	3" x 3"	(21 gm)	<1	4	98
Rice Krispie bar, with chocolate	3" x 3"	(50 gm)	5	11	228
Date bar, typical	2" x 2"	(59 gm)	3	6	188
Pumpkin bar, typical	2" x 2"	(47 gm)	5	8	164
Lemon bar, typical	2" x 2"	(37 gm)	6	6	140
Walnut Squares	1½" x 1½"	(14 gm)	tr.	1	40
Baklava	2" x 2"	(78 gm)	8	29	428

The abbreviation *tr.* stands for trace (less than (0.5); the symbol <1 stands for less than one (0.5 to 0.9). Recipes in **bold italics** can be found in Part III.

DESSERTS: FRUIT
(SELECT CSIs OF 1 OR LOWER PER SERVING)

	SERVING SIZE		CSI	FAT (GM)	CALORIES
Baked Apples	1 apple	(145 gm)	tr.	<1	125
Bananas en Papillote	1 banana	(128 gm)	tr.	<1	127
Berry Pavlova	3" x 3"	(114 gm)	tr.	<1	97
Berry Pavlova, typical	3" x 3¼"	(147 gm)	10	13	294
Fruit-Filled Dessert Cups	¼ recipe	(109 gm)	tr.	tr.	130
Fruit Salad Alaska	¼ recipe	(223 gm)	tr.	<1	164
Peach Cardinal	1 peach	(174 gm)	tr.	tr.	160
Peach and Berry Meringues	¼ recipe	(166 gm)	tr.	tr.	143
Pears in Wine	1 pear	(204 gm)	tr.	3	244
Apple Strudel	⅙ recipe	(64 gm)	tr.	2	133
Cherry Strudel	⅙ recipe	(76 gm)	tr.	2	148
Toasted Bananas	1/12 recipe	(125 gm)	1	4	226

188

DESSERTS: ICE CREAM AND OTHER FROZEN DESSERTS
(SELECT CSIs OF 3 OR LOWER PER CUP)

Food	Serving			
Soft-serve sorbet (Vitari)	1 cup	(153 gm)	0	0	160
Cranberry Sherbet	1 cup	(160 gm)	0	tr.	162
Sno-cone, Slushie, fruit ice, sorbet	1 cup	(193 gm)	0	0	255
Strawberry Ice	1 cup	(190 gm)	0	<1	240
Frozen yogurt, nonfat	1 cup	(184 gm)	tr.	tr.	224
Pumpkin Frozen Yogurt	1 cup	(234 gm)	tr.	tr.	208
Lite Lite Tofutti	1 cup	(238 gm)	<1	<1	180
Low, Lite 'n'Luscious (Baskin-Robbins)	1 cup	(208 gm)	2	3	214
Frozen yogurt, low-fat	1 cup	(150 gm)	3	4	227
Sherbet	1 cup	(193 gm)	3	4	270
Tofutti*	1 cup	(170 gm)	3	24	420
Ice Milk, typical soft-serve	1 cup	(175 gm)	4	5	224
Mocha Mix Frozen Dessert*	1 cup	(158 gm)	4	14	280
Frozen yogurt, cream added	1 cup	(167 gm)	6	7	240
Light ice cream (ice milk)	1 cup	(150 gm)	6	8	236
Ice cream, store brands (10% fat)	1 cup	(163 gm)	15	18	329
Ice cream, rich (12% fat)	1 cup	(208 gm)	19	24	480
Ice cream, extra rich (18% fat)	1 cup	(208 gm)	30	38	580
Popsicle	One	(75 gm)	0	0	99
Fudgesicle	One	(73 gm)	tr.	tr.	91

* Made with vegetable oil instead of butterfat.

The abbreviation *tr.* stands for trace (less than 0.5); the symbol <1 stands for less than one (0.5 to 0.9). Recipes in **bold italics** can be found in Part III.

189

DESSERTS: ICE CREAM AND OTHER FROZEN DESSERTS *(continued)*

	SERVING SIZE		CSI	FAT (GM)	CALORIES
Jell-O Pudding Pops	One	(1.8 fl. oz.)	2	2	80
Dreamsicle	One	(66 gm)	2	3	104
Ice cream sandwich	One	(62 gm)	4	5	173
Drumstick, Nutti-Buddie	One	(61 gm)	6	10	189
Ice cream bar (chocolate covered)	One	(85 gm)	12	13	224
Ice cream cone (cone only)	One	(12 gm)	tr.	tr.	45

DESSERTS: PIES AND COBBLERS
(SELECT CSIs OF 2 OR LOWER PER SERVING)

FILLING & CRUSTS					
Fruit/Nut:					
Swedish Pie	⅛ of recipe	(51 gm)	tr.	2	130
Cranberry Squares	1⁄12 of recipe	(46 gm)	tr.	3	125
Upside-Down Peach Cobbler	⅙ of recipe	(147 gm)	<1	4	226
Berry Cobbler	⅙ of recipe	(170 gm)	<1	5	233
Apple Crisp (crumb topping)	⅙ of recipe	(99 gm)	<1	4	153
Peach Almond Crisp	⅙ of recipe	(174 gm)	<1	5	158
Apple or cherry cobbler (biscuit topping)	1 cup	(144 gm)	2	8	272
Glazed fruit pie (single crust)	⅙ of 9″	(165 gm)	5	12	309

	Amount	Weight			
Mincemeat pie (single crust)	1/6 of 9"	(147 gm)	6	13	330
Fruit pie (double crust)	1/6 of 9"	(181 gm)	11	27	504
Pecan pie (single crust)	1/6 of 9"	(156 gm)	15	41	682
Cream:					
Berry Yogurt Pie (graham cracker crust)	1/6 of 9"	(151 gm)	1	4	196
Pumpkin Pie (graham cracker crust)	1/6 of 9"	(220 gm)	1	5	327
Pumpkin pie (single crust)	1/6 of 9"	(220 gm)	14	19	418
Lemon meringue pie (single crust)	1/6 of 9"	(178 gm)	14	20	452
Custard pie (single crust)	1/6 of 9"	(154 gm)	15	18	345
Banana cream pie (single crust)	1/6 of 9"	(173 gm)	20	26	447
Grasshopper pie (single crumb crust)	1/6 of 9"	(182 gm)	22	35	575
Chocolate cream pie (single crust)	1/6 of 9"	(192 gm)	23	30	491
Coconut cream pie (single crust)	1/6 of 9"	(179 gm)	25	29	455
PIE CRUSTS (SINGLE)					
Meringue	3"	(24 gm)	0	0	70
Graham cracker:					
Graham Cracker Crust	1/6 of 9"	(36 gm)	1	5	142
Commercial	1/6 of 9"	(45 gm)	6	15	237
Conventional:					
Made with oil	1/6 of 9"	(34 gm)	2	12	184
Made with shortening	1/6 of 9"	(33 gm)	4	14	189
Commercial	1/6 of 9"	(34 gm)	5	12	173
Made with lard	1/6 of 9"	(31 gm)	5	12	172

The abbreviation *tr.* stands for trace (less than (0.5); the symbol <1 stands for less than one (0.5 to 0.9). Recipes in **bold italics** can be found in Part III.

DESSERTS: PIES AND COBBLERS *(continued)*

	SERVING SIZE		CSI	FAT (GM)	CALORIES
Made with whole eggs	⅙ of 9"	(40 gm)	8	14	212
Chocolate Crumb	⅙ of 9"	(33 gm)	7	16	198
TURNOVERS AND TARTS					
Apple Strudel	⅙ recipe	(64 gm)	tr.	2	133
Cherry Strudel	⅙ recipe	(76 gm)	tr.	2	148
Turnover, fruit-filled, commercial	5" folded	(64 gm)	5	19	229
Pie tart, commercial	One	(86 gm)	7	15	275

DESSERTS: PUDDINGS
(SELECT CSIs OF 2 OR LOWER PER SERVING)

	SERVING SIZE		CSI	FAT (GM)	CALORIES
PUDDINGS FROM MIXES					
All flavors (with skim milk)	1 cup	(260 gm)	<1	1	251
All flavors (with whole milk)	1 cup	(260 gm)	6	8	307
PUDDINGS, HOMEMADE					
Chocolate Pudding	1 cup	(210 gm)	<1	<1	230
Lemon	1 cup	(200 gm)	4	2	114
Tapioca	1 cup	(200 gm)	15	9	255
Rice	1 cup	(265 gm)	17	11	365

BREAD PUDDINGS

Pumpkin Bread	1 cup	(300 gm)	<1	2	367
Bread puddings, typical	1 cup	(265 gm)	16	16	441

OTHER PUDDINGS

Gelatin, flavored (low-sugar)	1 cup	(240 gm)	0	0	16
Gelatin, flavored (Jell-O)	1 cup	(240 gm)	0	0	142
Pudding Pops	One	(52 gm)	2	2	80
Chocolate soufflé	1 cup	(59 gm)	8	8	127
Custard, baked	1 cup	(281 gm)	22	14	300
Chiffon, all flavors	1 cup	(165 gm)	25	12	414
Plum pudding	1 cup	(230 gm)	30	47	895
Chocolate mousse	1 cup	(191 gm)	33	31	380
Bavarian cream	1 cup	(152 gm)	37	35	388

DESSERTS: SAUCES
(SELECT CSIs OF 1 OR LOWER PER SERVING)

Yogurt Dessert Sauce	¼ cup	(64 gm)	<1	<1	61
Custard sauce	¼ cup	(68 gm)	9	5	93
Caramel or butterscotch (flavored sauce)	¼ cup	(85 gm)	0	0	264

The abbreviation tr. stands for trace (less than 0.5); the symbol <1 stands for less than one (0.5 to 0.9). Recipes in **bold italics** can be found in Part III.

193

DESSERTS: SAUCES *(continued)*

	SERVING SIZE		CSI	FAT (GM)	CALORIES
Caramel (homemade)	¼ cup	(82 gm)	2	7	291
Chocolate sauce (syrup type)	¼ cup	(76 gm)	<1	2	211
Chocolate sauce (fudge type)	¼ cup	(76 gm)	7	10	251
Fresh Rhubarb Sauce	¼ cup	(69 gm)	tr.	tr.	50
Strawberry or Raspberry Sauce	¼ cup	(44 gm)	0	tr.	31

The abbreviation *tr.* stands for trace (less than (0.5); the symbol <1 stands for less than one (0.5 to 0.9). Recipes in *bold italics* can be found in Part III.

Snacks (Including Beverages and Appetizers)

LOW-CSI SNACKING

Most people snack a lot, especially in the evenings and on weekends. Snacking is almost a natural thing to do and it can be healthy as we will explain, or it can be a direct route to overweight and heart disease. Think for a few minutes about what you eat in the way of snacks on any given day. Add up the CSIs—and calories—of those snacks using Table 27 at the end of this chapter. Many of you will be surprised, unpleasantly we're afraid, by your totals. Let's say you have a Danish roll mid-morning, some Wheat Thins in the afternoon, some vegetables with sour cream dip before dinner, a granola bar before bed-

time—and, somewhere in the course of the day, a couple cups of coffee with a little half-and-half. Those "modest" munchies will give you 842 Calories, 52 grams of fat (10+ teaspoons), and a CSI of 30!

Don't get the wrong idea. Just because typical snacks are loaded with CSIs, fat, and calories doesn't mean that there are no snacks involved in low-CSI eating. In fact snacks are an important part of low-CSI, low-fat eating. As you have already determined from the CSI tables, lower-CSI foods have fewer calories for the same serving sizes. For those who need to keep the calories up (growing youngsters and active young adults), snacks are essential to keep the "hungries" down and the weight appropriate.

Table 26 shows you our Phase One, Two,

and Three CSI goals for daily snacks. Men and teens should aim for a snack CSI of 5½ in Phase One, while women and children should try for 4. By Phase Three, the target CSIs are in the 2 to 3 range. So where does that leave us—or, more to the point, *what* does that leave us to snack on? Quite a lot. You just have to choose judiciously.

Table 27 shows you the CSIs of all snack foods. You'll find many delicious dips, with CSIs of 2 and under, that you can combine with vegetables to make great snacks/ appetizers. There are even 0 to trace-CSI candies (jelly beans, etc.) and some low-CSI candy bars. Even crackers with almost 0 to 2-CSIs are available, and Table 27 will enable you to distinguish them from their high-fat brethren. Note that while some sweets have low-CSIs, they are loaded with sugar and calories—so don't go overboard on those, either. Review the preceding chapter for guidelines on lowering sugar intake.

The Secret of Successful Low-CSI Snacking

One of the keys to healthy snacking is to have the *right kind* of snacks *on hand* at all times. When you're hungry, you will eat anything that's available. Purge your pantry (and your pockets) of high-fat snacks and stock up instead on the low-CSI variety. Don't tempt yourself needlessly—but don't deprive yourself, either. If you try to cut out snacks entirely, you'll probably be hungry between meals and eventually succumb to a "Snickers fit" or a "croissant craving" or otherwise trigger a high-CSI binge.

When you get your next snack attack, yield to it—but choose a low-CSI snack to help quell the assault. And *keep* those low-CSI snacks at the ready—so that you'll never be caught with your defenses down. We recommend low-fat homemade muf-

TABLE 26
THE CHOLESTEROL–SATURATED FAT INDEX (CSI) DAILY GOALS*

	BREAKFAST	LUNCH	DINNER	SNACKS	TOTAL
Women/Children	(2,000 Calories)				
CSI American Diet	5	12	28	**6**	51
CSI Phase One	4	9	20	**4**	37
CSI Phase Two	2	5	18	**3**	28
CSI Phase Three	1	3	11	**2**	17
Men/Teens	(2,800 Calories)				
CSI American Diet	8	18	35	**8**	69
CSI Phase One	5½	12½	24½	**5½**	48
CSI Phase Two	3	7	22	**4**	36
CSI Phase Three	1½	4	15½	**3**	24

* This is only one of many possible distributions.

fins, low-fat crackers, baked tortilla chips, fruit and vegetables (keep some cleaned and peeled), unsalted pretzels, cereals, breads, and popcorn.

Popcorn is an ideal snack since it has a CSI of nearly 0 if it is prepared without butter, margarine, or other fat. Air-popping is the way to go since this method of preparation requires absolutely no oil. A small amount of margarine can be used. Popcorn with one teaspoon of margarine has a CSI of 0.7, and with two teaspoons of margarine the CSI is 1.4. These quantities are still low and will take care of a whole popper (air-popped). Such preparations are quite appetizing and are eaten with relish by the authors. Also, a variety of no-salt seasonings can be used if desired. Some people who love popcorn rotate between white and yellow varieties. Either is great and both are very high in fiber and low in calories. Beware of the *microwave* popcorns. Check labels carefully. The ones we've examined contain anywhere from 1½ to 3 teaspoons (7½ to 15 grams) of fat per each 4-cup serving. They are also very high in salt. Avoid these.

Make your own microwave popcorn. Simply put a handful of popcorn kernels in a small brown paper bag; fold over the top. Put the bag in the microwave oven for three to five minutes on full power (high). You may have to experiment once or twice to get the right timing for your particular oven, but it is worth the initial effort. Brown-bag microwave popcorn is tasty, cheap, and healthy.

Invest in an air popper. The few dollars you'll spend on this type of popcorn machine are well worth the investment.

COMPARISON OF POPCORN (4 CUPS)

	FAT (GM)	SODIUM (MG)
Air-popped:		
plain	<1	1
"buttered" using 1 teaspoon margarine	5	44
Typical (Popped with Oil):		
plain (no extra fat added)	15	1
"buttered" using 2 tablespoons (6 teaspoons) margarine	39	250

The symbol <1 stands for less than one (0.5 to 0.9).

Try all of the low-fat crackers (CSI of 2 per serving) and very-low-fat crackers (CSI of nearly 0 per serving) to find those that suit your tastes. Bake your own tortilla chips (see our *Baked Corn Chips* recipe in Part III) to use as dippers for salsa and bean dip. Flour tortillas and thinly sliced bagels make good chips, and so does pita bread cut in triangles and baked (see our *Pita Chips* recipe in Part III). You can even buy pita chips and bagel chips—just make sure they are baked and not fried.

Don't forget the cereals. Most are nearly 0 in CSI, are very low in fat, and make for great snacks especially when eaten with skim milk. Some people munch on the dry cereals directly: puffed wheat, puffed rice, Cheerios, Grape-nuts, and Kashi. Be selective about granolas—look for those that contain no coconut, coconut oil, or palm oil. The fat content should be 6 grams of fat per cup or less. There are constantly new and lower-fat granolas appearing on the market. Again, read the labels.

Nonfat frozen yogurt and low-CSI cookies can be eaten for snacks. Look back in the previous chapter (Table 25) for guidelines.

Low-fat muffins are much better snack choices than cookies. Try our *Blueberry Bran Muffin* recipe (CSI of almost 0 per muffin), our *Pumpkin Oat Muffin* recipe (CSI of less than 1 per muffin), or one of the other recipes listed in Table 27. And you can't beat toast or bagels for a satisfying snack.

For a really substantial snack, keep some tortillas or pita (pocket) bread around and fill one with refried beans and salsa or some other low-CSI filling, such as our tasty *Chowchow* (CSI of almost 0 per ¼ cup), our *Hummous* recipe (CSI of almost 0 per ¼ cup), or our *Southern Caviar* (CSI of almost 0 per ¼ cup). The baby pocket bread is new and makes for great appetizers as well as for snacks. Keep cans of vegetarian refried beans on hand for these "heavy and filling" (but actually, low-calorie, low-CSI) snacks. Our bean salads make good fillings for "heavy and filling" snacks— *Spicy Black Bean Salad* (CSI of almost 0 per ¼ cup) and *Chili Bean Salad* (CSI of 0 per ¼ cup). Also *"Egg" Salad Sandwich Spread* (CSI of almost 0 per ¼ cup) on soda crackers makes for a very tasty snack. Toss in some fruits and vegetables for snacks and the assortment makes for very good low-CSI eating.

Table 27 shows you a number of low-CSI alternatives to typical high-CSI snacks. These substitutes will help you make the transition to a new, healthier way of snacking.

Candy

Candy is a special-occasion food—a treat. When you do have candy, select lower-CSI varieties and watch the *serving size* to avoid getting an overdose of calories. Candies made primarily from sugar have the lowest CSIs. These include gumdrops, hard candy, jelly beans, licorice, mints, taffy, and cracker jacks—CSIs of 0 or trace per ounce. Carob-coated raisins and peanuts have much lower CSIs than chocolate-coated raisins and peanuts (CSIs are 1 per ounce versus 3 per ounce)—but the fat and calories are not lower. For a 2-ounce candy bar, the CSIs range from 1 to 11, the fat from 3 to 22 grams, and the calories from 206 to 310!

Liquid Snacks

We have to add a few words of caution about some zero-CSI beverages we *don't* recommend, at least not as a regular thing. As you can see from Table 27, most alcoholic beverages and soft drinks have CSIs of zero. But alcohol, in excess, can have disastrous health consequences, not to mention many negative social ramifications. In addition, alcohol, though devoid of fat and cholesterol, is packed with calories and can contribute substantially to weight gain, high blood pressure, and obesity. We do not think that alcohol should be part of one's daily diet, rather—for those who enjoy an occasional drink—we suggest a limit of 1 to 2 drinks on any given day and no more than 2 to 3 drinks per week.

We also recommend cutting back on sodas, fruit drinks, sugared coffee and tea, and even fruit juice, as all have a lot of sugar and are calorically dense. Limit coffee and tea consumption to 3 cups a day, or less, and use low-fat or skim milk in it rather than cream, half-and-half, or non-dairy creamer.

To further cut calories, dilute wine, soft drinks, fruit drinks, and juices with salt-free seltzer or sparkling water. Routinely offer a tasty non-alcoholic alternative beverage and you may be surprised by the number of takers. Lemonade with pureed strawberries, raspberries, or blueberries is a treat for almost everyone. Offer iced tea with mint and lemon or a pitcher of iced water with lemon slices in addition to wine.

Appetizers

Webster's dictionary defines an appetizer as "a food or drink that stimulates the appetite and is usually served before a meal." The truth is that more often than not we eat so much of the appetizer that it becomes the meal. We call this "grazing"—not a good habit.

Appetizers are not something to eat every day. Rather, people with a low-CSI eating style serve them when they have company or eat them when they go out to friends' homes or to restaurants. Our recommendation, when serving them at home, is to keep them light, so they stimulate the appetite for the delicious *Peppered Salmon Steak* or the *Spicy Chicken with Peppers* (or other low-CSI entrée) that is to

come. If you are serving the latter, offer *Steamed Buns* as the appetizer. A nice starter for the salmon dinner is *Popeye's Spinach Dip* served in a hollowed-out loaf of sourdough rye bread with bread cubes for dipping. *Southern Caviar* served on low-fat crackers will delight you and your guests. Our appetizers range in CSI from almost 0 to 1 per serving. Compare this to typical appetizers, which range in CSI from 2 to 14 per serving.

When eating away from home and you find that there are no low-CSI appetizer choices, "just say no." Then you can enjoy the rest of the meal. Cheese and meat appetizers are just plain out, unless you want to put all your CSIs for the day on one small plate.

We've already discussed the use of nuts in Chapter 4 on fats, but, as a reminder, they do not make a good snack. The CSIs are low, but ½ cup of nuts has 6 to 10 teaspoons of fat. Macadamia nuts contain 49 grams (10 teaspoons) of fat in one handful! These, combined with a piña colada (which contains coconut), can be lethal while on a Hawaiian beach supposedly vacationing the heart!

We'll discuss eating in restaurants in Chapter 11. The best rule is to memorize the definition of appetizer—"to stimulate the appetite"—and choose accordingly.

Lower-CSI Snack Choices

Here are the snacks that go with the week of breakfasts, lunches, and dinners described in Tables 15, 18, and 22.

Phase One: ½ cup vanilla ice milk and 2 oatmeal cookies; bran muffin with 1 teaspoon soft margarine; 6 soda crackers (unsalted tops) with 2 tablespoons peanut butter; and 2 cups air-popped popcorn with 2 teaspoons soft margarine and 12 ounces of lemonade.

Phase Two: 6 ounces of low-fat raspberry yogurt, banana; and fresh fruit (½ cup peaches and ½ cup pears).

Phase Three: 3 cups air-popped popcorn with 1 teaspoon soft margarine; *Cereal Bran Muffin;* 4 ounces blueberry low-fat frozen yogurt on cone; banana; ¼ cup *"Egg" Salad Sandwich Spread* on 6 soda crackers (unsalted tops); 3 graham crackers and 1 cup skim milk; whole wheat cinnamon-raisin bagel; apple and 2 gingersnaps; and 3 cups

air-popped popcorn with 1 teaspoon soft margarine. Notice how many more snacks there are in Phase Three, which is typical of a lower-CSI eating pattern. Also the average CSI per snack for Phase One is between 3 and 4. The average CSI for the snacks in Phases Two and Three is about 1.

Sometimes, instead of snacking, *exercise.* Go for a walk or chew sugarless gum.

THE CSIs OF SNACKS, APPETIZERS, BEVERAGES

Table 27 lists the CSIs of individual snack foods, appetizers, and beverages.

TABLE 27
THE CSIs OF SNACK CHOICES

CHIPS, CRACKERS, AND POPCORN
(SELECT CSIs OF 2 OR LOWER PER SERVING)

	SERVING SIZE	CSI	FAT (GM)	CALORIES
CRACKERS				
Very Low–Fat Varieties: (average nutrient values)	(40 gm)	tr.	tr.	134
Armenian Crackerbread	1 large			
Breadsticks, plain	3½ sticks			
Cracklesnax	24			
Crispy Cakes (Squared Rice Cakes)	7 squares			
Crokine	8 slices			
Kavli	4 slices			
Matzo	1⅓			
Rice Cakes	4			
Ry Krisp, Natural	6			
Siljans Knacke (Swedish Crispbread)	½			
"Sunshine" Krispy (soda crackers)	14			
Wasa Lite Rye	5			
Low-Fat Varieties: (average nutrient values)	(40 gm)	2	5	172

The abbreviation *tr.* stands for trace (less than (0.5); the symbol <1 stands for less than one (0.5 to 0.9). Recipes in **bold italics** can be found in Part III.

CHIPS, CRACKERS, AND POPCORN (continued)

	SERVING SIZE		CSI	FAT (GM)	CALORIES
Soda crackers (most brands)	13				
Stoned Wheat Thins	6				
Ak Mak	7				
Melba Rounds	13				
Ry Krisp, Seasoned	6				
Carr's Table Water Crackers	12				
Bremner	17				
Pretzel Goldfish	60				
Harvest Crisps	18				
High-Fat Varieties:	(average nutrient values)	(40 gm)	3	9	192
Wheat Thins	20				
Triscuits	9				
Ritz	12				
Chicken in a Biskit	20				
Most "party" varieties	12–20				
Pretzels	20 twists/ 1 cup sticks	(40 gm)	1	2	156
POPCORN					
Air-popped (no fat)	3 cups	(18 gm)	tr.	<1	69
Air-popped (plus 1 teaspoon margarine)	3 cups	(23 gm)	<1	5	105
Microwave (selected brands):					
Redenbacher's Gourmet, Natural Flavor	3 cups	(28 gm)	<1	5	105
Betty Crocker Pop-Secret, Butter Flavor	3 cups	(28 gm)	1	8	140

Jolly Time, Natural Flavor	3 cups	(28 gm)	2	10	130
Cracker Jack	3 cups	(120 gm)	2	13	510
Commercially popped, plain- or cheese-flavored	3 cups	(28 gm)	5	6	116
Caramel corn	3 cups	(105 gm)	5	21	468

CHIPS

Baked Corn Chips	2 cups	(57 gm)	<1	5	228
Pita Chips	2 cups	(45 gm)	tr.	1	268
Tortilla chips:					
fried in vegetable oil	2 cups	(57 gm)	2	12	282
fried in lard	2 cups	(57 gm)	5	12	282
fried in palm or coconut oil	2 cups	(57 gm)	10	12	282
Cheese puffs	2 cups	(34 gm)	3	12	190
Corn chips	2 cups	(70 gm)	4	22	370
Potato chips	2 cups	(53 gm)	5	19	277
Pork rinds	2 cups	(28 gm)	5	9	150
Pringles	2 cups	(50 gm)	6	22	295

MISCELLANEOUS

Party mix, low-fat (cereal, pretzels, few nuts, oil)	1 cup	(59 gm)	2	14	185
Party mix, typical (cereal, nuts, butter)	1 cup	(64 gm)	8	23	334
Trail mix, commercial (peanuts, sunflower seeds, raisins, carob)	1 cup	(150 gm)	6	39	704
Cornnuts	1 cup	(92 gm)	6	14	419

The abbreviation *tr.* stands for trace (less than (0.5); the symbol <1 stands for less than one (0.5 to 0.9). Recipes in **bold italics** can be found in Part III.

CEREALS
(SELECT CSIs OF 2 OR LOWER PER CUP)

READY-TO-EAT	SERVING SIZE		CSI	FAT (GM)	CALORIES
Wheat Bran, unprocessed	1 tablespoon	(4 gm)	tr.	<1	7
All-Bran	1 cup	(85 gm)	tr.	2	212
Bran Buds	1 cup	(84 gm)	tr.	2	217
Branflakes	1 cup	(39 gm)	tr.	<1	127
Branflakes with Raisins	1 cup	(57 gm)	tr.	1	175
Cheerios/Wheaties	1 cup	(29 gm)	tr.	tr.	101
Chex, Corn & Rice	1 cup	(28 gm)	tr.	tr.	110
Corn Flakes/Rice Krispies	1 cup	(23 gm)	tr.	tr.	89
Grape-nuts	1 cup	(112 gm)	tr.	tr.	403
Grape-nut Flakes	1 cup	(32 gm)	tr.	tr.	115
Kashi	1 cup	(22 gm)	tr.	<1	74
Presweetened, variety of brands	1 cup	(28 gm)	tr.	<1	110
Puffed Rice	1 cup	(14 gm)	0	tr.	56
Puffed Wheat	1 cup	(12 gm)	tr.	tr.	44
Shredded Wheat	1 biscuit/25 bite-size	(24 gm)	tr.	<1	86
Special K	1 cup	(21 gm)	tr.	tr.	82
Captain Crunch	1 cup	(37 gm)	2	3	156
Muesli	1 cup	(84 gm)	tr.	2	280

Granola, low-fat commercial (Golden Temple)	1 cup	(57 gm)	<1	6	250
Granola, commercial with soy oil (Vita Crunch)	1 cup	(113 gm)	3	18	495
Granola, commercial with coconut oil	1 cup	(113 gm)	17	20	503
COOKED					
Farina, Cream of Wheat, Ralston, Roman Meal, Malt-O-Meal	1 cup	(233 gm)	tr.	tr.	126
Oat bran	1 cup	(240 gm)	tr.	2	103
Oatmeal, regular	1 cup	(234 gm)	tr.	2	145
Oatmeal, instant	1 cup	(207 gm)	tr.	3	217
MILK					
Milk, skim	1 cup	(245 gm)	<1	tr.	85
Milk, 1%	1 cup	(244 gm)	2	3	102
Milk, 2%	1 cup	(244 gm)	4	5	122
Milk, whole	1 cup	(244 gm)	7	8	149

The abbreviation *tr.* stands for trace (less than 0.5); the symbol <1 stands for less than one (0.5 to 0.9). Recipes in **_bold italics_** can be found in Part III.

BREADS AND TORTILLAS
(SELECT CSIs OF 1 OR LOWER PER SERVING)

	SERVING SIZE		CSI	FAT (GM)	CALORIES
YEAST BREADS					
White	1 slice	(25 gm)	tr.	<1	68
Whole wheat	1 slice	(29 gm)	tr.	<1	70
Raisin	1 slice	(23 gm)	tr.	<1	61
Rye	1 slice	(29 gm)	tr.	tr.	70
Pumpernickel	1 slice	(25 gm)	tr.	tr.	62
English muffin	One	(57 gm)	tr.	1	135
Whole Wheat French Bread	⅕ loaf	(38 gm)	tr.	<1	125
Grape-nut Bread	1 slice or roll	(42 gm)	tr.	1	99
French, Italian, sourdough	4¼" x 2¾" x 1"	(30 gm)	tr.	tr.	83
Pita or pocket	One	(64 gm)	tr.	<1	180
Boston brown	1 slice	(48 gm)	tr.	<1	101
Cinnamon swirl	1 slice	(22 gm)	tr.	<1	59
Egg	1 slice	(33 gm)	2	2	89
Cheese	1 slice	(29 gm)	2	3	87
Challah	1 slice	(33 gm)	2	2	89
Focaccia	⅙ loaf	(60 gm)	1	5	190
Boboli	⅙ loaf	(60 gm)	2	8	183
YEAST ROLLS					
Hard	1 small	(25 gm)	tr.	<1	77

Item	Serving	Weight			
Kaiser	One	(50 gm)	tr.	2	153
Caraway Dinner Roll	One	(48 gm)	tr.	<1	108
Pan or dinner-type	One	(28 gm)	<1	2	83
Poor boy or submarine	3" x 11½"	(135 gm)	1	4	385
Crescent	One	(28 gm)	3	6	101
Croissant	One	(55 gm)	9	12	167
TORTILLAS					
Corn, plain	5¾" diameter	(23 gm)	tr.	<1	52
Taco or tostada shell, fried	5½" diameter	(14 gm)	1	3	63
Flour, plain	7½" diameter	(38 gm)	1	3	118
Flour, fried	7½" diameter	(43 gm)	3	8	162
BAGELS					
Plain or flavored	One	(75 gm)	tr.	2	225
Egg	One	(75 gm)	2	4	225
MUFFINS AND SCONES					
Blueberry Bran Muffin	One	(89 gm)	tr.	<1	146
Cereal Bran Muffin	One	(59 gm)	<1	4	116
A Barrel of Muffins	One	(43 gm)	<1	4	105
Poppyseed Muffin	One	(62 gm)	<1	5	163
Nutty Orange Muffin	One	(63 gm)	<1	5	167
Mexican Cornbread Muffin	One	(74 gm)	<1	4	165
Pumpkin Oat Muffin	One	(82 gm)	<1	4	177

The abbreviation *tr.* stands for trace (less than 0.5); the symbol <1 stands for less than one (0.5 to 0.9). Recipes in ***bold italics*** can be found in Part III.

BREADS AND TORTILLAS (continued)

	SERVING SIZE	CSI	FAT (GM)	CALORIES
Applesauce Oatmeal Muffin	One (59 gm)	<1	5	157
Dutchy Crust Muffins or Coffee Cake	One (64 gm)	<1	5	181
Cinnamon Rhubarb Muffin	One (50 gm)	<1	4	140
Typical plain muffin	One (55 gm)	2	6	149
Oatmeal Raisin Muffin	One (47 gm)	<1	4	137
Oatmeal raisin muffin, typical	One (61 gm)	2	6	164
Yogurt Scone	One (60 gm)	<1	3	136
Fruit Scone	One (39 gm)	<1	4	107
QUICK BREADS				
Grandma Kirschner's Date Nut Bread	½" slice (61 gm)	tr.	4	209
Pumpkin Harvest Loaf	½" slice (38 gm)	<1	4	163
Lemon Nut Bread	½" slice (58 gm)	<1	5	153
Cornbread	2" x 4" x 2" (78 gm)	<1	6	180
Fruit Bread	½" slice (55 gm)	<1	4	151
Orange Walnut Bread	½" slice (55 gm)	<1	4	166
Banana Nut Bread	½" slice (66 gm)	<1	4	142
Whole Wheat Quick Bread	½" slice (36 gm)	<1	2	93
Nut bread	½" slice (58 gm)	2	10	199
Zucchini bread (no nuts)	½" slice (45 gm)	3	9	172
Pumpkin bread (no nuts)	½" slice (45 gm)	4	5	161
Cornbread, typical	3" x 3" x 1" (59 gm)	5	8	190

MISCELLANEOUS

Breadstick, plain	One 7½"	(11 gm)	tr.	tr.	30
Hamburger or hot dog bun	One	(40 gm)	<1	2	114
Breadcrumbs, commercial	½ cup	(50 gm)	<1	2	195
Lefse	1 serving	(38 gm)	1	3	78
Croutons, commercial	½ cup	(18 gm)	3	4	89
Popover	One	(40 gm)	5	4	92

BAKERY GOODS
(SELECT CSIs OF 2 OR LOWER PER SERVING)

SWEET ROLLS

Poptart	One	(50 gm)	2	6	196
Brioche	One	(30 gm)	4	6	119
Sweet roll, cinnamon	One 4"	(69 gm)	5	11	276
Maple bar	One	(42 gm)	6	12	192
Danish	One 4"	(58 gm)	8	18	235
Croissant	One	(55 gm)	9	12	167
Sunday Morning Sticky Buns	⅓ recipe	(60 gm)	<1	3	214
Sticky nut roll	One 4"	(102 gm)	13	20	444

The abbreviation *tr.* stands for trace (less than (0.5); the symbol <1 stands for less than one (0.5 to 0.9). Recipes in ***bold italics*** can be found in Part III.

BAKERY GOODS (continued)

	SERVING SIZE	CSI	FAT (GM)	CALORIES
DOUGHNUTS				
Baked Doughnut Holes				
Two	(40 gm)	tr.	3	118
Doughnut, cake (unfrosted)	One 3"	(36 gm)	4	6	153
Doughnut, cake (frosted)	One 3"	(67 gm)	5	10	279
Doughnut, cake (frosted, with coconut)	One 3"	(73 gm)	7	12	309
COFFEE CAKES				
Sunrise Cake				
1/16 of cake	(68 gm)	<1	4	161
Coffee cake, streusel topping	3" x 3" x 2"	(94 gm)	6	12	316
SPECIALTY ITEMS				
Twinkie, Hostess	One	(48 gm)	3	4	163
Ho Ho, Hostess	One	(25 gm)	4	6	118
Cupcake, Hostess	One	(57 gm)	4	7	219
Ding Dong, Hostess	One	(38 gm)	6	10	186
Eclair, chocolate	One 4" x 2"	(113 gm)	10	10	201
Cream puff	One 2½"	(87 gm)	12	8	173

APPETIZERS/SNACKS
(SELECT CSIs OF 2 OR LOWER PER SERVING)

DIPS AND SPREADS

Baba Ganouj	¼ cup	(61 gm)	tr.	1	18
Hummous	¼ cup	(65 gm)	tr.	3	106
Salmon Mousse	¼ cup	(47 gm)	1	4	70
Liver Pâté	¼ cup	(68 gm)	14	12	144
Bean Dip	¼ cup	(64 gm)	tr.	1	59
Bean dip	¼ cup	(69 gm)	2	3	82
Chowchow	¼ cup	(53 gm)	tr.	3	49
Chunky Avocado Dip	¼ cup	(61 gm)	<1	5	72
Guacamole	¼ cup	(60 gm)	1	5	62
Salsa	¼ cup	(63 gm)	tr.	tr.	24
Dill Dip	¼ cup	(52 gm)	1	3	66
Sour cream dip	¼ cup	(52 gm)	8	11	111
Popeye's Spinach Dip	¼ cup	(53 gm)	<1	1	37
Spinach dip	¼ cup	(54 gm)	4	13	138
Clam dip	¼ cup	(52 gm)	6	7	87
Cheese dip	¼ cup	(41 gm)	8	10	118
Shrimp dip	¼ cup	(47 gm)	8	8	99
"Egg" Salad Sandwich Spread	¼ cup	(53 gm)	tr.	3	55

POCKET BREAD FILLERS

The abbreviation *tr.* stands for trace (less than (0.5); the symbol <1 stands for less than one (0.5 to 0.9). Recipes in **bold italics** can be found in Part III.

APPETIZERS/SNACKS *(continued)*

	SERVING SIZE		CSI	FAT (GM)	CALORIES
Spicy Black Bean Salad	¼ cup	(43 gm)	tr.	1	57
Chili Bean Salad	¼ cup	(55 gm)	tr.	1	64
Southern Caviar	¼ cup	(52 gm)	tr.	1	68
Steamed Buns	1 bun	(41 gm)	<1	3	73
Eggroll (with shrimp and pork)	1 roll	(101 gm)	6	11	158
Marinated Mushrooms	1/10 recipe	(43 gm)	tr.	3	39
Snappy Clams	1/8 recipe	(50 gm)	<1	2	39
Zucchini Toast	2 toasts	(55 gm)	<1	2	51
Spinach Triangles	3 triangles	(22 gm)	1	2	54
Rumaki	3 pieces	(40 gm)	6	4	68
Oysters Rockefeller	3 oysters	(79 gm)	10	12	162
Swedish meatballs	3 meatballs	(131 gm)	12	21	287

CANDIES, CHOCOLATES, AND OTHER SWEETS
(SELECT CSIs OF 2 OR LOWER PER SERVING)

CANDY BARS					
Bit O' Honey	2 ounces	(57 gm)	1	3	206
Payday	2 ounces	(57 gm)	2	10	256
M & M's (peanut)	2 ounces	(57 gm)	2	10	268

Twix	2 ounces	(57 gm)	4	9	243
Zagnut	2 ounces	(57 gm)	4	9	254
Milky Way	2 ounces	(57 gm)	5	8	237
Baby Ruth	2 ounces	(57 gm)	5	13	283
Butterfinger	2 ounces	(57 gm)	5	11	264
Mars Bar	2 ounces	(57 gm)	5	8	237
M & M's (plain)	2 ounces	(57 gm)	5	11	266
Oh Henry	2 ounces	(57 gm)	5	13	283
Power House	2 ounces	(57 gm)	5	13	283
Snicker	2 ounces	(57 gm)	5	13	283
Three Musketeers	2 ounces	(57 gm)	5	8	237
Reese's Peanut Butter Cup	2 ounces	(57 gm)	6	16	296
Mounds	2 ounces	(57 gm)	7	10	250
Almond Joy	2 ounces	(57 gm)	8	15	274
Granola Bar	2 ounces	(57 gm)	9	10	254
Heath	2 ounces	(57 gm)	9	18	286
Hershey with almonds	2 ounces	(57 gm)	10	20	303
Krackel	2 ounces	(57 gm)	10	17	292
Mr. Goodbar	2 ounces	(57 gm)	10	22	310
Nestle (chocolate, almonds)	2 ounces	(57 gm)	10	20	303
Summit	2 ounces	(57 gm)	10	17	292
Hershey (plain) or Kisses	2 ounces	(57 gm)	11	18	296

The abbreviation *tr.* stands for trace (less than (0.5); the symbol <1 stands for less than one (0.5 to 0.9). Recipes in **bold italics** can be found in Part III.

CANDIES, CHOCOLATES, AND OTHER SWEETS (continued)

	SERVING SIZE		CSI	FAT (GM)	CALORIES
NUT-TYPE CANDY					
Divinity	2 ounces	(64 gm)	<1	8	235
Nut brittle	2 ounces	(57 gm)	2	15	302
Pecan praline	2 ounces	(57 gm)	3	9	243
Bridge mix	2 ounces	(57 gm)	3	9	252
Fudge with walnuts	2 ounces	(60 gm)	3	10	257
Rocky road (chocolate, nuts, and marshmallows)	2 ounces	(57 gm)	6	14	232
Almond Roca	2 ounces	(57 gm)	9	21	305
MISCELLANEOUS CANDY					
Gumdrops	1 ounce	(28 gm)	0	tr.	98
Hard candy	1 ounce	(28 gm)	0	tr.	109
Jelly beans	1 ounce	(28 gm)	0	tr.	104
Licorice	1 ounce	(28 gm)	tr.	tr.	100
Mints, non-chocolate	1 ounce	(28 gm)	tr.	1	103
Taffy	1 ounce	(28 gm)	tr.	2	103
Cracker Jack	⅔ cup	(28 gm)	0	3	120
Ayd's (diet candy)	1 ounce	(28 gm)	2	2	107
Toffee	1 ounce	(28 gm)	2	3	113
Sugar Babies	1 ounce	(28 gm)	3	5	116
Caramels, plain & chocolate	1 ounce	(28 gm)	3	5	116
Malted milk balls	1 ounce	(28 gm)	4	7	135
Carob-coated raisins	1 ounce	(28 gm)	<1	4	112

Food	Measure	Weight			Calories
Carob-coated peanuts	1 ounce	(28 gm)	1	8	140
Chocolate-covered cherries	1 ounce	(28 gm)	3	5	123
Chocolate-covered creams	1 ounce	(28 gm)	3	5	123
Chocolate-covered raisins	1 ounce	(28 gm)	3	5	120
Chocolate Easter eggs	1 ounce	(28 gm)	3	5	120
Yogurt-coated peanuts	1 ounce	(28 gm)	4	9	129
Yogurt-coated raisins	1 ounce	(28 gm)	4	5	101
OTHER SWEETS					
Honey	½ cup	(168 gm)	0	0	511
Honey	1 tablespoon	(21 gm)	0	0	64
Jam, jelly, typical	½ cup	(160 gm)	tr.	tr.	437
Jam, jelly, typical	1 tablespoon	(20 gm)	tr.	tr.	55
Jam, jelly, low-sugar	½ cup	(160 gm)	0	0	223
Jam, jelly, low-sugar	1 tablespoon	(20 gm)	0	0	30
Marshmallows, plain	½ cup	(25 gm)	0	0	80
Marshmallows, chocolate-covered	½ cup	(28 gm)	3	6	145
Marshmallow Creme	½ cup	(69 gm)	0	0	217
Molasses	½ cup	(160 gm)	0	0	371
Sugar, brown	½ cup	(110 gm)	0	0	410
Sugar, powdered	½ cup	(64 gm)	0	0	247
Sugar, granulated	½ cup	(96 gm)	0	0	370
Syrup, maple-flavored	½ cup	(168 gm)	0	0	487
Coconut, sweetened	½ cup	(37 gm)	12	13	185

The abbreviation *tr.* stands for trace (less than (0.5); the symbol <1 stands for less than one (0.5 to 0.9). Recipes in **bold italics** can be found in Part III.

BEVERAGES: ALCOHOLIC
(SELECT CSIs OF 0 PER SERVING)

	SERVING SIZE		CSI	FAT (GM)	CALORIES
Beer, light	12 ounces	(353 gm)	0	0	96
Beer or ale	12 ounces	(353 gm)	0	0	145
Wine, table (Chablis, Burgundy, Champagne)	4 ounces	(116 gm)	0	0	91
Wine, dessert or aperitif (port, sherry, sweet vermouth)	4 ounces	(116 gm)	0	0	158
Liquor (gin, whiskey, vodka, rum, cognac)	1½ ounces	(42 gm)	0	0	105
MIXED COCKTAILS					
Bloody Mary	6 ounces	(179 gm)	0	tr.	129
Gimlet	6 ounces	(184 gm)	0	0	335
Mai Tai	6 ounces	(171 gm)	0	0	374
Manhattan	6 ounces	(170 gm)	0	0	342
Martini	6 ounces	(170 gm)	0	0	363
Margarita, Daiquiri	6 ounces	(176 gm)	0	tr.	402
Old-Fashioned	6 ounces	(192 gm)	0	0	516
Brandy Alexander	6 ounces	(173 gm)	9	12	417
Crème de Menthe or Grasshopper	6 ounces	(197 gm)	9	12	537
Piña Colada	6 ounces	(191 gm)	13	14	323
LIQUEURS					
Cordials, fruit type	1 ounce	(28 gm)	0	0	80

Coffee-flavored (Kahlua)	1 ounce	(38 gm)	0	0	88
Irish Cream	1 ounce	(34 gm)	3	2	92

FRUIT-TYPE DRINKS

Apple cider	1 cup	(248 gm)	0	0	116
Lemonade	1 cup	(240 gm)	0	0	110110
Fruit juice, average	1 cup	(240 gm)	tr.	tr.	120110
Orange Iced Tea	1 cup	(240 gm)	tr.	tr.	67
Orange Frosty	1 cup	(239 gm)	tr.	tr.	168
Strawberry Banana Smoothie	1 cup	(390 gm)	1	1	102

MILK SHAKES

All flavors (McDonald's)	16 ounces	(231 gm)	5	7	304
All flavors (most restaurants including other fast-food restaurants)	16 ounces	(360 gm)	8	11	442
All flavors (specialty ice cream stores)	16 ounces	(384 gm)	32	39	671

POP DRINKS

Non-cola, sweetened	12 ounces	(360 gm)	0	0	111
Cola, sweetened	12 ounces	(360 gm)	0	0	155

The abbreviation *tr.* stands for trace (less than 0.5); the symbol <1 stands for less than one (0.5 to 0.9). Recipes in **bold italics** can be found in Part III.

BEVERAGES: COLD (continued)

	SERVING SIZE		CSI	FAT (GM)	CALORIES
Diet pop	12 ounces	(360 gm)	0	0	4
Root beer float	1½ cups	(307 gm)	6	7	241
MILK DRINKS					
Milk, skim	1 cup	(245 gm)	<1	tr.	85
Milk, 1%	1 cup	(244 gm)	2	3	102
Milk, 2%	1 cup	(244 gm)	4	5	122
Milk, whole	1 cup	(244 gm)	7	8	149
Buttermilk	1 cup	(245 gm)	2	2	98
Chocolate milk (2%)	1 cup	(250 gm)	5	7	194
Instant Breakfast, all flavors					
made with skim milk	1 cup	(285 gm)	1	1	215
made with whole milk	1 cup	(279 gm)	7	9	279
Egg Nog	1 cup	(246 gm)	tr.	tr.	200
Egg Nog, commercial (no alcohol)	1 cup	(254 gm)	16	19	340
OTHERS					
Club soda, carbonated water, seltzer	1 cup	(240 gm)	0	0	0
Gatorade	1 cup	(240 gm)	0	0	58
Tea, unsweetened	1 cup	(240 gm)	0	0	0

BEVERAGES: HOT
(SELECT CSIs OF 2 OR LOWER PER SERVING)

Quick Hot Spiced Cider	1 cup	(250 gm)	0	tr.	122
Postum	1 cup	(240 gm)	0	0	15
Tea, unsweetened	1 cup	(240 gm)	0	0	0
Coffee, black	1 cup	(240 gm)	0	tr.	5
Coffee with ½ ounce skim milk	1 cup	(255 gm)	<1	<1	10
Coffee with ½ ounce Mocha Mix	1 cup	(255 gm)	<1	2	24
Coffee with ½ ounce half-and-half	1 cup	(255 gm)	1	2	25
Coffee, specialty (cappuccino, mocha, Vienna, au lait)	1 cup	(249 gm)	3	3	85
Cocoa with skim milk, sugar-free	1 cup	(260 gm)	2	2	68
Cocoa with skim milk, (Swiss Miss, from vending machine)	1 cup	(264 gm)	2	2	154
Cocoa with whole milk	1 cup	(263 gm)	8	10	217

The abbreviation *tr.* stands for trace (less than 0.5); the symbol <1 stands for less than one (0.5 to 0.9). Recipes in ***bold italics*** can be found in Part III.

CHAPTER

11

How the CSI Can Help You Take the Hazards Out of Dining Out

THE HIGH-CSI HIGHWAY

If you eat "on the road" a lot, then chances are good you're on the high-CSI highway. Or maybe we should call it the freeway, since statistics show that Americans eat a third of all their meals out and spend fully 40 percent of their food budget in restaurants, delis, and fast-food outlets where high-fat, high-cholesterol fare typically abounds. Like most highways, this one is producing a lot of casualties. But you can continue to eat out and still be healthy; your safety belt is the CSI—*if* you remember to use it properly.

So let's buckle up and take an illuminating trip down the fast-food lane.

The Restaurant Choices Quiz

Start out by determining where you are right now when it comes to selecting foods in restaurants. The following quiz can go a long way—especially if your results aren't what you'd hoped for—in raising your CSI safety consciousness.

Give yourself 5 points for **each** *of the following choices you typically make when you eat in a restaurant.*

5 Select restaurants that offer low-fat choices and order those choices.

5 Order toast, muffins, cereal, pancakes, waffles for breakfast.

5 Order soup (not cream), salad, or other meatless, cheeseless entrées for lunch.

5 When ordering pizza choose vegetarian.

5 Avoid cheese, eggs, bacon bits on salads and avoid potato and macaroni salads.

5 Put garbanzo or kidney beans on salads at the salad bar.

5 Use a very small amount of salad dressing.

5 Order a fish, shellfish, chicken, or lean red meat entrée (but not fried).

5 Use no more than 1 pat of margarine at any meal.

5 Order fruit, sorbet, sherbet, frozen yogurt, or skip dessert.

SCORE _____ (The total of all of the above choices that reflect your typical eating-out habits.) NOTE: Give yourself a score of 50 points if you eat out less than once a month.

Analysis of Quiz (Women and Men)

Present American Diet	less than 20
CSI Phase One	20 to 25
CSI Phase Two	30 to 35
CSI Phase Three	40 to 45
My score of _____ classifies	
me as eating _____ .	

So how did you do? Room for improvement? If so, you've got plenty of company. Even many people who are very CSI-conscious at home let down their guards while on the road. The usual rationale is:

"Well, I don't do this very often, so it's okay." But stop and think: How often *do* you eat out? Add up those meals on the road. In most cases, it's more of a regular thing than the exception. The typical American is eating one in every three meals outside the home.

Restaurant Selection

One way to survive the hazards of dining out is to select restaurants that regularly offer lower-CSI choices or that are willing to make modifications in high-CSI fare. Once you've found and/or "educated" these restaurants, use them whenever possible.

Don't hesitate to call restaurants and ask about their fat/cholesterol "philosophy." Fortunately, there is a trend toward lower-fat, lower-cholesterol cooking in many restaurants, including even some fast-food outlets. Or, when you arrive at a restaurant, ask to see the menu *before* you are seated. And ask questions and make requests. Ask how foods are prepared and avoid, especially, deep-fried selections. Request salad dressings, butter, sour cream, and sauces "on the side," rather than have these arrive spread all over your food. This way *you* control how much of these high-CSI items you consume. You can also ask that these items be withheld entirely. Another way to control the CSIs is to be sure to eat plenty of nearly zero–CSI items— lots of rice (1½ to 2 cups), a large potato, and, of course, bread.

Ethnic restaurants are among your safest bets. Not only is the food varied and exciting, it's often lower in fat and cholesterol. Here are some tips when you try different ethnic restaurants.

Chinese, Vietnamese, Thai, Japanese

- Wonderfully tasty vegetable dishes abound. Served with rice, these make great low-CSI lunches and dinners. Plan to eat 1½ to 2 cups of the rice. Even stir-fried vegetable dishes with small amounts of meat, poultry, or fish served over steamed rice usually meet our low-CSI goals.
- Avoid *all* deep-fried dishes, such as sweet-and-sour pork and prawns, fried rice and noodles, egg preparations (such as egg foo yong), or Japanese tempura dishes.

Mexican

- Grains and beans are staples in many Mexican dishes, making them good low-CSI entrées. But set aside the sour cream and scrape off the heaps of cheese that often accompany Mexican dishes.
- "Fajitas" are a spicy stir-fried concoction of chicken, lean beef, or seafood with lots of peppers, onions, and tomatoes rolled into steamed flour tortillas. This is a "build-your-own" entrée available in many Mexican restaurants and is ideal since, again, *you* control the content.
- Bean tostadas and burritos do not contain meat, but watch out for the cheese. Request that it not be added.
- Another good choice is arroz con pollo, a spicy tomato/rice-based chicken dish that can be ordered without cheese or sour cream.
- If you order side dishes of refried beans, Spanish rice, steamed tortillas, and green

salad, you can make your own tostada. Add salsa to spice it up.
- Beware of tortilla chips! These innocent-looking little things are actually quite high in fat. And people typically consume them by the basketful while waiting for their entrées. *If* you can eat a few and then resist, fine; otherwise, have someone tie your hands behind your back until your main meal arrives. As for dips, use the salsa and the bean variety, rather than the guacamole, which has significant amounts of fat.
- "Just say no" to all *huevos* (eggs).

Middle Eastern (Lebanese)

- For appetizers, enjoy the exotic and pungent flavors of tabouli (a great mixture of cracked wheat, olive oil, mint, and parsley), hummous (made with garbanzo beans and tahini—sesame "butter"), baba ganouj (an eggplant and tahini mixture), and rice-filled grape leaves.
- For entrées, try chicken or vegetable shish kabobs.
- Dilute meatier dishes with large servings of rice or bulgur (cracked wheat). And be sure to eat plenty of the wonderful pocket (pita) bread.

French

- Yes, it *is* possible to dine in a French restaurant without ending up in a CSI pileup. But it does demand some "defensive dining." Though the French worship at the altar of eggs, cream, and butter, *you* can snub these and still enjoy many of the distinctive flavors of French cuisine. Here are some tips to help you:

- Indulge in that great French bread (without butter) all through your meal. French and Italians eat their bread without spread.
- In place of fatty appetizers, order a platter of "crudités," fresh vegetables.
- Ask for vegetables to be steamed and sauces, if any, to be served on the side.
- Avoid all "au gratin" dishes, as these are prepared with a lot of cheese and butter.
- Best entrée choices are poached fish dishes without sauces, bouillabaisse (which is the famous fish soup from Marseille), and chicken and veal dishes with tomato or other vegetable sauces.
- For dessert, ask for a poached fruit or a sorbet.

Italian

- Many think of Italian foods as the most fattening of all. Not true. There *are* high-CSI Italian dishes, but, as a rule, Italian cuisine is among your better choices. Pastas, provided they aren't smothered in cheese and cream sauces, are excellent, low-CSI, non-fattening choices.
- One of the best, low-CSI dishes you can eat is a plate of spaghetti with a marinara (tomato) sauce. Marsala sauce made with wine and clam sauce is another good choice to top off your pasta dishes. But avoid the white sauces.
- A bowl of minestrone soup, crisp Italian bread, and a green salad served with a low-calorie or small amount of regular Italian salad dressing make an irresistible lunch or light dinner.
- Cannelloni, ravioli, and manicotti filled with spinach and ricotta cheese or

chicken are other good selections, provided the sauce is tomato-based, rather than cheese-based. Request that cheese toppings, if any, be omitted.
- Avoid "scallopine" and "Parmigiana" dishes as these are very high in cheese and other fat.
- Pollo cacciatore—chicken prepared with a mushroom and tomato sauce—is a good selection. Do not eat the chicken skin.
- Choose your pizzas *carefully*. Order thick crust pizzas topped with vegetables, shrimp, or Canadian bacon. Avoid pepperoni and sausage toppings. Never go for the "extra cheese" selections. In fact, you should always ask for "half the amount of cheese you normally use." See Table 31 at the end of the chapter for the CSIs of various pizzas. If you order the home-delivered pizza, ask for one-third or one-half less cheese. Serve the pizza with salad, baked potato (yes, you read correctly), and fruit to help keep the CSI down.
- For dessert, try a fruit ice (sorbet) or non-fat frozen yogurt.

American Well, you can't eat in ethnic restaurants all the time—so how does American fare compare? Okay, provided you, once again, take precautions. Here are some tips:

- Put a meal together at the salad bar. Add variety to your salad by including some beans, a few sunflower seeds, and a low-calorie, low-CSI dressing. Side dishes can include coleslaw made with oil and vinegar and German-style potato salad (without bacon). Bread or rolls and fresh sliced fruit complete the meal. Stay away from the meat and cheese trays, salads containing mayonnaise, fruit salads with whipped cream, and salad toppings such as chopped egg, cheese, croutons, and bacon. Use only a *little* of the regular salad dressing. French and Italian are your best choices if lower-calorie selections aren't available. Or use lemon wedges.

- For an entrée, fish is an excellent choice—steamed, baked, poached, or broiled, rather than fried.
- A baked potato, even with a modest amount of margarine, beats French fries.

- Choose a fruit sorbet or sherbet for dessert.
- Table 28 compares a number of high-fat, high-CSI menu items with several lower-fat, low-CSI alternatives.

Fast Foods

Cheeseburger, fries, and milk shake. Sound familiar? That "little" order adds up to a CSI catastrophe of 19. Table 31 at the end of the chapter provides you with the CSIs

TABLE 28
COMPARISONS OF LOW-CSI AND HIGH-CSI MENU CHOICES

HIGHER-CSI CHOICE				LOWER-CSI CHOICE			
FOOD	CSI	FAT (GRAMS)	CALORIES	FOOD	CSI	FAT (GRAMS)	CALORIES
Fried rice, 1 cup	18	14	338	Steamed rice, 1 cup	tr.	tr.	223
Spaghetti with meat sauce, 1½ cups	6	11	356	Spaghetti with marinara sauce, 1½ cups	tr.	3	251
Combination pizza ¼ of 14″	20	38	676	Green pepper-mushroom-onion pizza, ¼ of 14″	9	14	419
Cream of broccoli soup, 1 cup	14	18	230	Minestrone soup, 1 cup	1	3	83
Quarter pounder, cheese, 1 serving	18	32	525	Hamburger, 1 serving	9	11	263
Green salad with ¼ cup blue Cheese dressing	6	32	287	Green salad with 2 tablespoons low-cal blue cheese dressing	1	2	30
French fries, large serving	10	24	440	Baked potato with 1 teaspoon margarine	<2	5	205
Deep-fried fish, 6 ounces fish	21	52	725	Fish, poached, 6 ounces	5	2	141

The abbreviation tr. stands for trace (less than 0.5).

of many familiar fast foods, including hamburgers, fries, shakes, breakfast selections, and pizza.

About the only way to avoid a high-CSI head-on collision in a fast food restaurant is to order the *smallest* and *plainest* hamburger in the joint (or avoid hamburgers altogether); throw in some onions and tomatoes but hold the mayo and cheese. And if you *do* order a hamburger, even the smallest and plainest, *don't* have a shake and fries, as well. Instead, have a salad (with low-calorie salad dressing or oil and vinegar), iced tea, water, or soda.

Many fast-food places now have expanded salad bars. (Follow tips under "American" in the preceding section when making your salad bar selections.)

Other reasonable choices include tacos, tostadas, and bean burritos (provided they aren't deep-fried). For tips on selecting pizza, review "Italian" section earlier in this chapter. And see Table 31 for their CSIs.

Entrées and Desserts

People are always very interested in seeing how the CSIs stack up for entrée and dessert choices in restaurants. Many of these are provided in Tables 29 and 30. Ideally, you should select a dinner entrée that has a CSI of 9 or lower per serving. If the goal is to have a daily CSI of 17 (women/children) or 24 (men/teens), several of these entrées do not fit—unless you plan to have almost

0 CSI days before and after eating out. Eventually, you'll want to make some of these selections once-a-year treats—filet mignon, prime rib, lamb chops, deep-fried fish, etc., if you still want them and haven't lost your taste for these items. When you eat out for lunch, you need to eat very-low-CSI for dinner. Ditto for the weekend brunch—this is your big CSI meal for the day.

The CSI lineup of desserts is actually shocking. It is immediately clear that selecting prime rib (CSI of 45 per 9 ounces) and chocolate mousse (CSI of 33 per cup) sends you into CSI outer space—CSI of 78! Choosing fried chicken (CSI of 17 per 3 pieces) and strawberry shortcake (CSI of 19 per piece) produces a CSI of 36! Instead, consider ordering chicken cacciatore (CSI of 8 per piece) and blackberry cobbler (CSI of 2 per cup) for a total CSI of 10. How about bouillabaisse (CSI of 4 per 2 cups) and glazed apple pie (CSI of 5 per piece) for a total CSI of 9? Perhaps you would like a fast-food hamburger (CSI of 9 for one) and nonfat frozen yogurt (CSI of almost 0); add to it a salad with low-calorie dressing and a piece of fruit.

It may be tempting to select a low-CSI entrée, such as spaghetti with marinara sauce (CSI of almost 0), and then reward yourself with a piece of cheesecake (CSI of 22 for one piece). Or, you might order a delicious poached halibut (CSI of 5 per 6 ounces) and finish up with chocolate mousse (CSI of 33 per cup) for a total of 38. *Not* a good plan. These choices do not fit in with a dinner CSI goal of 11 for women and 15½ for men—at least not on a regular basis.

Even choosing with the best of inten-

TABLE 29
THE CSIs, FAT, AND CALORIES IN TYPICAL RESTAURANT ENTRÉES
(Select CSIs of 9 or lower per serving)

	CSI	FAT(GM)	CALORIES
Spaghetti with marinara sauce, 1½ cups	tr.	3	251
Bouillabaisse, 2 cups	4	4	164
Chicken chow mein, 1 cup	4	9	224
Grilled fish (no added fat), 6 ounces	5	2	141
Poached fish, 6 ounces	5	2	141
Plain chicken or turkey hot dog, 1	6	10	216
Cioppino, 2 cups	7	6	266
Chicken enchilada, 1	7	10	197
Plain beef hot dog, 1	8	15	259
Chicken cacciatore, 1 piece	8	16	298
Green pepper-mushroom-onion pizza, ¼ of 14″	9	14	419
Fast-food hamburger, 1	9	11	263
Barbecued chicken with skin, 3 pieces	14	24	501
Fried chicken, 3 pieces	17	35	647
Quarter pounder with cheese, 1	18	32	525
Combination pizza, ¼ of 14″	20	38	676
Batter-coated deep-fried fish, 6 ounces fish	21	52	725
Lamb chops, 9 ounces	36	51	714
Prime rib, 9 ounces	45	81	969
Filet mignon, 9 ounces	45	81	969

The abbreviation *tr.* stands for trace (less than 0.5).

tions, one can be surprised by the size of the dish when it arrives. Some plates of spaghetti, Mexican combinations, Chinese noodles, etc., can be enormous. That's what those take-home boxes are for—make good use of them. Eat a reasonable amount and stop there.

THE CSIs OF FAST-FOOD DISHES

Table 31 provides the CSIs of many fast foods, including breakfast selections, sandwiches and hamburgers, pizzas, and side orders.

TABLE 30
THE CSIs, FAT, AND CALORIES IN TYPICAL RESTAURANT DESSERTS
(Select CSIs of 5 or lower per serving)

	CSI	FAT(GM)	CALORIES
Sorbet, 1 cup	0	0	255
Poached fruit, 1 serving	tr.	tr.	160
Nonfat frozen yogurt, 1 cup	tr.	tr.	224
Rice Krispie bar, 3″ x 3″	<1	4	98
Fruit cobbler, 1 cup	2	8	272
Sherbet, 1 cup	3	4	270
Glazed fruit pie, ⅙ of 9″	5	12	309
Pound cake, 5″ x 3″ x ½″	7	9	178
Baklava, 2″ x 2″	8	29	428
Chocolate eclair, 2″ x 4″	10	10	201
Apple pie, ⅙ of 9″	11	27	504
Lemon meringue pie, ⅙ of 9″	14	20	452
Carrot cake, 3″ x 3¼″	14	29	662
Chocolate chip cookie, 5¼″	14	30	637
Pecan pie, ⅙ of 9″	15	41	682
German chocolate cake, 3″ x 3″ x 2″	17	24	472
Strawberry shortcake, ⅙ of 8″	19	31	616
Brownie, frosted 3″ x 3″	20	42	721
Cheesecake, ¹⁄₁₂ of 10″	22	25	355
Grasshopper pie, ⅙ of 9″	22	35	575
Ice cream (extra rich), 1 cup	30	38	580
Chocolate mousse, 1 cup	33	31	380

The abbreviation *tr.* stands for trace (less than 0.5); the symbol <1 stands for less than one (0.5 to 0.9).

TABLE 31
THE CSIs OF FAST-FOOD DISHES AND PIZZAS

FAST-FOOD DISHES

	SERVING SIZE	CSI	FAT (GM)	CALORIES
BREAKFAST				
English muffin (with butter)	One	(63 gm)	3	5	186
Hash brown potatoes	1 serving	(55 gm)	3	9	144
Hot cakes (with butter and syrup)	1 serving	(214 gm)	6	10	500
Danish:				
Raspberry	One	(117 gm)	5	16	414
Apple	One	(115 gm)	5	18	389
Cinnamon-raisin	One	(110 gm)	6	21	445
Iced cheese	One	(110 gm)	8	22	395
Biscuit:				
with spread	One	(85 gm)	8	18	330
with sausage	1 serving	(121 gm)	14	31	467
with bacon, egg, & cheese	1 serving	(145 gm)	23	32	483
with sausage & egg	1 serving	(175 gm)	29	40	585
Sausage, pork	1 serving	(53 gm)	9	19	210
Sausage McMuffin	1 serving	(138 gm)	13	26	427
Egg McMuffin	1 serving	(138 gm)	19	16	340
Sausage McMuffin with egg	1 serving	(165 gm)	27	33	517
Eggs, scrambled	1 serving	(98 gm)	31	13	180
SANDWICHES				
Chicken McNuggets	1 serving	(109 gm)	8	20	323
Filet o' Fish	1 sandwich	(143 gm)	8	26	435

228

Hamburger	1 serving	(100 gm)	9	11	263
Cheeseburger	1 serving	(114 gm)	9	16	318
Quarter Pounder	1 serving	(160 gm)	13	24	427
Big Mac	1 serving	(200 gm)	16	35	570
Quarter Pounder, cheese	1 serving	(186 gm)	18	32	525
Mc DLT	1 serving	(254 gm)	20	44	680
SIDE ORDERS					
Soft-serve/cone	1 cone	(115 gm)	3	5	189
Sundae:					
strawberry	1 serving	(164 gm)	5	9	320
caramel	1 serving	(165 gm)	5	10	361
hot fudge	1 serving	(164 gm)	7	11	357
French fries	1 serving	(68 gm)	5	12	220
Apple pie	1 serving	(85 gm)	5	14	253
Cookies, McDonaldland	1 serving	(67 gm)	5	11	308
Choclaty Chip	1 serving	(69 gm)	9	16	342
Milk shake:					
vanilla	16 fl. ounces	(231 gm)	5	7	287
strawberry	16 fl. ounces	231 gm)	5	7	279
chocolate	16 fl. ounces	(231 gm)	5	7	304

The abbreviation *tr.* stands for trace (less than (0.5); the symbol <1 stands for less than one (0.5 to 0.9). Recipes in **bold *italics*** can be found in Part III.

MAIN ENTRÉES: PIZZAS
(SELECT CSIs OF 9 OR LOWER PER SERVING)

	SERVING SIZE		CSI	FAT (GM)	CALORIES
THIN CRUST PIZZA					
Spicy Cheese Pizza	¼ of 14" pizza	(357 gm)	5	9	390
Green pepper-mushroom-onion	¼ of 14" pizza	(292 gm)	9	14	419
Canadian bacon	¼ of 14" pizza	(229 gm)	10	16	446
Pepperoni	¼ of 14" pizza	(229 gm)	13	23	509
Cheese	¼ of 14" pizza	(257 gm)	16	24	552
Combination	¼ of 14" pizza	(279 gm)	20	38	676
THICK CRUST PIZZA					
Spicy Cheese Pizza	¼ of 14" pizza	(417 gm)	4	7	565
Green pepper-mushroom-onion	¼ of 14" pizza	(360 gm)	6	9	574
Canadian bacon	¼ of 14" pizza	(334 gm)	7	12	611
Pepperoni	¼ of 14" pizza	(334 gm)	10	19	674
Cheese	¼ of 14" pizza	(343 gm)	11	16	664
Combination	¼ of 14" pizza	(384 gm)	17	33	842
Quick-and-Easy Pan Bread Pizza	⅙ of recipe	(251 gm)	2	11	339
Pita Pizza	1 pizza	(149 gm)	3	5	255
Baguette with Vegetable Filling	½ of recipe	(354 gm)	2	10	500
Vegetable Calzone	¼ of recipe	(301 gm)	5	11	437

The abbreviation *tr.* stands for trace (less than (0.5); the symbol <1 stands for less than one (0.5 to 0.9). Recipes in **bold italics** can be found in Part III.

Using the CSI for Weight Loss and Control

THE BEST WEIGHT-LOSS DIET IS A LOW-CSI DIET

The CSI makes it much easier to design an optimal weight-loss, weight-control program. A reduced-calorie intake that emphasizes low-CSI foods is the key to success. If you normally eat 2,000 or 3,000 or 4,000 Calories a day and cut down to 1,000 Calories, you *will* lose weight, no doubt about it. But if those 1,000 Calories are high in fat, you will still have an unhealthy diet. The CSI for 1,000 Calories of high-fat food can easily be 25 instead of the 9 that we consider optimal for weight loss.

If those 1,000 Calories are derived, in significant part, from low-CSI fare, you will

be eating much healthier foods. You will be eating foods high in complex carbohydrates and fiber—and those foods have very low CSIs. Thanks to the greater bulk of these foods, you'll feel fuller and more satisfied—and you will avoid one of the problems of high-fat dieting—constipation. In general, the lower the CSI of your weight-loss regimen, the better your chances will be of preserving your muscle tissue as you lose weight and the better your chances will be of keeping the weight off over the long term—because you will have adapted to a permanent low-CSI way of eating.

The old, still persistent idea that carbohydrates are fattening is one we have to correct right now. Obviously, if you eat too many calories derived from *anything* you'll gain weight—but it's much more difficult to "overdose" on bulky, high-fiber carbohydrates than on fat (which goes down fast and easy—and then sticks). You simply feel fuller with far fewer calories after eating high-fiber "carbos."

The very *worst* dietary results come from the so-called "starvation" diets that are very low in carbohydrate and high in fat. These very-low-calorie, high-CSI diets certainly do result in rapid weight loss, it's true, but what's lost tends to be lean body mass (muscle, including water and salts), as well as fat. Such regimens leave dieters needing even fewer calories later to maintain their weight and, in almost every case, the weight is regained. This regained weight is largely fat, with the result that the dieter has more body fat and less lean tissue than *before* the diet was started. Since fat is less active metabolically than muscle, it takes fewer calories to maintain weight the fatter you get. The bottom line is that you end up having to eat less than ever before in order to avoid gaining still more

weight. Sound familiar? *Avoid high-CSI "crash" diets. They are fattening in the long run.*

The idea that eating fat begets greater hunger was further confirmed recently in a scientific study from Canada. Subjects were allowed to eat as much as they wanted from two different regimens. Those on the high-fat fare consumed, on average, 4,100 Calories per day, while those on a somewhat lower-fat regimen consumed about 3,000 Calories per day. Both groups felt equally full after their meals.

We have found the diet program that is most effective in reducing fat, rather than lean body mass, is a *balanced low-CSI diet of 1,000 to 1,200 Calories per day for women and 1,800 to 2,000 Calories per day for men.* Table 32 shows you the different results, in terms of composition of body tissue lost, on different short-term weight-loss programs. Note that on the starvation/ ketogenic diets (typically very-low-carbohydrate diets

TABLE 32
COMPOSITION OF TISSUE LOST ON DIFFERENT DIETS

	LEAN BODY MASS	FAT
	(PERCENT OF WEIGHT LOSS)	
Starvation or fasting	68	32
Ketogenic diets (less than 1,000 Calories)	65	35
Mixed-food diets (less than 1,000 Calories)	40	60
Mixed-food diets (more than 1,000 Calories)	32	68
Mixed-food diets plus mild exercise (more than 1,000 Calories)	21	79

TABLE 33
REDUCED-CALORIE DAILY GUIDELINES FOR MEN AND WOMEN

	FOR WOMEN 1,000 TO 1,200 CALORIES	FOR MEN 1,800 TO 2,000 CALORIES
Lean meat, fish, poultry (ounces/day)	3	3
Low-fat dairy products (servings/day)*	1 to 2	2 to 3
Bread or grain products (servings/day)†	6 to 7	13 to 14
Fruit (pieces/day)	3	4
Vegetables (cups/day)	2	2
Fat, visible and hidden (servings/day)††	2	5

*One low-fat dairy product serving = about 75 Calories. (1 cup skim milk or nonfat yogurt; ½ cup 2 percent milk, low-fat plain yogurt, or low-fat cottage cheese; or 1½ to 2 ounces of these cheeses: Lite-line, Lite n' Lively, Weight Watchers, part-skim ricotta, Reduced Calories Laughing Cow).

†One bread serving = about 80 Calories (½ large baked potato, ½ cup macaroni or other pasta, ⅓ cup rice, ⅓ cup cooked beans, 1 slice bread, 1 corn tortilla, ½ flour tortilla, ½ bagel, ½ cup cooked cereal, 1 cup dry cereal, one 4" pancake).

††One fat serving = about 40 Calories (1 teaspoon or pat of margarine, oil, mayonnaise, or Miracle Whip; 2 teaspoons imitation or light mayonnaise, salad dressing, peanut butter, or diet margarine; 1 tablespoon low-calorie salad dressing).

of fewer than 1,000 Calories per day), a whopping 65 to 68 percent of the weight loss is in the form of lean body mass and only 32 to 35 percent is from fat. These diets are usually extremely restrictive in terms of what you can eat and soon become tedious and monotonous—not the kind of eating style you can sustain for very long.

But note—again referring to Table 32—that when you move to more balanced diets, consisting of a much broader mixture of foods, better results are obtained—even when calories are still quite restricted. And when you go to a *mixed* diet that provides *more than* 1,000 Calories per day, even better results are obtained. Combining a mixed diet of 1,000 Calories or more with mild exercise is the best program of all, resulting in weight loss that is 79 percent fat and only 21 percent lean body mass.

9 and 18 are the Magic Numbers

Construct a balanced diet of 1,000 Calories per day (women) with a daily CSI of no more than 9, and it will be difficult for you to go wrong. For men on a 2,000-Calorie diet, the magic number is double that: 18. Table 34 at the end of the chapter shows you five days of sample meal plans that provide CSIs of 9 or less per 1,000 Calories. Men can double the portions to arrive at a 2,000-Calorie regimen with daily CSIs of 18 or less.

To ensure that you achieve these goals and get a good mixed (balanced) diet, generally stick to the guidelines provided in Table 33. Choose from *each* of the food groups every day. Don't try to make exchanges from one group to the other. For example, if you give up one of your bread or vegetable servings, don't think that you can replace it with an extra fat serving. That won't work. Look at the five days of menus (Table 34) to see how these guidelines translate to food.

Follow this plan, and you *will* lose weight—and your chances of keeping the weight off will be better than ever. This is a plan that will fill you up without filling you out and will provide a wide range of foods so that monotony won't defeat you. Weight loss will be more in the form of fat and less in the form of lean body mass. You'll have more energy and feel far happier and more alert than you would on a starvation-type diet.

And don't forget that regular exercise is a very important part of any weight-loss program. Not only has exercise been shown to be a key factor for successful weight *loss*, but studies also make it clear that exercise is a crucial part of any successful weight *maintenance* program. It takes a two-prong approach—a low-fat eating style *plus* exercise—to maximize weight loss *and* maintain the loss over time.

It takes somewhat longer to lose weight on our regimen than it does on a starvation diet. You're likely to lose 1 to 2 pounds per week on our program. On some starvation diets you might lose twice as fast. But—and this is the all-important "but"—you're far less likely to regain the weight on our program or to suffer negative health consequences while losing the weight in the first place. The choice is yours.

TABLE 34
FIVE LOW-CSI WEIGHT-LOSS MEAL PLANS*

	CSI	FAT(GM)	CALORIES
Day One			
Breakfast			
3 **Oatmeal Buttermilk Pancakes**	1	3	228
½ cup berries	tr.	tr.	30
1 cup black coffee or tea	0	tr.	5
Lunch			
1 flour tortilla	1	3	118
½ cup refried beans	<1	2	124
2 tablespoons salsa	tr.	tr.	12
1 medium apple	tr.	tr.	60
Dinner			
1 piece **Portland Fried Chicken**	3	3	94
½ cup **Skinny "French Fries"**	<1	2	67
1 cup cooked carrots	tr.	tr.	50
1 cup green salad with 2 tablespoons low-calorie French dressing	tr.	2	51
1 dinner roll	<1	2	83
Evening Snack			
3 gingersnaps	1	2	88
1 cup skim milk	<1	tr.	85
TOTALS	**10**	**19**	**1,095**
Day Two			
Breakfast			
½ grapefruit	tr.	tr.	30
½ cup oatmeal	tr.	1	73
½ cup skim milk	½	tr.	43
Lunch			
1 cup minestrone soup	1	3	83
6 soda crackers	1	2½	86
1 medium pear	tr.	tr.	60
Snack			
3 cups air-popped popcorn	tr.	<1	69
Dinner			
1½ cups spaghetti with **Marinara Sauce**	tr.	3	251
1 cup steamed broccoli	tr.	tr.	50
1 cup green salad with 2 tablespoons low-calorie Italian dressing	1	3	39
2 pieces French bread	tr.	tr.	166
Evening Snack			
1 cup honeydew melon	tr.	tr.	60
TOTALS	**3½**	**13½**	**1,010**

* The goals of each day's meal plan are a CSI of 9, with 22½ grams of fat in a caloric range of 1,000 to 1,200.
Recipes in **bold italics** can be found in Part III.
The abbreviation *tr.* stands for trace (less than 0.5); and symbol <1 stands for less than one (0.5 to 0.9).

	CSI	FAT(GM)	CALORIES
Day Three			
Breakfast			
½ cup orange juice	tr.	tr.	60
1 cup bran flakes with raisins	tr.	1	175
½ cup skim milk	½	tr.	43
Lunch			
1 pita or pocket bread filled with	tr.	<1	180
½ cup *Chili Bean Salad*	<1	3	128
1 cup strawberries	tr.	tr.	60
Dinner			
2 pieces *Parmesan Yogurt Chicken*	7	10	235
1 cup cooked brown rice	tr.	<1	179
1 cup green beans	tr.	tr.	50
1 cup carrot and celery sticks	tr.	tr.	25
Evening Snack			
1 peach	tr.	tr.	60
TOTALS	**8½**	**16**	**1,195**
Day Four			
Breakfast			
1 orange, sliced	tr.	tr.	60
1 slice whole wheat toast	tr.	<1	70
1 tablespoon low-sugar jam	0	0	30
Snack			
1 rice cake	tr.	tr.	34
Lunch			
Sandwich:			
2 slices whole wheat bread	tr.	1	140
2 slices thin, pressed turkey	tr.	tr.	12
1 tablespoon mustard	tr.	<1	11
lettuce and tomato	tr.	tr.	13
1 cup tomato soup (skim milk)	1	2	128
1 cup grapes	tr.	tr.	60
Snack			
1½ cups air-popped popcorn	tr.	<1	35
Dinner			
3 ounces *Baked Herbed Fish*	2	2	81
1 baked potato	<1	<1	170
¼ cup nonfat yogurt with dillweed	tr.	tr.	32
1 cup green salad with 2 tablespoons low-calorie Italian dressing	1	3	39
1 serving *Apple Crisp*	<1	4	153
TOTALS	**6**	**16**	**1,053**

Recipes in **bold italics** can be found in Part III.

The abbreviation *tr.* stands for trace (less than 0.5); and symbol <1 stands for less than one (0.5 to 0.9).

DAY FIVE

Breakfast

1 **Barrel of Muffins**	<1	4	105
1 cup strawberry nonfat yogurt	<1	tr.	200
1 cup black coffee	0	tr.	5

Lunch

1 medium baked potato	<1	<1	170
½ cup 1-percent-fat cottage cheese	<1	1	81
¼ cup salsa	tr.	tr.	24
1 banana	tr.	tr.	120

Dinner

1½ cups **Beef-Tomato Chow Yuk**	3	7	211
1 cup steamed rice	tr.	tr.	223
1 cup steamed broccoli	tr.	tr.	50
1 cup lettuce salad with raspberry vinegar	tr.	tr.	10
TOTALS	**7**	**13**	**1,200**

Recipes in **bold italics** can be found in Part III.
The abbreviation *tr.* stands for trace (less than 0.5); and symbol <1 stands for less than one (0.5 to 0.9).

CSI Goals for Children

Atherosclerosis, the basic cholesterol disorder that leads to coronary artery disease, typically begins to develop in childhood in the United States, Western Europe, and the rest of the "developed" world. By their early twenties, Americans not infrequently have considerable atherosclerosis, a fact made clear by autopsy studies of young servicemen killed in Korea and Vietnam. Children dying of accidents in Louisiana already had demonstrable atherosclerosis; they had consumed a high-CSI diet.

It's particularly important to establish sound dietary and related health goals early in life because the risk factors for coronary heart disease have their roots in childhood. These are associated with the typical lifestyle of Americans: a high-CSI, high-salt, low-fiber diet excessive in calories, lack of physical activity, cigarette smoking—a lifestyle that contributes to obesity, high blood pressure, and heart disease, among other ailments.

What Is a Normal Blood-Cholesterol Level for a Child?

We are born with concentrations of cholesterol in umbilical cord blood from 60 to 80 milligrams per deciliter (mg/dl). In *all* cultures from around the world the blood cholesterol ranges from 120 to 140 mg/dl during breast feeding. The nervous system and the retina of the eye need a certain amount of dietary fat, including essential fatty acids (see Chapter 4 earlier in Part II), in order to mature and develop properly. In fact, milk is about 50 percent fat and has a relatively high CSI. Thus, human milk, which is particularly rich in CSI (and in two essential fatty acids, omega-6 and omega-3, also needed by the developing nervous system), is ideal during the first 1½ to 2 years of life. But beyond that point a high-fat milk diet with a high-CSI is no longer needed. And in the cultures of the developing world, once the child has been weaned at about age two, the child's blood cholesterol level declines a bit to about 110 to 130 mg/dl, where it stays for the rest of that individual's lifetime. The diets of these children are typically low in fat. A good example are the Mexican Indians we have studied over a fifteen-year period. Healthy Tarahumara school children have blood cholesterol levels of 110 mg/dl, and their parents and grandparents are little different (average values of 122 mg/dl). The CSI of the Tarahumara diet after weaning is 15 for women and children and 20 for men and teens.

This is, unfortunately, not true in American children. Here, blood cholesterol levels gradually *rise* to the 160–180 mg/dl range during the school years. Worse yet, much of this rise is due to an increase in LDL cholesterol, the "bad cholesterol" that contributes the most to atherosclerosis. Again, the risk factors discussed above, especially the very high-fat, high-CSI, high-salt fare children are fed and then tend to

favor, are to blame. The CSI of the diet of U.S. women and children is 51 and for men and teens is 69. The stage is set for further escalation in blood cholesterol levels, typically to the 200–220 mg/dl range between the ages of 25 and 40 and to 220–240 mg/dl range by fifty-five to sixty years of age, as is shown in Figure 7 from our family study.

So what *should* the blood cholesterol level of a school-age child be? In our Lipid

AGE-RELATED CHOLESTEROL CHANGES

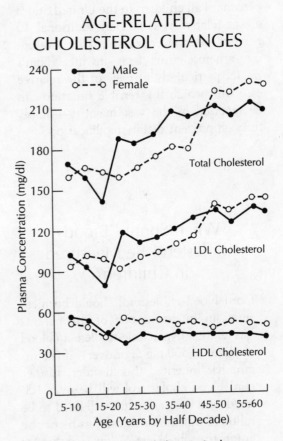

FIGURE 7. The age-related changes in the plasma concentrations of total cholesterol and the high- and low-density lipoprotein (LDL and HDL) in males and females aged 6 to 65 years.

Clinic, we have set the goal for childhood blood cholesterol levels in the 140–160 mg/dl range. And we like to see LDL cholesterol levels at 100 mg/dl *or lower*. Healthy, well-fed Tarahumara Indian children have blood cholesterol levels below 120 mg/dl and LDL cholesterol levels well below 100 mg/dl. So it can be done—and without any real deprivation.

As things stand now, however, one in three American children fail to meet the goals we have established. Some 20 to 25 percent of all children in the United States are at relative risk, and an additional 10 percent are at more severe risk of developing atherosclerosis later in life. That's tragic, particularly in view of the relative ease with which this terrible situation can be reversed in the vast majority—simply through prudent dietary modification.

When Should Blood Cholesterol Be Measured in Children?

- Cord blood cholesterol should be measured in infants if one of the parents has familial hypercholesterolemia (blood cholesterol 300 mg/dl or over). If the infant has inherited this disorder, his/her cord blood cholesterol will be over 100 mg/dl and such an infant will need to be followed much more closely as he or she enters the school age. A low-CSI diet for such a child is then especially important.
- All school-age children whose parents have abnormally high blood cholesterol

levels and/or who have had coronary heart disease should have their blood cholesterol level checked.
- Cholesterol should be measured whenever blood is drawn (for *any* other reason) from children.
- Cholesterol should be measured at least once by age eighteen as a component of an overall health examination, just like the blood pressure should be checked.
- LDL and HDL cholesterol levels and triglyceride level should be measured if the blood cholesterol of a child is 180 mg/dl or greater. Such children require intensified low-CSI counseling and should have blood levels retested annually.

What Should Children Eat?

Many people mistakenly believe that a high-fat diet is "normal" and "healthy" during childhood. As previously noted, there is only one period when we require a relatively high-fat diet—up to the age of two when growth is extremely rapid and when the nervous system is completing its maturation. After that, numerous studies have shown, balanced low-fat fare is ideal for children, just as it is for adults. By "low-fat," we mean a diet in which only 20 to 30 percent of calories come from fat. As preceding chapters have made evident, our recommended fare is *not* strictly vegetarian or fat-free, by any means. It still includes entirely adequate—in fact, optimal—amounts of calories, protein, fat, and other nutrients.

When to Start Feeding Your Child Low-Fat Foods

Your infant needs high-fat milk as long as milk is supplying the majority of calories—breast milk or formula and later whole milk. The baby begins to eat more table food between the ages of one and two. During this time the majority of calories ceases to come from milk and comes from an ever-widening variety of foods. When this occurs, it is then appropriate to switch to a lower-fat milk. Two years of age is generally a good time for making this switch. If your child is eating and growing well, switching to skim or 1-percent-fat milk is in order. If your child is a picky eater and is on the slim side, move to a lower-fat milk more cautiously. Switch to a 2-percent-fat milk, then to 1-percent-fat milk, and on to skim milk. The lower-fat milks have just as much calcium and protein as whole milk. Other foods should also be low-CSI. The earlier good eating habits are taught and learned, the easier it will be for the child (and eventually the adult) to stick with and enjoy a healthy nutritional life-style.

Obesity in Children

Since American children are becoming increasingly obese, moving to a low-CSI way of eating early in childhood makes good sense. Obesity, once developed, is notoriously difficult to treat, whether it be in children or adults. Prevention of obesity is the preferred goal. The Tarahumara school children we observed were not obese; they consumed a low-CSI, high-carbohydrate diet with lots of fiber. While we are not recommending their diet of largely corn and beans for Americans north of the border, we can learn from them about the value of a low-CSI diet to help prevent obesity. It must be admitted also that the word Tarahumara means "fleet of foot" or runner. Tarahumara children had no TVs or computer games. They had a lot of exercise. The prevention of childhood obesity clearly must encourage both a low-CSI eating style and much more physical activity.

Children *Need* Snacks and Desserts—of the *Right* Kind

What's the first thing most people do when they learn they or their child has high blood cholesterol? They typically call a halt to the snacks, desserts, and fast foods. This is not a good idea. Lower-fat foods are also lower in calories. In many children the result of eliminating snacks and desserts is weight loss or a slowing down of growth. For adults who tend to be chubby this is not bad. For children who are supposed to be growing, this *is* bad. They really need snacks and desserts when eating low-fat fare—but they need different snacks and desserts and they need to learn how to make low-fat choices in fast-food places. Parents can benefit from this also. Read on for further guidelines.

Desserts

The rule of thumb for desserts is to use fat-modified recipes and cut the serving size in half. The size of the portion is important even in recipes which have been modified to be lower in CSI and fat. In Table 35, look at comparable sizes of two zucchini cakes—a typical recipe and a lower-fat one. For that portion size, the amounts of fat and calories per serving are high, even in the fat-modified cake. Only when the portion is small is the cake really low-fat. Look in Chapter 9 on desserts for other recipes that have a CSI of 5 or less and contain no more than 5 grams (1 teaspoon) of fat per serving.

Snacks

Be sure to offer your child snacks. Snacking or nibbling is a good way to eat, in any event, and children do not always adapt well to a pattern of three fixed meals a day. Our primate ancestors ate frequently throughout the day, and children need to do this also. More frequent, small and light meals place less stress on the metabolic machinery of the body and often result in lower blood cholesterol levels when compared with three heavy meals (gorging).

Expand your horizons and your child's by trying new and different snacks. Some will take and some will not. Here are some ideas:

Beans. Kids usually like beans, so try them. Start with bean dip—the regular kind made from refried beans or try the Middle Eastern bean dip *Hummous.* Roll refried beans up in a flour tortilla. Put bean mixtures in tiny pocket breads.

Pizzas. Make pizzas using pocket bread, English muffins, or the popular Italian pan bread (focaccia) for a crust. Top with vegetables, thin-pressed lunch meat, and a small amount of imitation or part-skim mozzarella.

Cereal. Don't forget cereals. They are almost always low in fat. Always have six or seven varieties on hand plus lots of skim milk. Be selective about granolas—look for ones that contain no coconut, coconut oil, or palm oil. The CSI should be less than 1 and the fat content should not be greater than 3 grams per ½ cup.

Dried Fruit. These make great snacks.

TABLE 35
SELECT LOW-FAT DESSERTS AND SMALLER SERVING SIZES

ITEM	SERVING SIZE	CSI	FAT		CALORIES
			grams	teaspoons	
Zucchini cake	¹⁄₁₂ of cake	6	9	2	285
Chocolate Zucchini Cake	¹⁄₁₂ of cake	2	10	2	284
Chocolate Zucchini Cake	¹⁄₂₄ of cake	<1	5	1	142

Recipes in **bold italics** can be found in Part III. The symbol <1 stands for less than one (0.5 to 0.9).

Apricots, apples, raisins, pears, peaches—the list is long. They taste great and provide lots of fiber.

Chips, Crackers, and Popcorn. Here you'll want to try different kinds until you find the ones that suit you. Make your own tortilla chips and dippers—especially bean dip. Flour tortillas work well also and so do bagels (sliced thin) and pita bread (cut in triangles). You can even buy pita chips and bagel chips—just make sure they are baked. Offer the low-CSI crackers on our list and serve plenty of popcorn with just a smidgen of melted margarine.

Sandwiches. Peanut butter and jelly sandwiches are great. Or you can make a sandwich using bread, a light mayonnaise or Light Miracle Whip, 2 slices of thin-pressed lunch meat, and lettuce. See our snack chapter for other ideas.

Fast-Food Restaurants

The biggest problem with fast-food restaurants is the lack of choices. Mostly you choose from sandwiches and fries and drinks. The selection of fruit, vegetables, grains, and beans is usually zero. You can handle this problem in three ways: (1) You can select the lowest-fat items—the plain hamburger or the salad bar with a tiny amount of dressing (no cheese and other fatty foods)—and a soft drink (instead of a shake); (2) Be sure your children (and you) eat vegetables and fruit in addition to the foods purchased; and (3) If your family is eating low-fat at home, an occasional trip to the fast-food restaurant will not wipe out a low-CSI eating pattern (by occasionally we mean once a month).

Eating Patterns Are Set Early

It takes some effort to try enough recipes and food products to change your family's eating from higher to lower CSI. Look to the other chapters in this book and to your dietitian and physician and even to your grocery store for new ideas. And remember, the dietary patterns of adults are set in childhood. Once established, dietary patterns are difficult to change, so it is really important that our children learn how to eat correctly to avoid coronary heart disease and the other diseases of overconsumption. A low-CSI diet throughout life will help them a great deal. This is not to say that an individual who has consumed a high-CSI diet for decades of his life cannot make the change to a lower-CSI with benefit. This can certainly happen. Changing to a low-CSI diet will have benefits at any time in life. The maximal benefit, however, will come as a result of a low-CSI diet being consumed *throughout* life.

Lifetime Goals for Children

Follow the CSI guidelines for women and children discussed in preceding chapters. These will help you achieve daily CSIs, per 2,000 Calories, for school-age children as follows:

CSI Phase One: 37
CSI Phase Two: 28
CSI Phase Three: 16

For teens, the goals are, per 2,800 Calories:

CSI Phase One: 49
CSI Phase Two: 36
CSI Phase Three: 23

If your children are eating a wide variety of foods from every food group (grains, fruits, vegetables, beans, fats, and low-fat animal foods) and are progressing along normal growth curves for height and weight, one can generally assume that nutritional requirements are being met.

Controlling Your Child's Blood Cholesterol

The most important thing we parents can do for our children is to promote a healthy life-style by setting a good example ourselves. We can best achieve this if we

- have a low-CSI eating style
- exercise regularly
- never smoke.

Talk with your children about why these things are important to you and why it is important for them.

Putting It All Together: The *Lifetime* Cholesterol Cure

Congratulations! You've come to the end of our CSI "revolution"—to the *end* of learning what the CSI can do to improve your health and to the *beginning* of actually putting it to work for you and your family. You've learned the enormous value of making positive changes in your eating life-style and now you have a powerful new tool with which to implement those changes: the CSI. It's time now to take what you've learned and put it all together. With the CSI, you've got what it takes to achieve the *lifetime* cholesterol/saturated fat cure.

How Far Are You Going?

As we've pointed out many times, *any* progress you make toward a lower-CSI life-style is valuable progress. How far you decide to travel along the CSI trail is up to you. We've spelled out the benefits you'll reap each step of the way. Most of you, we're confident, will achieve Phase One CSI goals, and many will make it to the Phase Two CSI goals. Don't feel badly if you stop short of Phase Three. The benefits you'll enjoy from Phases One and Two are very significant. But we would like to point out that Phase Three really isn't that different from Phase Two—and it *does* deliver important added benefits. The difference really comes down to *consistency*. In Phase Three, you do *every day* what you do, in Phase Two, only once, twice, or three times a week.

Thinking It Through

Over the years we've found that those who are the most successful in adopting a lower-CSI way of eating are those who carefully consider each change they make. Their decisions are thoughtful and deliberate, not spur-of-the moment or impulsive. And they don't bite off more than they can chew (or less than they want to chew). They go one step at a time. They set realistic goals for given time periods and then they make sure they have all of the support and supplies at hand that they will need to achieve those goals.

Next week, next month, next year—whatever you set out to accomplish in a given time period, the choice is yours. We hope you will continue to choose good food, good eating, good exercise, good health—for the rest of your life. Thanks for journeying with us this far. We feel you're now part of "the family," a family of Americans committed to taking charge of their lives and ensuring their own good health.

Help Us Help You

Wouldn't it be wonderful if the CSI of foods were listed on food labels? It isn't listed at this time but it could be and *should* be. If you agree, please request that the CSI be required on food labeling. Do this by writing to:

Commissioner
Food and Drug Administration
200 Independence Avenue, S.W.
Washington, D.C. 20201

PART III

The CSI Cookbook: 350 Great Food/Healthy Heart Recipes

Developed under direction of
Sonja L. Connor, M.S., R.D., and
William E. Connor, M.D.

Produced by the Lipid-Atherosclerosis
Research Nutrition Staff

Joyce R. Gustafson, B.S., R.D.

Sabine M. Artaud-Wild, B.S., R.D.
Sandra R. Bacon, R.N.
Dianne L. Carville, M.S., R.D.
Reba J. Clow, B.S., R.D.
Carolyn J. Classick-Kohn, M.S., R.D.
Donna P. Flavell, B.A., R.D.
Lauren F. Hatcher, M.S., R.D.
Martha P. McMurry, M.S., R.D.

We wish to express our appreciation to the following publications, which have provided inspiration for several recipes that we modified to meet our nutritional guidelines: *Laurel's Kitchen, Joy of Cooking, Sunset* magazine and cookbooks, *Betty Crocker's Cookbook, Diet for a Small Planet,* and *Oregon Trawl Fish and Shrimp Story.*

SPECIAL THANKS

This cookbook would not have been possible without the help of many people.

We are especially grateful to:

Family, friends, and colleagues who were willing to experiment and who ate many a strange-looking meal on the way to our ultimate development of some great recipes. These recipes reflect years of experimentation in both adapting family favorites and trying new foods.

We also wish to thank:
Typists—Marcia Hindman and Patricia McCormick

Cooks who prepared recipes for testing:
Clinical Research Center Metabolic Kitchen Staff—

Mary E. Miller
David L. Belknap
Teresa A. Murray, B.S.
Lisa Feringa, A.S.

THE CSI COOKBOOK
CONTENTS

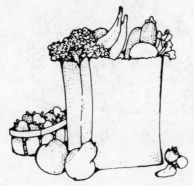

INTRODUCTION

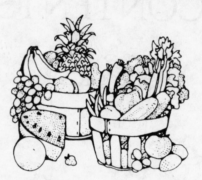

We love to cook as well as eat and are proud to offer new recipes as well as repeats from *The New American Diet*. As we developed the CSI tables over the last three years we became inspired to test hundreds of new recipes. As in our earlier book, our sources have been many and reflect the varied tastes and food experience of our own families, the families of our colleagues who now live all over the United States, and our patients.

We selected the following guidelines to determine which recipes would be suitable for inclusion in this book. The values represent upper limits for one serving. If you look closely at our recipes, you will note that we exceed these guidelines here and there. Most often this decision was made in favor of using a convenience product or two in the recipe. These recipes will be changed in future editions the minute better choices become available.

Recipes often had to go through many testings and modifications before they met both our taste and nutritional criteria. Some recipes didn't make it. The good news is that we were able to achieve success with the majority of recipes that we wanted to include.

There are some cooking techniques and food products that we have found to be very useful. We want to share them with you in order to help you with your shopping and cooking.

1. We never use egg yolks in our cooking. Instead we use 3 whites for 2 whole eggs; or 1 white and 1 to 2 tablespoons egg substitute for each single egg; or egg substitute alone

(commercial or our *Homemade Egg Substitute* recipe in the "Breakfasts and Brunches" section). This saves CSIs for meat, cheese, frozen desserts, etc.

2. We always use the lowest-fat dairy products that taste good and are widely available. You'll note that we have changed from low-fat to nonfat plain yogurt because it tastes great and is available in most supermarkets. Try the different brands—some are very mild (Dannon) and others are more bitey (Nancy's—an Oregon product—and Weight Watchers). There are uses for each kind. We like to use the mild yogurt to make frozen yogurts and the bitey yogurts in our salad dressings. We always cook with skim milk. By low-fat cheese we mean cheeses that contain five or fewer grams of fat per ounce if they are made from skim milk and butterfat—these are generally referred to on the label as "part-skim." Our current favorite is Olympia's Sharp Cheddar, which delivers the most flavor for the least amount of cheese. You'll find that higher-fat cheeses (5 to 9 grams fat per ounce) that are made from skim milk and vegetable oil, such as Scandic's Mini Chol or Dorman's Light, melt very nicely and have low CSIs.

3. In keeping up with the latest in food products, we now use light mayonnaise or Miracle Whip Light, both of which are also cholesterol-free.

4. When we call for lemon juice, we mean juice squeezed from a fresh lemon. Lemon juice from the bottle does not taste good!

5. In the ground-meat category, we use either 10-percent-fat ground beef and/or ground turkey. If you have the butcher grind the turkey, you can eliminate the skin before grinding.

6. We always cook our grains (pasta, rice, macaroni, oatmeal, and other cereals) and potatoes in unsalted water, and we never add oil to the water.

7. Whenever possible, we use canned

THE CHOLESTEROL–SATURATED FAT INDEX, AND FAT, CALORIE, AND SODIUM GUIDELINES FOR ONE SERVING OF MAIN DISHES AND OTHER DISHES*

	ONE SERVING			
	CSI	FAT GM	CALORIES	SODIUM MG
Main dishes	9	10	300 or 500†	600
Other dishes:				
Appetizers, salads, side dishes, soups, desserts, etc.	5	5	300	500

*These guidelines represent upper limits.
†If dish contains pasta, rice, or beans.

products labeled "no salt added." The no-salt-added tomatoes and tomato sauce work very well. And we use lower-salt cream-style corn and canned beans when we can find them, such as S&W's beans with 50 percent less salt.

8. We have changed from using chicken broth in recipes in our previous book to using lower-salt chicken broth in our current recipes. We like Swanson's Natural Goodness Clear Chicken Broth, which has 30 percent less salt.

9. We have continued to use lower-sodium soy sauce and Lite Salt, the latter being a fifty-fifty mixture of sodium chloride and potassium chloride. If you use Lite Salt in place of regular salt, you will reduce the sodium from salt—teaspoon for teaspoon—by 50 percent. If you use Lite Salt and cut the amount in half, the sodium from salt will be reduced by 75 percent. If we have gone a bit below your salt threshold, do add a little Lite Salt rather than give up on a recipe.

10. We have included some ingredients you will undoubtedly have never heard of—tamarind paste, Thai chili sauce, black bean sauce with chili, and balsamic vinegar, to name a few. Believe us, it is worth the effort to get these ingredients into your kitchen as the recipes that use them are among our favorites.

11. The nutrient content of each and every recipe has been computed using Version 1.2, Nutrient Calculation System, Nutrition Coordinating Center, University of Minnesota. The nutrients for one serving are listed at the bottom of each recipe. When there is more than one choice given for an ingredient, we have used the first one listed in the nutrient analysis. Therefore, if dried beans are listed first and canned beans are listed second, the sodium content will be higher if you use canned beans. The different choices given for an ingredient do not alter the CSI, fat, or calories significantly. When "optional" is listed after an ingredient, we did not include that ingredient in the nutrient analysis.

Many recipes have been labeled "Quick" and "Easy." If a dish can be prepared in thirty minutes or less it has earned the "Quick" label. "Easy" identifies the recipes that can be assembled in a short time with a minimum of effort.

You won't like every product or recipe we suggest. Not all of us like every one, either. But the recipe one of us doesn't like is the same recipe that another among us probably makes every Monday night. We have produced 155 new recipes and remodeled many of the 191 repeats from *The New American Diet*. This has been very inspirational and each of us has added a whole new assortment to our cooking repertoire. Our wish is for you to do the same.

Bon appétit!

APPETIZERS AND HORS D'OEUVRES

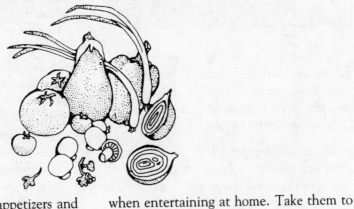

Our selection of recipes for appetizers and hors d'oeuvres will stimulate the appetite but not expand the waistline if you pay attention to the serving sizes. Serve them when entertaining at home. Take them to potlucks so others can discover that low-CSI foods are very tasty.

Dips
  Bean Dip—*Easy*
  Chunky Avocado Dip
  Dill Dip
  Popeye's Spinach Dip

Fish and Fancier
  Onion Squares (see "Side Dishes" section)
  Salmon Mousse
  Snappy Clams—*Easy*
  Spinach Triangles
  Steamed Buns
  Zucchini Toast

Bean or Vegetable Combos
  Baba Ganouj
  Chowchow
  Hummous—*Easy*
  Marinated Mushrooms
  Southern Caviar—*Quick*

Chips
  Baked Corn Chips
  Pita Chips

DIPS

BEAN DIP—*EASY*

This dip makes a marvelous burrito filling. To prepare, simply spoon bean dip inside a warm flour tortilla and roll up. (For an easier bean dip, combine several tablespoons of salsa with refried beans.)

¼ cup diced green chiles
¼ cup unsalted tomato sauce
4 green onions, chopped
¼–½ teaspoon ground cumin
½ teaspoon garlic powder
1 can (30 ounces) refried beans*

Combine chiles, tomato sauce, onions and seasonings in a saucepan and cook until onions are tender. Add beans and simmer until warmed through. Serve either hot or cold; may be topped with grated low-fat cheese.

Makes about 4 cups.

*Use low-sodium beans if available.

PER ¼ cup:
CALORIES 59   FIBER 6 gm
CSI trace   SODIUM 243 mg
FAT 1 gm

CHUNKY AVOCADO DIP

A creamy avocado dip, full of chopped vegetables and zapped with a touch of Tabasco sauce.

1 large, ripe avocado, peeled
1 tablespoon freshly squeezed lemon juice
¼ package (0.7 ounce) Italian salad dressing mix
½ cup plain nonfat yogurt
1 cup grated carrot (1 medium)
1 green onion, finely chopped (use all of the green, too)
¼ cup finely chopped broccoli
¼ cup finely chopped celery
¼ cup finely chopped cauliflower
¼ teaspoon Tabasco sauce

Mix avocado, lemon juice, dry salad dressing mix, and yogurt until smooth. (A food processor works well for this.) Stir in prepared raw vegetables and Tabasco sauce until mixed. Cover and refrigerate. Serve with low-fat crackers or raw vegetables.

Makes 2 cups.

PER ¼ cup:
CALORIES 72   FIBER 2 gm
CSI <1   SODIUM 161 mg
FAT 5 gm

DILL DIP

Very attractive when served in a hollowed-out red cabbage.

- 2 cups low-fat cottage cheese
- 4 tablespoons buttermilk
- 1½ teaspoons freshly squeezed lemon juice

Mix above ingredients in blender until very smooth. Remove from blender and add:

- ½ cup light mayonnaise or ¼ cup mayonnaise
- 1 tablespoon finely chopped parsley
- 1 tablespoon finely chopped onion
- ¾ teaspoon Beau Monde seasoning
- 1½ teaspoons dill weed

Chill until very cold. To serve in hollowed-out cabbage, flatten bottom of the cabbage head by slicing off a piece so it will sit straight. Surround with fresh vegetables on a large platter.

Makes 3 cups.

PER ¼ cup:

CALORIES 66	FIBER 0 gm
CSI 1	SODIUM 311 mg
FAT 3 gm	

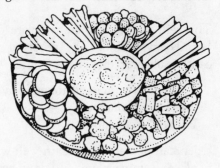

POPEYE'S SPINACH DIP

Serve in a round loaf of bread that has been hollowed out!

- 1 package (10 ounces) frozen, chopped spinach, thawed and squeezed dry
- ¼ package dry vegetable-soup mix
- 1¾ cups plain nonfat yogurt
- ¼ cup light mayonnaise
- 1 can (8 ounces) water chestnuts, drained and chopped
- 2 tablespoons chopped chives or green onions

Thaw spinach, drain, and squeeze until fairly dry. Stir dry soup mix before measuring, to ensure that it is evenly mixed. Mix all ingredients together when spinach is ready. Chill and serve with raw vegetables.

For an unusual serving dish, slice top off a round loaf of unsliced sourdough bread and hollow out inside. Fill with cold dip. Save insides to use for bread crumbs, or cube and use for dipping.

Makes 4 cups.

PER ¼ cup:

CALORIES 37	FIBER <1 gm
CSI <1	SODIUM 108 mg
FAT 1 gm	

FISH AND FANCIER

SALMON MOUSSE

This versatile recipe is quickly prepared in a blender. It can be served in many attractive ways as described below.

    1 tablespoon unflavored gelatin
    2 tablespoons freshly squeezed lemon
      juice
    ¼ small onion, cut in chunks
    ½ cup boiling water
    ½ cup light mayonnaise
    ¼ teaspoon paprika
    1½ cups low-fat cottage cheese
    1 can (16 ounces) salmon, drained,
      with skin and bones removed or 2 cups
      leftover cooked salmon
    ½ teaspoon Tabasco sauce
    1 tablespoon capers (optional)

Empty gelatin into blender container. Add lemon juice, onion, and boiling water. Cover and blend on high speed 40 seconds. Add light mayonnaise, paprika, and cottage cheese. Cover and blend on high speed for 30 seconds or until well blended. Remove cover and add salmon or leftover cooked salmon, Tabasco sauce, and capers. Blend well for 30 seconds.

Pour into a lightly oiled 1½-quart mold (use a fish-shaped mold if possible), 8 individual molds or an attractive pottery bowl, depending on how you want to serve it. Refrigerate until set.

SERVING IDEAS

—For an attractive buffet entrée, unmold and decorate with lemon wedges and thin cucumber slices. Serve with *Cucumber-Dilly Sauce* (page 453). Bring it to a potluck and you will be thanked warmly. Makes 10 servings.
—For individual servings, unmold on lettuce leaves and top with a dollop of *Cucumber-Dilly Sauce.* Serve with crusty French bread. It will make an unusual entrée. Makes 8 individual servings.
—As an appetizer, serve directly from a pottery dish and sprinkle with dill weed or paprika. It can be offered as a dip with vegetables or low-fat crackers. Makes 10 servings.

PER ⅒ recipe (½ cup):
CALORIES 140   FIBER trace
CSI 3   SODIUM 466 mg
FAT 7 gm

SNAPPY CLAMS—*EASY*

This will be the first empty plate on the hors d'oeuvre table! Baby oysters or shrimp can be substituted for the clams.

    1 can (3¾ ounces) smoked baby clams
    24 cherry tomatoes
    Parsley, to decorate

Open can of clams and drain well with lid in place. Remove clams and drain again on several layers of paper towels. Slit the top of each cherry tomato (not the stem side) and insert a small clam. Arrange on a bed of parsley. Serve cold.

Makes 8 servings.

PER serving:
CALORIES 39   FIBER 1 gm
CSI <1   SODIUM 56 mg
FAT 2 gm

SPINACH TRIANGLES

These pastry triangles are some work but really worth the effort. They can be made ahead and frozen.

    1 package (10 ounces) frozen chopped
      spinach, thawed
    1 teaspoon oil
    ½ cup minced green onions
    3 ounces (¾ cup) feta cheese, finely
      crumbled
    ½ cup bread crumbs, divided
    ½ cup minced parsley
    4 egg whites
    2 teaspoons oregano leaves
    ¼ teaspoon pepper
    5 sheets phyllo*
    1½ tablespoons melted margarine

*Phyllo (or filo) can be found in the freezer section of most supermarkets. Thaw the unwrapped frozen dough in the refrigerator for 3–4 hours and work with it while it is cold. The remainder of the pastry keeps well in refrigerator if wrapped tightly.

Thaw spinach and squeeze dry. Pour oil in a small skillet and sauté onion until tender. Remove from heat. Combine onion, feta cheese, 2 tablespoons bread crumbs, parsley, egg whites, oregano, and pepper with spinach and blend well.

Preheat oven to 375°. Lightly spray baking sheet with nonstick spray. Cut 5 sheets of phyllo into strips about 2 inches wide. (Scissors work well for the cutting.) Lay one strip phyllo on flat surface and brush very lightly with melted margarine and sprinkle lightly with bread crumbs. Place a rounded teaspoon of filling in one corner. Fold phyllo over filling at an angle; continue to fold at an angle to form a triangle. Brush finished "triangle" with margarine. Place on baking sheet. When all dough is folded, bake about 15 minutes or until golden brown. (To freeze, place in single layer on cookie sheet. Then transfer to storage container with a tight lid and return to freezer.)

Makes 60 triangles.

PER 3 triangles:
CALORIES 54   FIBER 1 gm
CSI 1   SODIUM 114 mg
FAT 2 gm

STEAMED BUNS

"Homemade Hom Bow"—a real dazzler. This meatless version is very good.

SAUCE FOR FILLING

2 teaspoons cornstarch
2 tablespoons water
½ teaspoon vinegar
½ teaspoon sesame oil
2 teaspoons lower-sodium soy sauce
¼ teaspoon sugar

FILLING FOR BUNS

1 clove garlic, minced
1 teaspoon peeled and minced fresh ginger root
½ teaspoon black bean sauce with chili*
1 teaspoon oil
3 green onions, minced
½ cup finely chopped, drained water chestnuts
2½ cups chopped Chinese cabbage

3 cans (7.5 ounces each) refrigerated buttermilk biscuits (makes 30 biscuits)

To prepare sauce for filling: Dissolve cornstarch in water in small bowl and add remaining sauce ingredients. Set aside.

*Available in Oriental specialty stores.

To prepare filling: Mix garlic, ginger, and black bean sauce with chili. Heat 1 teaspoon oil in skillet or wok. Add garlic mixture and stir until very hot. Add green onions, water chestnuts, and Chinese cabbage. Stir-fry until cabbage is limp. Add cornstarch sauce and stir until thickened. This filling can be made ahead and refrigerated.

Roll out one of the canned biscuits on a floured board with a small glass or cup, until it is about 3 inches in diameter. Roll the edges out so that the center is slightly thicker. Place 2 teaspoons of the filling in the center. Bring up the edges of the biscuit so that they meet in the center and pleat them together, then press down on top so that the biscuit is an enclosed shell around the filling, with fluting around the top. Repeat this process with each of the 30 biscuits, then place them on waxed paper squares in a steamer. Steam as many as will fit in the steamer for 6 minutes.

Makes 30 steamed buns.

PER bun:
CALORIES 73   FIBER <1 gm
CSI <1   SODIUM 179 mg
FAT 3 gm

ZUCCHINI TOAST

A delicious appetizer that can be popped in the oven for a quick bake and served warm.

2 cups shredded zucchini, well drained
¼ cup light mayonnaise
½ cup plain nonfat yogurt
3 tablespoons grated Parmesan cheese
¼ cup finely minced green onions
1 teaspoon Worcestershire sauce
¼ teaspoon garlic powder
⅛–¼ teaspoon Tabasco sauce
32 small, thinly sliced pieces of rye bread

Preheat oven to 375°. Place all ingredients except rye bread in a small bowl and mix well. Place a tablespoon full of mixture on one side of the rye bread. Bake on a non-stick baking sheet 10–12 minutes or until slightly bubbly.

Makes 32 toasts.

PER 2 toasts:
CALORIES 51   FIBER 1 gm
CSI <1   SODIUM 123 mg
FAT 2 gm

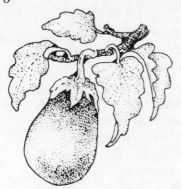

BEAN OR VEGETABLE COMBOS

BABA GANOUJ

A Middle Eastern appetizer—eggplant pâté. Surround with fresh vegetables or pita bread triangles to use as dippers.

2 medium eggplants (2 cups pulp)
2 tablespoons freshly squeezed lemon juice
¼ cup tahini*
2 medium cloves garlic
1 teaspoon Lite Salt or less

Preheat oven to 400°. Cut off the stem-ends of the eggplants. Prick the eggplants all over with a fork. Place them on a baking sheet and cook 45–60 minutes or until very soft. Cool. Slice in half lengthwise, scoop the pulp out, and mash with a potato masher or a fork. While eggplants are baking, place all other ingredients in a blender and process until smooth. Stir the mixture into the mashed eggplant pulp. Chill before serving.

Makes 2 cups.

*Tahini is sometimes labeled "sesame seed butter" and can be found in the specialty food section of most supermarkets.

PER ¼ cup:
CALORIES 18   FIBER 1 gm
CSI trace   SODIUM 124 mg
FAT 1 gm

CHOWCHOW

From Phoenix, Arizona, where the sun does shine and shine and shine . . . Make this when tomatoes are nice and ripe.

2 tomatoes, finely chopped
3–4 green onions, finely chopped
1 can (4 ounces) diced green chiles (or less if a milder product is preferred)
1 can (2.2 ounces) black olives, sliced
1 tablespoon olive oil
1 tablespoon vinegar
½ teaspoon garlic powder

Combine ingredients and serve with the *Baked Corn Chips* (page 262).
Makes 8 servings (2 cups).

PER ¼ cup:
CALORIES 49   FIBER <1 gm
CSI trace   SODIUM 74 mg
FAT 3 gm

HUMMOUS—EASY

2 cups cooked and drained garbanzo beans (canned beans* can be used)
¼ cup tahini†
2–5 tablespoons freshly squeezed lemon juice
1 garlic clove, chopped fine
¼–½ cup water
1 tablespoon chopped parsley

Combine above ingredients (except parsley) in the blender and blend until smooth,

adding water as necessary. Remove from blender and add chopped parsley.
Makes 2½ cups.

SERVE AS DIP WITH:
Low-fat crackers
Pieces of Middle Eastern bread

OR AS A SANDWICH WITH:
Middle Eastern bread (also called pocket or pita bread)
Alfalfa sprouts

*Use low-sodium beans if available.

†Tahini is sometimes labeled "sesame seed butter" and is usually available in supermarkets in the specialty food section.

PER ¼ cup:
CALORIES 106   FIBER 3 gm
CSI trace   SODIUM 125 mg
FAT 3 gm

MARINATED MUSHROOMS

Spicy and juicy, these appeal to everyone.

2 pints fresh mushrooms *or* 2 cans (6 ounces each) mushroom crowns, drained
⅔ cup tarragon vinegar
1 onion, sliced and separated into rings
1 clove garlic, minced
1 tablespoon sugar
½ teaspoon Lite Salt or less
2 tablespoons water
2 tablespoons oil
Pepper and dash cayenne

Remove stems of mushrooms if using fresh ones. Wash and pour boiling water over mushroom crowns. Stir 2–3 minutes. Drain and marinate in remaining ingredients overnight. When ready to serve, drain most of marinade off, and place mushrooms and onions in shallow serving dish. Serve with wooden picks for spearing.

Makes 10 servings.

PER serving:
CALORIES 39   FIBER <1 gm
CSI trace   SODIUM 25 mg
FAT 3 gm

Combine black-eyed peas or black beans, green pepper, onion, jalapeños, pimiento, and garlic. Add salad dressing and mix gently to combine. Cover and chill overnight, if you have the time. The longer it stands the better it tastes. It will keep well refrigerated for about a week.

When ready to serve, drain "caviar" and place in bowl. Serve with low-fat crackers, *Baked Corn Chips,* or *Pita Chips.*

Makes 2 cups.

PER ¼ cup:
CALORIES 68   FIBER 2 gm
CSI trace   SODIUM 238 mg
FAT 1 gm

SOUTHERN CAVIAR—*QUICK*

A pretty and festive-looking appetizer or an excellent filling for pocket bread for lunch.

1 can (16 ounces) black-eyed peas or black beans,* drained and rinsed
⅓ cup diced green bell pepper
¼ cup diced onion
1–4 tablespoons seeded and diced jalapeño peppers (they can be hot)
2 tablespoons diced pimiento
1 clove garlic, minced
⅓ cup oil-free Italian salad dressing

Low-fat crackers, *Baked Corn Chips* (page 262) *or Pita Chips* (page 262).

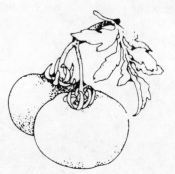

*Use low-sodium beans if available.

CHIPS

BAKED CORN CHIPS

20 corn tortillas*
Margarine (not more than 2 teaspoons)

Scrape each tortilla with a small amount of soft margarine. Cut tortillas, several at a time, into 8 pie-shaped wedges using kitchen shears. Arrange in a single layer on cookie sheet. Bake at 350° until crisp and slightly browned (10 minutes). Store in an airtight container.

Makes approximately 8 cups.

*Use thin tortillas (e.g., Diane's Corn Tortillas).

PER cup:
CALORIES 114   FIBER 2 gm
CSI trace   SODIUM 97 mg
FAT 3 gm

PITA CHIPS

These are good with bean dip, and soups, and in lunches.

Preheat oven to 325°. Split each of 6 pita breads into 2 round pieces (whole wheat pita bread has more fiber, 2 gms per ½ cup chips). Cut each half into 6 triangles with kitchen scissors. Arrange in single layers on cookie sheets. Sprinkle lightly with garlic powder, if desired. Bake for 8 minutes until chips are lightly browned and very crisp. Store in tight container.

Makes 8 cups.

PER ½ cup:
CALORIES 67   FIBER trace
CSI trace   SODIUM 135 mg
FAT trace

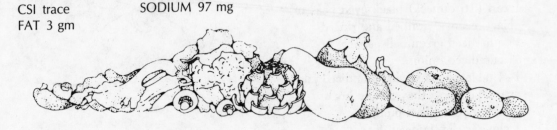

BREADS AND MUFFINS

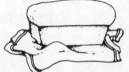

We recommend that breads be included in every meal. They also make great snack foods. You may find that our muffins, scones, and biscuits are not as moist as those you buy. This is probably because commercial muffins, biscuits, and scones are made with even more fat and sugar than the traditional recipes. Many people have come to expect muffins to have the texture and taste of cakes. Likewise, they expect biscuits and scones to taste like pastries. Do develop a taste for our breads and muffins. And remember our motto: "If it has fat in it, don't put any on it."

Quick Breads
Banana Nut Bread
Cornbread
Fruit Bread
Grandma Kirschner's Date Nut Bread
Lemon Nut Bread
Orange Walnut Bread
Pumpkin Harvest Loaf
Whole Wheat Quick Bread

Yeast Breads
Caraway Dinner Rolls
Grape-nut Bread
Whole Wheat French Bread

Muffins
A Barrel of Muffins
Applesauce Oatmeal Muffins

Blueberry Bran Muffins
Cereal Bran Muffins
Cinnamon Rhubarb Muffins
Dutchy Crust Muffins (see page 281 in "Breakfasts and Brunches" section)
Mexican Cornbread Muffins
Nutty Orange Muffins
Oatmeal Raisin Muffins
Poppyseed Muffins
Pumpkin Oat Muffins

Biscuits, Scones, and Specialties
Baking Mix
Fruit Scones
Old-Style Wheat Biscuits
Pizza Crusts
Yogurt Scones

QUICK BREADS

BANANA NUT BREAD

A moist bread loaded with fiber.

1 cup All-Bran cereal
½ cup skim milk
¼ cup margarine, softened
½ cup sugar *or* ⅓ cup honey
2 egg whites
1 teaspoon vanilla
2 cups mashed ripe bananas (4 medium bananas)
1½ cups whole wheat flour
2 teaspoons baking powder
½ teaspoon baking soda
¼ cup chopped walnuts

Preheat oven to 350°. Soak cereal in milk and set aside. Combine margarine and sugar or honey. Beat until light and fluffy. Add egg whites and vanilla. Beat well. Mix in mashed bananas and the cereal/milk mixture. Add flour, baking powder, baking soda, and nuts, mixing only until just combined. Pour batter evenly in lightly oiled 9-by-5-inch loaf pan. Bake 50–60 minutes or until wooden pick inserted in center comes out clean. Cool 10 minutes before removing from pan.

Makes 1 loaf (16 slices).

PER slice:
CALORIES 142   FIBER 3 gm
CSI <1   SODIUM 171 mg
FAT 4 gm

CORNBREAD

Our motto is: "If it has fat in it, don't put any on it!"

1 cup cornmeal
1 cup flour
1 tablespoon sugar
1 tablespoon baking powder
3 tablespoons oil
2 egg whites
1 cup skim milk

Heat oven to 400°. Combine dry ingredients in bowl and mix well. Beat oil, egg whites, and milk together. Mix with dry ingredients until just blended. Pour into lightly oiled 8-by-8-inch pan. Bake 15 minutes or until done.

Makes 8 servings.

PER serving (2 by 4 inches):
CALORIES 180   FIBER 2 gm
CSI <1   SODIUM 154 mg
FAT 6 gm

FRUIT BREAD

This French fruit bread is excellent for toasting and makes an attractive gift. It is not meant to be as moist or as sweet as other breads.

½ cup raisins, presoaked in warm water (*or* rum, if you like the flavor)
1 cup egg substitute
½ cup sugar
1½ cups flour
1½ teaspoons baking powder
½ teaspoon cinnamon
½ teaspoon Lite Salt or less
¼ cup melted margarine
¼ cup chopped walnuts *or* almonds
4 ounces dried figs, cut into small pieces
2 ounces candied pineapple, diced

Cover raisins with warm water or rum; soak for 1 hour or so and drain. Preheat oven to 350° (after raisins have soaked).

Beat egg substitute and sugar until well blended. Mix together flour, baking powder, cinnamon, and Lite Salt. Add to the egg/sugar mixture. Add melted margarine, nuts, figs, citron, and raisins. Blend thoroughly. Pour into a lightly oiled 9-by-5-inch loaf pan. Bake for 50–60 minutes. Cool slightly in the pan, then remove and cool on a rack.

Makes 1 loaf (16 slices).

PER slice:
CALORIES 151   FIBER 2 gm
CSI <1   SODIUM 128 mg
FAT 4 gm

GRANDMA KIRSCHNER'S DATE NUT BREAD

This bread is so good it does not need a spread and can be served as dessert!

1 package (8 ounces) dates
¾ cup coarsely chopped walnuts
1 cup raisins
1 teaspoon baking soda
1 cup boiling water
2 cups flour
1 cup sugar
1 teaspoon baking powder
2 egg whites

Preheat oven to 350°. Chop dates. Combine dates, nuts, and raisins in bowl. Sprinkle baking soda over date-nut-raisin combination. Pour 1 cup boiling water over all of bowl's contents. Cover the bowl and set aside while mixing rest of ingredients.

In another bowl mix flour, sugar, baking powder, and egg whites. Mix together with pastry blender or two knives held together. Combine ingredients of both bowls; mix well. Bake in lightly oiled 9-by-5-inch loaf pan for 1 hour.

Makes 1 loaf (16 slices).

PER slice:
CALORIES 209   FIBER 3 gm
CSI trace   SODIUM 83 mg
FAT 4 gm

LEMON NUT BREAD

⅓ cup margarine
⅔ cup sugar
3 egg whites
2 teaspoons baking powder
¾ cup whole wheat flour
1½ cups white flour
1 cup skim milk
1½ teaspoons dried lemon rind
3 tablespoons chopped nuts

GLAZE

⅓ cup powdered sugar
3 tablespoons freshly squeezed lemon
  juice

Preheat oven to 350°. Cream together margarine and sugar. Add egg whites and mix thoroughly. Combine dry ingredients and add the above alternately with milk. Stir in lemon rind and nuts. Bake in a lightly oiled 9-by-5-inch loaf pan for 60 minutes or until wooden pick inserted in center comes out clean. Remove bread from oven. Mix powdered sugar with lemon juice until smooth and pour over warm bread. Allow to sit for 20 minutes, then remove bread from pan.

Makes 1 loaf (16 slices).

PER slice:
CALORIES 153   FIBER 1 gm
CSI <1   SODIUM 113 mg
FAT 5 gm

ORANGE WALNUT BREAD

1½ cups white flour
1 cup whole wheat flour
1¼ cups sugar
2 teaspoons baking powder
½ teaspoon baking soda
3 egg whites, beaten
¼ cup melted margarine
½ cup orange juice
2 tablespoons grated orange peel
2 tablespoons water
¼ cup coarsely chopped walnuts

Preheat oven to 350°. Mix flours, sugar, baking powder, and baking soda. Combine beaten egg whites, melted margarine, orange juice, orange peel, and water. Add liquid ingredients all at once to flour mixture. Stir quickly until dry ingredients are moistened. Stir in nuts. Turn into lightly oiled and floured 9-by-5-inch loaf pan.

Bake 1 hour or until wooden pick inserted in center comes out clean. Cool in pan 10 minutes. Remove from pan and cool on wire rack.

Makes 1 loaf (16 slices).

PER slice:
CALORIES 166   FIBER 1 gm
CSI <1   SODIUM 110 mg
FAT 4 gm

PUMPKIN HARVEST LOAF

Take the time to add the *Lemon Glaze* on top as it makes the bread very special! Freezes well.

1¾ cups pumpkin
½ cup egg substitute (commercial *or Homemade Egg Substitute,* page 283)
2 egg whites
¼ cup oil
1 cup sugar
2 cups flour
2 teaspoons baking powder
1 teaspoon baking soda
1¼ teaspoons cinnamon

Preheat oven to 350°. Beat together pumpkin, egg substitute, egg whites, and oil. Add sugar, flour, baking powder, baking soda, and cinnamon. Combine all ingredients and pour into 9-by-5-inch loaf pan that has been sprayed with nonstick spray, then floured. Bake 60 minutes or until wooden pick inserted in center comes out clean.

LEMON GLAZE

½ cup powdered sugar
3 tablespoons freshly squeezed lemon juice
½ teaspoon lemon rind

If a glaze is desired, mix the ingredients and pour over warm bread while in pan. Let cool slightly and remove from pan. Dust with powdered sugar.
Makes 1 loaf (16 slices).

PER slice:
CALORIES 163   FIBER 1 gm
CSI <1   SODIUM 119 mg
FAT 4 gm

WHOLE WHEAT QUICK BREAD

A moist, great-tasting quick bread.

3 cups whole wheat flour
1 cup sugar
½ teaspoon Lite Salt or less
1 teaspoon baking soda
2 cups buttermilk
1 cup raisins
½ cup chopped walnuts

Preheat oven to 325°. Mix together flour, sugar, Lite Salt, and baking soda. To this mixture add the buttermilk followed by the raisins and walnuts. Place in two lightly oiled and floured 9-by-5-inch loaf pans.

Bake 1 hour or until wooden pick inserted in center comes out clean. Cool in pans 10 minutes. Remove from pans and serve.
Makes 2 loaves (32 slices).

PER slice:
CALORIES 93   FIBER 1 gm
CSI <1   SODIUM 59 mg
FAT 2 gm

YEAST BREADS

CARAWAY DINNER ROLLS

These lovely dinner rolls can also have dill flavoring. They can be made early in the day and reheated at mealtime.

> 2 tablespoons yeast
> ½ cup warm water
> 2 tablespoons caraway seeds *or* dill weed
> 2 cups low-fat cottage cheese
> ¼ cup sugar
> ½ teaspoon Lite Salt
> ½ teaspoon baking soda
> 3 egg whites
> 2⅔ cups white flour
> 2 cups whole wheat flour

Dissolve yeast in warm water. Add caraway seeds *or* dill weed. Heat cottage cheese, just until lukewarm. Mix cottage cheese, sugar, Lite Salt, baking soda, and egg whites into yeast mixture. Slowly add flours, mixing until dough cleans bowl.

Cover and let rise in warm place until double, about 1 hour. Stir down dough. Place in 24 lightly oiled muffin tins. Cover and let rise again until double, about 45 minutes.

Preheat oven to 350°. Bake about 25 minutes. Remove from muffin tins while warm.

Makes 24 rolls.

PER roll:
CALORIES 108   FIBER 2 gm
CSI trace   SODIUM 111 mg
FAT <1 gm

GRAPE-NUT BREAD

If you are a bread maker, you'll like this one!

> 1 cup Grape-nuts cereal
> 2 cups boiling water
> 2 tablespoons sugar
> 2 tablespoons margarine
> 1 tablespoon yeast
> ½ teaspoon Lite Salt or less
> 4 cups flour

Combine cereal with boiling water, sugar, and margarine. Cool until lukewarm. Add the yeast and stir until dissolved. Blend in Lite Salt and flour. Cover the dough and let rise until doubled in volume. Punch dough down and turn onto a floured board. Knead the dough; adding flour, if necessary, to make a firm dough that can easily be shaped. Shape the dough into 24 rolls or into 2 loaves. To make round loaves, shape into two round balls, flatten slightly, and place on cookie sheet.

Makes 2 loaves or 24 rolls.

ROLLS
Place rolls in lightly oiled round cake pans,

cover, and let rise again until doubled in volume. Bake at 400° for 20 minutes.

LOAVES

Place loaves in lightly oiled 9-by-5-inch loaf pans or on cookie sheet. Cover and let rise again until doubled in volume. Bake at 350° for 30 minutes or until lightly browned.

PER roll:
CALORIES 99   FIBER 1 gm
CSI trace   SODIUM 65 mg
FAT 1 gm

WHOLE WHEAT FRENCH BREAD

A special "baguette pan" gives this bread a crunchy, crispy crust.

1 tablespoon yeast
1 tablespoon sugar
1 teaspoon Lite Salt
2½ cups lukewarm water
3 cups white flour
2–3 cups whole wheat flour
1 egg white mixed with 1 tablespoon cold water

Combine yeast, sugar, Lite Salt, and water in a large bowl. Gradually add the flours and mix well (hands work best). At first the dough will be very sticky; add enough flour to transfer it to a lightly floured board. Knead until the dough is no longer sticky

(about 10 minutes), adding more flour as necessary. Place in lightly oiled bowl. Cover with a damp cloth and let rise in warm place until doubled in volume (1½–2 hours).

Punch dough down. Transfer to a floured board and cut into four equal parts. Roll and shape each part into a long loaf. Place loaves into lightly oiled, special long-loaf pans (baguette pans). Slash the top of each loaf diagonally in three or four places and brush with the egg white and water mixture. Let dough rise another hour or until doubled in volume.

Preheat oven to 350°. Bake the loaves until browned and hollow-sounding when thumped, about 25 minutes.* Halfway through baking, it may be necessary to cover the loaves with foil to prevent scorching the tops. Let cool on rack.

Makes 4 loaves, about 18 inches long.

* If planning to freeze bread, underbake, i.e., bake in oven only 15 minutes. Wrap in foil when cool. When ready to serve, remove from freezer. Leave wrapped in foil. Place in 350° oven for 10 minutes. Remove foil and continue to bake for 5 minutes, until crisp.

PER ⅕ loaf:
CALORIES 125   FIBER 3 gm
CSI trace   SODIUM 52 mg
FAT <1 gm

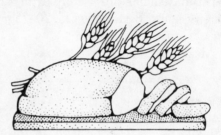

MUFFINS

A BARREL OF MUFFINS

This recipe makes a large amount—the batter can be stored in the refrigerator for up to 4 weeks and the muffins freshly baked when you are ready for them.

  5 teaspoons baking soda
  2 cups boiling water
  1 cup oil
  1 cup sugar
  6 egg whites
  4 cups All-Bran cereal
  2 cups Bran flakes
  5 cups white flour (or part whole wheat)
  1 quart buttermilk

Mix baking soda and water. Set aside to cool. Cream oil and sugar. Add egg whites and mix well. Combine bran cereals and flours. Add to creamed mixture and stir in buttermilk. Add water and baking soda and mix. Store the batter in a covered container in the refrigerator.

When ready to bake, preheat oven to 375° and spoon batter into lightly oiled or paper-lined muffin tins. Return extra batter to refrigerator. Bake muffins for 20–25 minutes.

Makes 60 muffins.

PER muffin:
CALORIES 105
CSI <1
FAT 4 gm
FIBER 2 gm
SODIUM 166 mg

APPLESAUCE OATMEAL MUFFINS

As a change from cooked cereal . . .

  1¼ cups uncooked oatmeal
  1 cup whole wheat flour
  2 teaspoons cinnamon
  1 teaspoon baking powder
  ¾ teaspoon baking soda
  ¾ cup unsweetened applesauce
  ½ cup honey
  3 tablespoons oil
  2 egg whites
  1 teaspoon vanilla
  2 tablespoons chopped nuts

Preheat oven to 375°. In small bowl, combine oatmeal, flour, cinnamon, baking powder, and baking soda. In another bowl, combine applesauce, honey, oil, egg whites, and vanilla. Stir in dry ingredients; mix well. Stir in nuts. Divide batter among 12 lightly oiled or paper-lined muffin tins. Bake 15 minutes or until golden brown.

Makes 12 muffins

PER muffin:
CALORIES 157
CSI <1
FAT 5 gm
FIBER 2 gm
SODIUM 86 mg

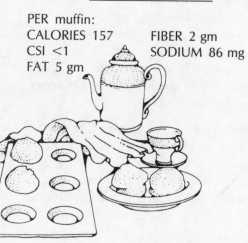

BLUEBERRY BRAN MUFFINS

These muffins contain no fat at all and are surprisingly good!

2⅔ cups **All-Bran cereal**
1½ cups **skim milk**
4 **egg whites**
1 tablespoon **vanilla**
2 cups **flour**
⅔ cup **brown sugar**
2 tablespoons **baking powder**
¾ teaspoon **baking soda**
1½ teaspoons **cinnamon**
2 cups **blueberries, fresh or frozen**

Preheat oven to 325°. Combine bran cereal, milk, egg whites, and vanilla—let stand 5 minutes. Stir together flour, brown sugar, baking powder, baking soda, and cinnamon in large bowl. Add cereal-milk mixture and mix. Add blueberries and stir carefully. Spoon into lightly oiled or paper-lined muffin tins. Bake for 30 minutes.

Makes 16 muffins.

————————————

PER muffin:
CALORIES 146   FIBER 5 gm
CSI trace   SODIUM 354 mg
FAT <1 gm

CEREAL BRAN MUFFINS

A breakfast staple or coffee break treat.

1½ cups **Bran Buds** *or* **All-Bran cereal**
1¼ cups **skim milk**
2 **egg whites**
3 tablespoons **oil**
½ cup **white flour**
¾ cup **whole wheat flour**
1 tablespoon **baking powder**
1 tablespoon **sugar**

Preheat oven to 400°. Measure cereal and milk into mixing bowl. Stir to combine. Add egg whites and oil. Let stand 1 to 2 minutes to soften cereal. Mix flours, baking powder, and sugar. Beat liquid-cereal mixture with wire whisk. Add dry ingredients to cereal mixture, stirring *only until combined*. Spoon batter gently into lightly oiled or paper-lined muffin tins. Bake for 25 minutes.

Makes 12 muffins.

————————————

PER muffin:
CALORIES 116   FIBER 4 gm
CSI <1   SODIUM 171 mg
FAT 4 gm

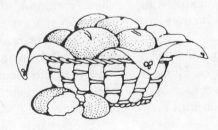

CINNAMON RHUBARB MUFFINS

A delightful treat that works well with fresh *or* frozen rhubarb.

⅔ cup brown sugar
2 tablespoons oil
1 egg white
1 teaspoon vanilla
⅔ cup buttermilk
¾ cup diced rhubarb (very small pieces)
2 tablespoons chopped walnuts *or* almonds
¾ cup white flour
½ cup whole wheat flour
½ teaspoon baking soda
½ teaspoon baking powder

TOPPING

3 tablespoons sugar
1½ teaspoons melted margarine
½ teaspoon cinnamon

Preheat oven to 400°. In a bowl combine sugar, oil, egg white, vanilla, and buttermilk; beat well. Stir in rhubarb and nuts.

In a separate bowl combine flours, baking soda, and baking powder. Stir the dry ingredients into the rhubarb mixture just until blended. Mix topping mixture together and set aside.

Spoon batter into muffin tins that have been sprayed with nonstick spray, filling ⅔ full. Sprinkle sugar topping over each muffin and bake 15–20 minutes or until muffins are lightly browned.

Makes 12 muffins.

PER muffin:
CALORIES 140   FIBER <1 gm
CSI <1   SODIUM 75 mg
FAT 4 gm

MEXICAN CORNBREAD MUFFINS

A sweet cornbread. Green chiles and red pimiento give these muffins a very festive look. A nice accompaniment for *Northwest Gumbo* (page 375).

1¼ cups flour
1 cup cornmeal
⅓ cup sugar
1 tablespoon baking powder
¾ cup skim milk
2 egg whites
¼ cup melted margarine
1 small can (8 ounces) cream-style corn
⅛–¼ cup diced green chiles (How hot do you like it?)
1 tablespoon diced pimiento

Preheat oven to 375°. In a large bowl mix flour, cornmeal, sugar, and baking powder. In a separate bowl beat milk, egg whites, and melted margarine. Add cream of corn, green chiles, and pimiento. Fold milk/corn mixture into flour/cornmeal ingredients. Stir just until lightly blended; batter should be lumpy.

Spoon batter into lightly oiled or paper-lined muffin tins and bake about 18 minutes or until wooden pick inserted in center comes out clean. Let cool 5 minutes and serve warm.

Makes 12 muffins.

PER muffin:
CALORIES 165   FIBER 2 gm
CSI <1   SODIUM 234 mg
FAT 4 gm

NUTTY ORANGE MUFFINS

2¼ cups flour
½ cup sugar
2½ teaspoons baking powder
½ teaspoon baking soda
¼ cup sliced almonds
½ cup skim milk
½ cup orange juice
¼ cup melted margarine
2 egg whites
1 teaspoon grated orange peel

Preheat oven to 375°. In a large bowl, mix flour, sugar, baking powder, and baking soda until blended. Stir in almonds. In a small bowl, combine milk, orange juice, melted margarine, egg whites, and orange peel; beat to blend. Pour liquid mixture into flour mixture, mixing lightly to blend. Batter should be lumpy.

Spoon mixture equally into lightly oiled

or paper-lined muffin tins. Bake 15–20 minutes.

Makes 12 muffins.

PER muffin:
CALORIES 167   FIBER 1 gm
CSI <1   SODIUM 160 mg
FAT 5 gm

OATMEAL RAISIN MUFFINS

We have modified a traditional oatmeal muffin recipe and think you will like the results. As with all low-fat muffins, they are best fresh from the oven.

1 cup buttermilk
1 cup uncooked oatmeal
½ cup raisins
½ cup white flour
½ cup whole wheat flour
1 teaspoon baking powder
½ teaspoon baking soda
3 tablespoons oil
¼ cup packed brown sugar
2 egg whites

In a small bowl, combine buttermilk, oatmeal, and raisins. Let the mixture stand until the liquid is absorbed (about ½ hour or overnight).

Preheat oven to 400°. In another bowl, combine the flour, baking powder, and baking soda. In a large mixing bowl beat the oil and sugar until mixture is light. Beat in the egg whites. In alternating batches,

(continued)

add flour mixture and oatmeal mixture to the sugar/oil mix, stirring only to moisten the dry ingredients after each addition. Spoon batter into 12 lightly oiled or paper-lined muffin tins. Bake 20–25 minutes.
 Makes 12 muffins.

PER muffin:
CALORIES 137   FIBER 1 gm
CSI <1   SODIUM 92 mg
FAT 4 gm

POPPYSEED MUFFINS

This recipe also makes forty-eight small muffins, which make excellent treats for school, church, etc.

    2½ cups flour
    ½ cup uncooked oatmeal
    ¼ cup poppyseeds
    ¾ cup sugar
    ½ teaspoon Lite Salt or less
    4 teaspoons baking powder
    ½ cup egg substitute (commercial or Homemade Egg Substitute, page 283)
    1⅓ cups buttermilk or skim milk
    ¼ cup oil
    ½–1 teaspoon almond extract

Preheat oven to 400°. Mix flour, oatmeal, poppyseeds, sugar, Lite Salt, and baking powder. Form a well in center and add egg substitute, milk, oil, and almond extract. Stir only until dry ingredients are moistened. Fill lightly oiled or paper-lined muf-

fin tins. Bake for 15 minutes or until done.
 Makes 16 muffins.

PER muffin:
CALORIES 163   FIBER 1 gm
CSI <1   SODIUM 134 mg
FAT 5 gm

PUMPKIN OAT MUFFINS

A fun way to eat oatmeal. Make ahead, freeze, and reheat for breakfast or snacks.

    1⅓ cups oat bran
    1 cup uncooked oatmeal
    1¼ cups skim milk
    ¾ cup whole wheat flour
    ½ cup brown sugar
    1 tablespoon baking powder
    2 teaspoons cinnamon
    ½ teaspoon nutmeg
    ½ teaspoon ginger
    1 cup cooked or canned pumpkin
    2 egg whites or ¼ cup egg substitute (commercial or Homemade Egg Substitute, page 283)
    2 tablespoons oil
    ½ cup raisins

Preheat oven to 400°. Combine oat bran, oatmeal, and milk in a bowl. In a separate bowl mix flour, brown sugar, baking powder, and spices. Blend pumpkin, egg whites or egg substitute, oil, and raisins in a third bowl and then add to oat/milk mixture. Add in the flour/sugar mixture and stir contents until moist. Spoon into lightly oiled or paper-lined muffin tins. Bake 20–25 minutes, or until lightly browned.

Makes 12 muffins.

PER muffin:
CALORIES 177   FIBER 4 gm
CSI <1   SODIUM 101 mg
FAT 4 gm

BISCUITS, SCONES, AND SPECIALTIES

BAKING MIX

Homemade "Bisquick"—more fiber, less salt.

4 cups whole wheat flour
4 cups white flour
1 cup powdered nonfat milk
2 teaspoons cream of tartar
¼ cup baking powder
2½ teaspoons Lite Salt or less
¾ cup shortening

Measure dry ingredients into bowl. Sift together 3 times. Put into large bowl; cut in shortening with pastry blender (or two knives) until size of small peas. Store in tightly covered container. (Recipe may be easily doubled.)

Makes 11 cups.

FOR PANCAKES

2 egg whites
1½ cups water
2 cups *Baking Mix*

Combine egg whites and water; stir into *Baking Mix* until well blended. Spoon onto a lightly oiled grill and cook, turning when bubbles appear.

Makes 12–15 medium pancakes.

PER cup dry mix:
CALORIES 491   FIBER 7 gm
CSI 4   SODIUM 738 mg
FAT 17 gm

FRUIT SCONES

Whipped Honey Orange Spread (page 455) is great served with these scones.

3 cups flour
½ cup sugar
1 tablespoon baking powder
½ teaspoon baking soda
⅓ cup margarine, cut into small pieces
1 cup chopped fresh or frozen cranberries *or* ¾ cup chopped dates
¼ cup chopped walnuts
1½ teaspoons grated orange peel
1 cup buttermilk
1 tablespoon skim milk
1 tablespoon sugar
¼ teaspoon cinnamon
⅛ teaspoon allspice

Preheat oven to 400°. In a large bowl, stir together flour, ½ cup sugar, baking pow-

(continued)

der, and baking soda. Using a pastry blender or your fingers, cut margarine into flour mixture until coarse crumbs form; stir in cranberries (or dates), walnuts, and orange peel. Add buttermilk and mix with a fork just until dough is evenly moistened.

Gather dough into a ball and place on a floured board. Roll or pat into a ¾-inch thick circle. Using a 2-inch-diameter cutter, cut into rounds. Place on a nonstick 12-by-15-inch baking sheet, about 1½ inches apart. Brush tops of scones with milk. Mix 1 tablespoon sugar, cinnamon, and allspice and sprinkle over the top. Bake until tops are lightly browned, 14–16 minutes. Serve warm.

Makes 24 (2-inch) scones.

PER scone:
CALORIES 107   FIBER 1 gm
CSI <1   SODIUM 99 mg
FAT 4 gm

OLD-STYLE WHEAT BISCUITS

1 cup white flour
1 cup whole wheat flour
2 teaspoons baking powder
¼ teaspoon Lite Salt or less
¼ teaspoon baking soda
¼ cup oil
2 tablespoons vinegar
1 cup skim milk

Preheat oven to 475°. Sift together flours, baking powder, Lite Salt, and baking soda.

Cut in oil until mixture looks like coarse cornmeal. Put vinegar and milk together in a cup and stir. Stir enough milk into flour mixture until soft dough is formed. Sprinkle flour on countertop and knead dough. Roll out dough to 1-inch thick. Cut with biscuit cutter or glass. Place on baking sheet. Bake about 12 minutes.

Makes 16 (2-inch) biscuits.

PER biscuit:
CALORIES 86   FIBER 1 gm
CSI <1   SODIUM 81 mg
FAT 4 gm

PIZZA CRUSTS

Choose a thin yeast crust or a quicker thick crust and create your own masterpiece.

THIN PIZZA CRUST
(Makes enough for two crusts.)

1½ tablespoons yeast
1¾ cups warm water
1 tablespoon honey *or* sugar
1 tablespoon oil
2 cups whole wheat flour
2 cups white flour

Dissolve yeast in warm water and add honey or sugar. Blend in oil and flours. Knead on lightly floured surface, adding more flour if needed. Spread and pat dough out onto two large pans (pizza or jelly roll pans, or cookie sheets). Roll edge slightly. Top with pizza sauce, vegetables, and grated imitation mozzarella cheese. Bake at 425° for 25–30 minutes.

Makes 30 pieces (3½ by 3½ inches each).

THICK PIZZA CRUST
(One crust very quickly made. No rising necessary.)

2 cups white flour
1 cup whole wheat flour
1 tablespoon baking powder
12 ounces beer

Mix all ingredients and spread in a 9-by-13-inch baking pan. Top with pizza sauce, vegetables, and grated imitation mozzarella cheese. Bake at 425° for 25–30 minutes.

Makes 12 pieces (3 by 3 inches each).

PER thin piece (crust only):
CALORIES 64   FIBER 2 gm
CSI trace   SODIUM <1 mg
FAT <1 gm

PER thick piece (crust only):
CALORIES 107   FIBER 2 gm
CSI trace   SODIUM 90 mg
FAT trace

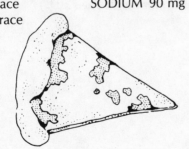

YOGURT SCONES

These scones require no rolling and are dropped like cookies on a baking sheet.

1½ cups white flour
1½ cups whole wheat flour
2 teaspoons baking powder
2 teaspoons baking soda
¼ cup cold margarine
2 tablespoons brown sugar
1¼ cups plain nonfat yogurt
2 egg whites
½ cup raisins *or* currants
3 tablespoons skim milk

Preheat oven to 400°. Lightly spray a baking sheet with nonstick spray. Mix flours, baking powder, and baking soda. Cut in cold margarine and brown sugar using a food processor, pastry cutter, or two forks until blended and the consistency of cornmeal.

Mix yogurt and egg whites. Add to flour mixture along with raisins or currants and mix in quick strokes only until blended. Drop by ¼-cup amounts onto baking sheet. Brush the top with skim milk. Bake 12–15 minutes. Serve warm with jam or preserves.

Makes 16 scones.

PER scone:
CALORIES 136   FIBER 2 gm
CSI <1   SODIUM 201 mg
FAT 3 gm

BREAKFASTS AND BRUNCHES

These recipes can make weekend breakfasts delightful as well as delicious. We particularly like the pancakes, waffles, hash browns, and sticky buns.

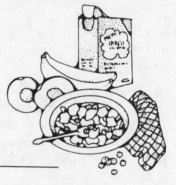

Cinnamon Waffles
Cornmeal Pancakes—*Easy*
Crepe Blintzes
Crepes
Dutchy Crust Muffins or Coffee Cake
"Eggs" Benedict
French Toast—*Quick*
German Oven Pancake
Homemade Egg Substitute
Oatmeal Buttermilk Pancakes

Orange Waffles
Skinny Hash Browns
Spanish Omelet
Sunday Morning Sticky Buns
Sunrise Cake
Vegetable Frittata

(Also see "Breads and Muffins" section, beginning on page 263.)

CINNAMON WAFFLES

Serve with warm applesauce. For a crunchy version, sprinkle each waffle with one tablespoon Grape-nuts cereal before baking.

- 3 egg whites
- 2 cups buttermilk
- 2 cups white flour (*or* 1 cup white flour and 1 cup whole wheat flour)
- 2 teaspoons baking powder
- 1 teaspoon baking soda
- 1 teaspoon cinnamon
- ½ teaspoon vanilla
- ¼ cup oil

Heat waffle iron. Lightly beat egg whites until frothy; fold in remaining ingredients until smooth.

Pour ½ cup batter onto center of hot waffle iron. Bake about 5 minutes or until steaming stops. Remove waffle carefully.

Makes 8 waffles (7 inches each).

PER waffle:
CALORIES 197   FIBER 1 gm
CSI 2   SODIUM 259 mg
FAT 8 gm

CORNMEAL PANCAKES—*EASY*

An unusual breakfast treat. Maple syrup or *Fresh Rhubarb Sauce* (page 455) are delicious with these pancakes.

- ½ cup flour
- 1 teaspoon baking soda
- ½ teaspoon Lite Salt or less
- 1 cup yellow cornmeal
- ½ cup egg substitute (commercial *or Homemade Egg Substitute,* page 283)
- 2 cups buttermilk
- 1 tablespoon melted margarine

Combine flour, baking soda, Lite Salt, and cornmeal. In a separate bowl combine egg substitute and buttermilk. Stir egg/buttermilk mixture into the other ingredients just enough to moisten. Add melted margarine and lightly fold into the batter. Bake on a hot, lightly oiled griddle.

Makes 12 pancakes (5 inches each).

PER pancake:
CALORIES 89   FIBER 1 gm
CSI trace   SODIUM 184 mg
FAT 1 gm

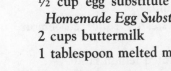

CREPE BLINTZES

A nice weekend breakfast idea: crepes with a cheese filling that are lightly browned and served warm with fresh fruit or other toppings.

Crepes (below)
1½ cups low-fat cottage cheese
3 ounces Neufchâtel cheese (lower-fat cream cheese)
⅓ cup sugar
1 teaspoon vanilla
1 tablespoon freshly squeezed lemon juice
½ teaspoon grated lemon rind
1 tablespoon oil
1 cup plain nonfat yogurt
4 cups sliced fruit *or* berries
2 tablespoons powdered sugar

Prepare *Crepes.*

Mix cottage cheese, Neufchâtel cheese, sugar, vanilla, lemon juice, and lemon rind. Fill each crepe. Fold. Sauté in oil until slightly browned.

Serve with nonfat yogurt, fresh berries, or fruit and sprinkle with powdered sugar.

Makes filling for 8 crepes.

PER blintz:
CALORIES 239   FIBER 2 gm
CSI 4   SODIUM 281 mg
FAT 7 gm

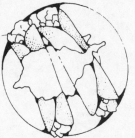

CREPES

The following basic recipe is a low-fat, low-cholesterol version of the original one, which called for whole eggs, whole milk, and butter.

1 cup cold water
1 cup cold skim milk
6 egg whites
½ teaspoon Lite Salt or less
2 cups flour
2 tablespoons oil

Put liquids, egg whites, and Lite Salt into blender jar; add flour, then oil. Blend at top speed, scraping any flour adhering to the sides of the jar. Cover, refrigerate 2 hours. This is an important step—it allows the flour particles to expand in the liquid and ensures a tender, thin crepe. The batter should be a very light, creamy texture—just thick enough to coat a wooden spoon.

For each crepe, heat a 6-inch nonstick skillet over moderately high heat. When hot, pour a scant ¼ cup of the batter into skillet; immediately rotate pan until batter covers bottom. Cook until light brown; turn and brown on other side. Slide onto warm plate and proceed in same manner with the rest of the batter. Put waxed paper between crepes. Keep covered, as they cool, to prevent them from drying out. The crepes are now ready to be filled.

Makes 20 crepes (6 inches each).

PER crepe:
CALORIES 62   FIBER trace
CSI trace   SODIUM 41 mg
FAT 2 gm

DUTCHY CRUST MUFFINS OR COFFEE CAKE

Blueberries, fresh pitted cherries, fresh chopped apple—or no fruit at all—work equally well. This also makes a great coffee cake.

DUTCHY CRUST

- 2 tablespoons margarine, softened
- ¼ cup packed brown sugar
- ¼ cup uncooked oatmeal
- ¼ cup flour
- 1 teaspoon cinnamon

MUFFIN/CAKE BASE

- ¾ cup white flour
- ¾ cup whole wheat flour
- ½ cup uncooked oatmeal
- ½ cup packed brown sugar
- 2 teaspoons baking powder
- 1 teaspoon baking soda
- 1 cup fresh or partially thawed frozen blueberries *or* other fruit
- 3 egg whites
- ⅔ cup buttermilk
- 2 tablespoons melted margarine

Preheat oven to 400°. Prepare Dutchy Crust by mixing all ingredients until crumbly and set aside.

In large bowl mix flours, oatmeal, sugar, baking powder, and baking soda. Add fruit; stir carefully to coat. In small bowl beat egg whites with fork; beat in buttermilk and margarine. Add to flour mixture; stir just until blended.

If making muffins, pour into 12 paper-lined muffin tins and top with Dutchy Crust. Bake 20 minutes or until wooden pick inserted in center comes out clean. For a coffee cake, bake in a lightly oiled 9-inch square pan for 25–30 minutes.

Makes 12 servings.

PER muffin:
CALORIES 181   FIBER 2 gm
CSI <1   SODIUM 200 mg
FAT 5 gm

"EGGS" BENEDICT

Similar to typical Eggs Benedict. For a meatless and lower-salt version, serve a tomato slice in place of the Canadian bacon.

- 1 cup *Mock Hollandaise Sauce* (page 451)
- 2 tablespoons chopped onion
- 2 tablespoons chopped green bell pepper
- 1 cup egg substitute (commercial *or Homemade Egg Substitute,* page 283)
- 2 English muffins
- 4 slices Canadian bacon *or* turkey ham *or* 4 thick slices tomato

Make 1 cup *Mock Hollandaise Sauce* and set aside. Steam onions and green pepper in a little water until soft, add egg substitute to make "scrambled eggs." Split and toast English muffins, heat *thin* slices of Canadian bacon, and place one slice of meat on each muffin. Top with scrambled egg mixture

(continued)

and 4 tablespoons of *Mock Hollandaise Sauce.*

Makes 4 servings.

PER serving:
CALORIES 238   FIBER 1 gm
CSI 4   SODIUM 840 mg
FAT 11 gm

FRENCH TOAST—*QUICK*

This is the traditional form of the old standby. Be adventurous and sprinkle with cinnamon or use sourdough rye bread or thick sliced French bread.

2 egg whites
¼ cup egg substitute (commercial *or* Homemade Egg Substitute, page 283)
½ teaspoon sugar
½ cup skim milk
4 slices day-old bread *or* 12 slices (¾-inch thick) baguette bread

Stir egg whites and egg substitute together with a fork. Add sugar and skim milk and mix well. Dip bread into egg mixture and cook on nonstick griddle until golden brown on each side. Serve with warm syrup or fruit sauce.

Makes 4 servings.

PER serving:
CALORIES 95   FIBER trace
CSI trace   SODIUM 197 mg
FAT 1 gm

GERMAN OVEN PANCAKE

A puff pancake that is very simple to make and so attractive!

½ cup flour
¾ cup egg substitute (commercial *or* Homemade Egg Substitute, page 283)
½ cup skim milk
5 teaspoons melted margarine
2 cups sliced fruit*
2 tablespoons powdered sugar
Lemon wedges

Preheat oven to 450°. Gradually add flour to egg substitute, beating with rotary beater or in blender. Stir in milk and melted margarine. Lightly oil or spray with nonstick spray a 9-inch or 10-inch ovenproof skillet. (A round cake pan works well.) Pour batter into prepared pan. Bake for 20 minutes. (Pancake will form a well in the center and sides will puff up.) Spoon fruit into the center of the pancake.

Loosen pancake from pan with wide spatula and cut into wedges with sharp knife. Serve immediately with powdered sugar and lemon wedges.

Makes 2 servings.

*Any fresh fruit works well (berries, bananas, or peaches).

PER ½ pancake:
CALORIES 373   FIBER 3 gm
CSI 2   SODIUM 355 mg
FAT 10 gm

HOMEMADE EGG SUBSTITUTE
(¼ CUP = 1 WHOLE EGG)

This can be used in place of commercial egg substitute and is considerably cheaper!

  6 egg whites
  ¼ cup powdered nonfat milk
  1 tablespoon oil

Combine all ingredients in a mixing bowl and blend until smooth. Store in jar in refrigerator up to 1 week. Also freezes well.

To prepare as scrambled egg: Fry slowly over low heat in a nonstick skillet.
  Makes 1 cup.

PER ¼ cup:
CALORIES 70   FIBER 0 gm
CSI <1   SODIUM 99 mg
FAT 4 gm

OATMEAL BUTTERMILK PANCAKES

If you have time, premix part of batter and refrigerate overnight. These are truly a breakfast treat, especially with fresh fruit or warm syrup.

  1½ cups uncooked oatmeal
  2 cups buttermilk
  3 egg whites
  1 cup whole wheat flour
  2 teaspoons baking soda
  2 tablespoons brown sugar

Combine oatmeal, buttermilk, and egg whites and let stand for at least ½ hour or refrigerate up to 24 hours. Add remaining ingredients, and stir the batter just until the dry ingredients are moistened. Bake on a hot, lightly oiled griddle.
  Makes 16 pancakes (4 inches each).

PER pancake:
CALORIES 76   FIBER 2 gm
CSI trace   SODIUM 145 mg
FAT 1 gm

ORANGE WAFFLES

Serve with *Orange Sauce* (page 419), or hot maple syrup.

  3 egg whites
  1½ cups buttermilk
  ½ cup orange juice
  2 cups white flour (*or* 1 cup white flour and 1 cup whole wheat flour)
  1 tablespoon grated orange rind
  2 teaspoons baking powder
  1 teaspoon baking soda
  ¼ cup oil

Heat waffle iron. Lightly beat egg whites until frothy; fold in remaining ingredients until smooth.

(continued)

Pour ½ cup batter onto center of hot waffle iron. Bake about 5 minutes or until steaming stops. Remove waffle carefully. Makes 8 waffles (7 inches each).

PER waffle:
CALORIES 197   FIBER 1 gm
CSI 1   SODIUM 243 mg
FAT 8 gm

SKINNY HASH BROWNS

A small amount of oil makes crispy hash browns—you can indeed have these!

4 cups shredded baked potatoes
4 teaspoons oil
¼ teaspoon Lite Salt or less
Pepper to taste

Bake potatoes. Allow to cool or use leftover cold ones and shred them. Heat oil in skillet. Tilt skillet so oil covers bottom of pan. Add shredded potatoes. Sprinkle with Lite Salt and pepper. Cover and cook until brown on bottom. Carefully turn with a spatula. Cook until brown on bottom again. Serve hot.
Makes 4 cups.

PER cup:
CALORIES 174   FIBER 3 gm
CSI <1   SODIUM 130 mg
FAT 5 gm

SPANISH OMELET

Yes, you can have an omelet!

1 teaspoon oil
¾ cup chopped onion
1½ cups chopped fresh tomatoes
1½ cups frozen peas
¼ teaspoon pepper
1½ cups egg whites (about 12)
⅔ cup egg substitute (commercial *or* *Homemade Egg Substitute*, page 283)

Sauté onions in oil. Stir in tomatoes and simmer uncovered for 4 to 5 minutes. Add peas and pepper to the tomato mixture and simmer until done.
Combine the egg whites and egg substitute in a mixing bowl. Beat on high speed with an electric mixer until foamy.
Heat a nonstick skillet over low heat. Pour in egg mixture and cook slowly until mixture begins to set. Loosen the edges from pan. Pour tomato filling in the center of the omelet. Fold one half over the other and tip onto a plate. Serve hot with whole-grain toast.
Makes 6 servings.

PER serving:
CALORIES 93   FIBER 2 gm
CSI trace   SODIUM 170 mg
FAT 1 gm

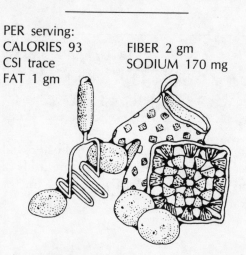

SUNDAY MORNING STICKY BUNS

Start the evening before for this wonderful treat.

- 1 loaf (16 ounces) frozen bread dough
- 1 tablespoon melted margarine
- ½ cup brown sugar
- 2 tablespoons light corn syrup
- 3 tablespoons skim milk
- 1 teaspoon cinnamon
- 1 tablespoon slivered almonds

Partially thaw frozen bread and cut into 1-inch cubes. Pour melted margarine in bottom of 9-by-9-inch pan. Add remaining ingredients and mix in pan. Arrange dough cubes in a single layer over sauce. Cover and refrigerate overnight.

Next morning: Remove from refrigerator, cover loosely, and let rise 1 hour at room temperature*. Preheat oven to 350°, and when dough has doubled in volume, bake 30 minutes. Loosen edges and immediately invert onto serving plate. (The sauce will drizzle over the bread.) Serve warm.

Makes 9 servings.

VARIATION:
Reduce brown sugar to 2 tablespoons and omit corn syrup. Add 1 package (3⅝ ounces) butterscotch pudding mix (not instant). Prepare as directed above.

*If your kitchen is not too warm, let dough rise inside microwave with a large bowl of hot water under it. *Do not turn on heat.*

PER serving:
CALORIES 214   FIBER 1 gm
CSI <1   SODIUM 282 mg
FAT 3 gm

SUNRISE CAKE

One of the few low-fat coffee cakes we've found. The texture seems to be best when baked in a tube pan.

- ¼ cup margarine
- 2 egg whites
- Grated rind of 1 small lemon
- 2 teaspoons freshly squeezed lemon juice
- ¾ cup brown sugar
- 1 cup whole wheat flour
- 1 cup white flour
- 1 teaspoon baking soda
- ¼ teaspoon Lite Salt or less
- 1 cup plain nonfat yogurt
- 2 cups chopped fruit*

TOPPING

- 1 tablespoon margarine
- 1 tablespoon wheat germ
- ¼ cup white flour
- ¼ cup brown sugar
- 1 teaspoon cinnamon
- ½ teaspoon allspice

*Apples, peaches, blueberries, rhubarb, etc. (a combination is nice); if canned fruit is used, drain well.

(continued)

Preheat oven to 350°. Cream margarine, egg whites, lemon rind, juice, and brown sugar until smooth. Sift together dry ingredients and add alternately with yogurt to egg white mixture. Fold in fruit, and spread into a tube pan that has been sprayed with nonstick spray.

Combine all topping ingredients (it works well to use the same bowl and incorporate the "scrapings" from the batter) and sprinkle over coffee cake. Bake for about 35 minutes until wooden pick inserted in center comes out clean. Serve topped with yogurt, if desired.

Makes 16 servings.

PER serving:
CALORIES 161   FIBER 2 gm
CSI <1   SODIUM 132 mg
FAT 4 gm

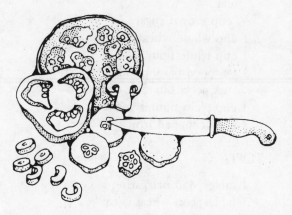

VEGETABLE FRITTATA

An Italian version of the omelet. Makes a nice brunch or luncheon dish for two.

1 clove garlic
2 teaspoons oil
1–1½ cups leftover, cooked vegetables
½ teaspoon thyme leaves
½ teaspoon basil leaves
½ teaspoon rosemary leaves
Freshly ground black pepper to taste
¾ cup egg substitute (commercial *or* Homemade Egg Substitute, page 283)
2 egg whites
2 tablespoons grated Parmesan cheese

Mince garlic and sauté in oil in a 7-inch skillet until softened. Add vegetables and seasonings and cook very briefly, just to heat. Beat egg substitute and egg whites together; stir in Parmesan cheese. Pour over vegetable mixture and cook until golden on the bottom. Turn over with a broad spatula and cook until other side is golden, or, without turning, place under broiler until top is set and very lightly browned. Serve from skillet.

Makes 2 servings.

PER serving:
CALORIES 232   FIBER 6 gm
CSI 2   SODIUM 410 mg
FAT 7 gm

SALADS

We are especially proud of our salad recipes. A number of them make good pocket bread or tortilla fillers for lunch. We have a green salad that contains figs. There are two molded salads that are less sweet than typical molded salads and contain no sour cream.

Fruit and Vegetable Salads
Absolutely Delicious Molded Salad
Carrot Raisin Salad
Confetti Appleslaw
Crunchy Vegetable Salad
Greek Salad—*Easy*
Green Bean, Mushroom, and Tomato Salad
Holiday Wreath Salad
Lemony Beets—*Easy*
Orange Yogurt Fruit Slaw
Salad Athene
Sesame Slaw
Snowbird Salad
Sunshine Spinach Salad
Vinaigrette Salad Dressing with Greens—*Quick*
Waldorf Salad—*Quick*

Pasta, Rice, and Potato Salads
Alphabet Seafood Salad (see page 364 in "Fish and Shellfish" section)
Crunchy Confetti Salad—*Quick*
Curried Rice and Artichoke Salad
Four-Star Pasta Salad with Green Sauce
Fruit and Rice Salad
Montana Pasta Salad
Moroccan Salad
Orange Bulgur Salad
Potato Salad
Tabouli

Bean Salads
California Beans—*Easy*
Chili Bean Salad
Spicy Black Bean Salad—*Easy*
Summer Bean Salad

Other Salads
Chicken Salad with Yogurt-Chive Dressing (see page 393 in "Chicken and Turkey" section)
Curried Chicken and Peanut Salad (see page 394 in "Chicken and Turkey" section)
Simply Wonderful Turkey Salad (see page 394 in "Chicken and Turkey" section)
Taco Salad (see page 411 in "Beef and Pork" section)

FRUIT AND VEGETABLE SALADS

ABSOLUTELY DELICIOUS MOLDED SALAD

1 large package (6 ounces) raspberry-flavored Jell-O
1 small package (3 ounces) lemon-flavored Jell-O
2 cups boiling water
1 cup orange juice
2 packages (12 ounces each) frozen raspberries, unsweetened (thawed)
1 can (20 ounces) crushed pineapple, undrained
2 bananas, mashed
16 ounces plain or vanilla nonfat yogurt

Mix Jell-O powders with boiling water to dissolve. Stir in orange juice and fruit. Pour ½ mixture into mold or 13-by-9-inch dish. Chill until firm, keeping remaining half at room temperature. When set spread yogurt over fruit and top with remaining mixture. Chill until firm. Cut into squares to serve.
Makes 15 servings.

PER serving:
CALORIES 150   FIBER 3 gm
CSI trace   SODIUM 80 mg
FAT trace

CARROT RAISIN SALAD

An old standby and colorful lunchtime treat. Add a grated unpeeled apple for an unusual change.

4 cups shredded raw carrots
1 cup raisins
¾ cup plain nonfat yogurt
1 tablespoon light mayonnaise

Combine carrots and raisins. Toss with yogurt and light mayonnaise.
Makes 5⅓ cups.

PER cup:
CALORIES 166   FIBER 5 gm
CSI <1   SODIUM 80 mg
FAT 2 gm

CONFETTI APPLESLAW

2 tablespoons undiluted orange juice concentrate
1½ cups diced unpeeled red apple
4 cups finely shredded cabbage
2 tablespoons finely chopped red onions
1¼ cups thinly sliced red or green bell pepper
3 tablespoons raisins
1 tablespoon light mayonnaise
½ cup plain nonfat yogurt
½ teaspoon dry mustard
Paprika
Pepper to taste

Stir orange juice concentrate and diced apple together. Combine with remaining ingredients in a large mixing bowl and toss well. Refrigerate until serving time.

Makes 8 servings (1 cup each).

PER cup:
CALORIES 55   FIBER 2 gm
CSI trace   SODIUM 25 mg
FAT 1 gm

CRUNCHY VEGETABLE SALAD

1 package (10 ounces) frozen peas
1 cup sliced celery
1 cup chopped cauliflower
¼ cup diced green onions
2 tablespoons sliced pimiento
¾ cup *Hearty Ranch Salad Dressing* (page 303)
¾ teaspoon Dijon mustard
1 small clove garlic, minced
3 tablespoons coarsely chopped cashews

Combine vegetables. To *Hearty Ranch Salad Dressing* add mustard and garlic; pour over salad. Toss carefully and chill. At serving time, add nuts and gently stir in.

Makes 4 servings.

PER serving:
CALORIES 136   FIBER 5 gm
CSI 1   SODIUM 392 mg
FAT 5 gm

GREEK SALAD—*EASY*

1 large green bell pepper
1 can (2.2 ounces) sliced black olives, drained
1 small head cauliflower, separated into flowerets
1 clove garlic, minced
1 cup plain nonfat yogurt
1 tablespoon olive oil
2 tablespoons freshly squeezed lemon juice
Pepper

Toss green pepper, olives and cauliflower together. Combine garlic, yogurt, olive oil, and lemon juice. Pour over vegetables and stir. Season with pepper and chill.

Makes 12 servings (1 cup each).

PER cup:
CALORIES 55   FIBER 2 gm
CSI <1   SODIUM 86 mg
FAT 3 gm

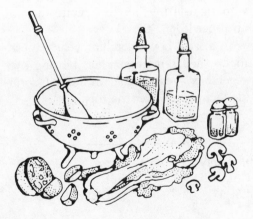

GREEN BEAN, MUSHROOM, AND TOMATO SALAD

1 pound fresh green beans
¼ cup red wine vinegar
2 tablespoons olive oil
2 teaspoons egg substitute (commercial or *Homemade Egg Substitute*, page 283)
1½ tablespoons red wine
¼ teaspoon oregano leaves
¼ teaspoon Lite Salt or less
1½ cups sliced fresh mushrooms
1 pint cherry tomatoes
1 ounce crumbled feta cheese (optional)

Steam or cook beans in a small amount of water until just tender. Drain. Cool under running cold water.

In a blender combine vinegar, oil, and egg substitute. Process until thick and creamy. Add red wine, oregano, and Lite Salt. Process 10 seconds. Pour into a jar with tight-fitting lid. Refrigerate dressing until needed.

In a salad bowl, combine beans, mushrooms, and tomatoes. Pour dressing over vegetables. Toss to coat. If desired, sprinkle feta cheese over the top.

Makes 8 servings.

PER serving:
CALORIES 67   FIBER 3 gm
CSI 1   SODIUM 83 mg
FAT 4 gm

HOLIDAY WREATH SALAD

A beautiful dish you will be proud to serve to friends or to take to a party. If you are serving fewer than twenty people, cut the amount to a half or a third and mold in a smaller pan.

To prepare salad, start day before serving: Combine ingredients for either cranberry or raspberry layer as directed. Refrigerate until slightly thickened and pour in bottom of 10-inch tube, Bundt, or springform pan. Chill until almost set. Prepare creamy layer, and when it is cool and slightly thickened, spoon into mold over berry layer. Chill until set.

To serve: Unmold onto a large glass plate. Decorate with greens and frosted berries or holly.

CRANBERRY LAYER

2 envelopes unflavored gelatin
¾ cup sugar
1½ cups boiling water
1 cup chilled ginger ale
1½ cups ground cranberries

OR

RASPBERRY LAYER

1 large package (6 ounces) raspberry Jell-O
2 cups boiling water
1½ cups cold water
1 bag (12 ounces) frozen raspberries, unsweetened

If using cranberries: Mix gelatin powder with ¾ cup sugar. Add boiling water and stir until dissolved. Stir in ginger ale and ground berries.

If using raspberries: Dissolve Jell-O in boiling water, add remaining cold water and raspberries.

CREAMY LAYER

- 3 envelopes unflavored gelatin
- 6 tablespoons sugar
- 1¼ cups boiling water
- 2 cups lemon custard low-fat yogurt (three 6-ounce cartons)
- 1½ cups plain nonfat yogurt
- 2 cups lemon sherbet
- ½ cup chopped walnuts

Mix 3 envelopes of gelatin powder with 6 tablespoons of sugar. Add boiling water and stir until dissolved. With wire whisk, mix in yogurt, 1 cup at a time. Then mix in the sherbet, also 1 cup at a time until mixture is smooth. Stir in nuts. Refrigerate for a few minutes until mixture is slightly thickened. Spoon over the berry layer. Chill until set.

Makes 10 cups (twenty ½-cup servings).

———————

PER ½ cup of cranberry version:
CALORIES 137   FIBER 1 gm
CSI <1   SODIUM 40 mg
FAT 3 gm

———————

PER ½ cup raspberry version:
CALORIES 112   FIBER 1 gm
CSI <1   SODIUM 43 mg
FAT 3 gm

LEMONY BEETS—*EASY*

- 1 can (16 ounces) sliced beets, drained
- 1 clove garlic, minced
- 2 tablespoons freshly squeezed lemon juice
- ½ teaspoon Dijon mustard
- 2 tablespoons olive oil
- ¼ teaspoon Lite Salt or less
- Freshly ground pepper
- 2 tablespoons chopped fresh parsley, for garnish

Place beets in a shallow bowl. In a small jar, combine garlic, lemon juice, and mustard. Gradually add the oil. Season with Lite Salt and pepper. Shake well to blend. Pour vinaigrette over beets. Refrigerate for several hours or serve immediately.

Arrange beets on lettuce-lined salad plates, in an attractive bowl as a side dish or arrange with other salad ingredients. Sprinkle chopped parsley over top of beets and serve.

Makes 6 servings.

———————

PER serving:
CALORIES 66   FIBER 2 gm
CSI <1   SODIUM 150 mg
FAT 5 gm

ORANGE YOGURT FRUIT SLAW

An incredibly easy dressing adds a nice orange flavor to the fruit and cabbage.

1 cup seedless red grapes
1 can (11 ounces) mandarin oranges, drained
½ cup sliced celery
3 cups shredded cabbage
1 carton (8 ounces) orange-flavored low-fat yogurt
1 small apple, chopped
1 tablespoon sunflower seeds

Combine grapes, oranges, and celery with the shredded cabbage in a bowl. To prepare dressing combine yogurt with chopped apple. Spread dressing over cabbage, cover well, and chill.

At serving time, toss salad, and sprinkle with sunflower seeds. Serve on cabbage-lined plates.

Makes 7 cups.

PER cup:
CALORIES 96   FIBER 2 gm
CSI trace   SODIUM 33 mg
FAT 2 gm

SALAD ATHENE

Greens with interesting additions . . .

SALAD

6 cups romaine, torn into bite-size pieces
1 cup slivered figs (8-ounce bag)
½ cup thinly sliced red onion
1½ cups chopped tomato (quartered cherry tomatoes work well)
¼ cup sliced ripe olives, drained
¼ cup crumbled feta cheese

CAPER DRESSING

2 tablespoons olive oil
1 tablespoon red wine vinegar
1 teaspoon sugar
1 tablespoon capers
2 teaspoons Dijon mustard
¼ teaspoon paprika
¼ teaspoon thyme leaves
¼ teaspoon oregano leaves

Add dressing to prepared vegetables. Sprinkle feta cheese over top of salad and serve immediately.

Makes 10 cups.

PER cup:
CALORIES 103   FIBER 4 gm
CSI 1   SODIUM 102 mg
FAT 4 gm

SESAME SLAW

An outstanding salad—try it, you'll like it!

DRESSING

¼ cup sugar
1 teaspoon fresh ground black pepper
6 tablespoons rice vinegar
1 clove garlic, crushed
1 tablespoon grated fresh ginger root
2 teaspoons sesame oil
½ teaspoon Lite Salt or less

SALAD

4 cups shredded green cabbage (about 1 small head)
1 cup shredded red cabbage
1 cup sliced fresh mushrooms
1 cup diagonally sliced pea pods
1 can (8 ounces) sliced water chestnuts, drained
½ cup diagonally sliced green onions
¼ cup sliced almonds, toasted

Prepare dressing by combining sugar, pepper, vinegar, garlic, grated ginger, sesame oil, and Lite Salt. Set aside. Toss together salad ingredients. Add dressing and toss to mix. Cover well and chill.

Makes 8 cups.

PER cup:
CALORIES 91
CSI trace
FAT 3 gm

FIBER 3 gm
SODIUM 73 mg

SNOWBIRD SALAD

A very nice fresh spinach salad.

3 cups packed, chopped fresh spinach (½ pound or 1 bunch)
3 cups finely chopped cauliflower (½ of medium)
2 cups sliced fresh mushrooms
½ cup peeled, pitted, and sliced avocado

OLIVE OIL DRESSING

2 tablespoons olive oil
3 tablespoons white wine vinegar
1 clove garlic, minced
½ teaspoon dry mustard
½ teaspoon dried basil leaves or 1½ teaspoons fresh basil
¼ teaspoon pepper
¼ teaspoon Lite Salt or less
Dash nutmeg

Wash and dry spinach. Stack leaves and slice into ¼-inch strips. Mix cauliflower and spinach and refrigerate if the salad is made ahead of time. Combine dressing ingredients.

At serving time: Add mushrooms to cauliflower and spinach; pour *Olive Oil Dressing* over all and toss. Garnish with avocado and serve immediately.

Makes 9 cups.

PER cup:
CALORIES 58
CSI <1
FAT 5 gm

FIBER 2 gm
SODIUM 48 mg

SUNSHINE SPINACH SALAD

Beautiful *and* tasty!

4 cups torn lettuce or other salad greens
4 cups torn fresh spinach
1 fresh orange, sliced, *or* 1 can (11 ounces) mandarin orange sections, drained
1 can (8 ounces) sliced water chestnuts, drained
1 cup sliced fresh mushrooms
1 small red onion, sliced and separated into rings
½ cup low-calorie Italian dressing

In large bowl, combine all ingredients except dressing. Chill until serving time. Toss with dressing.

Makes 6 servings (2 cups each).

PER 1 cup:
CALORIES 51   FIBER 2 gm
CSI trace   SODIUM 175 mg
FAT 2 gm

VINAIGRETTE SALAD DRESSING WITH GREENS—*QUICK*

A quick dressing made directly in the salad bowl. When you toss the salad this way, not much dressing is required. A simple salad of romaine becomes very elegant.

1 clove garlic
1 tablespoon olive oil
1 tablespoon garlic-flavored wine vinegar
1 teaspoon Dijon mustard
6 cups torn lettuce, preferably romaine
Pepper

Rub a large salad bowl with the whole garlic clove, then mince it. Add minced garlic, oil, vinegar, and mustard and stir well to combine. Cover bowl until ready to serve. Remove cover and add lettuce. Mix until all pieces are very well coated. Grind fresh pepper over the salad.

Makes 6 cups of salad.

OPTION
For special treats, add up to 1 teaspoon grated Parmesan cheese before tossing.

PER cup:
CALORIES 31   FIBER <1 gm
CSI trace   SODIUM 15 mg
FAT 2 gm

WALDORF SALAD—*QUICK*

A low-fat version of an old standby.

1 cup diced celery
1 cup diced unpeeled apple
⅓ cup chopped walnuts
⅓ cup raisins
½ cup nonfat yogurt (use plain *or* combination of vanilla or orange and plain)

Combine diced celery, apples, chopped nuts, and raisins. Blend yogurt into the mixture.

Makes 6 servings (½ cup each).

PER ½ cup:
CALORIES 98   FIBER 2 gm
CSI <1   SODIUM 41 mg
FAT 5 gm

PASTA, RICE, AND POTATO SALADS

CRUNCHY CONFETTI SALAD—QUICK

Very quick—an unusual and colorful vegetable salad.

2 cups tomatoes, coarsely chopped
1 cup uncooked couscous*
1 medium zucchini, cut into small strips
1 cup shredded carrots (2 medium)
⅓ cup sliced green onions (4 pieces)
¼ cup sliced ripe olives, drained
2 tablespoons oil
3 tablespoons white wine vinegar
1 teaspoon Dijon mustard
½ teaspoon dried basil leaves *or* 1½ teaspoons fresh basil
¼ teaspoon Lite Salt or less
¼ teaspoon pepper
½ cup thinly sliced radishes

*Found in the macaroni/rice department of most supermarkets.

Stir together tomatoes, uncooked couscous, zucchini, carrots, green onions, and olives.

In a jar with a tight lid combine oil, vinegar, mustard, basil, Lite Salt, and pepper. Cover and shake well. Pour dressing over couscous mixture; toss to coat. Cover salad and chill.

Stir in radishes just before serving.

Makes 6 cups.

PER cup:
CALORIES 170   FIBER 3 gm
CSI <1   SODIUM 117 mg
FAT 6 gm

CURRIED RICE AND ARTICHOKE SALAD

¾ cup white rice cooked in 1 cup lower-salt chicken broth and 1 cup water *or* 1 package (6 ounces) MJB chicken-flavored rice mix (use ¼ seasoning packet)
1 package (10 ounces) frozen artichoke hearts *or* 1 can (14 ounces), drained
8 stuffed green olives, sliced
½ cup minced green onions
½ cup plain nonfat yogurt
1 tablespoon light mayonnaise
½–1 teaspoon curry powder

Prepare rice and artichokes according to package directions (without adding fat). Cool both rice and artichokes and add olives and green onions. Mix together yo-

(continued)

gurt, light mayonnaise, and curry powder and add to rice mixture. Mix well and chill. (Save a small amount of dressing to add at serving time to keep salad from becoming dry.)

Makes 4 cups.

PER cup:
CALORIES 206   FIBER 4 gm
CSI <1   SODIUM 471 mg
FAT 3 gm

FOUR-STAR PASTA SALAD WITH GREEN SAUCE

A beautiful and unusual salad that really deserves ten stars! It is served with a pungent *Green Sauce*. Some preparation is needed the day before serving.

1 package (16 ounces) pasta (curled, short pasta works well)
¼ pound shrimp meat (optional)

MARINADE

2 tablespoons oil
¼ cup white vinegar
½ teaspoon Lite Salt or less
⅛ teaspoon pepper
1 tablespoon sherry (optional)
1 clove garlic, minced

GREEN SAUCE
(Double this sauce if you wish to have lots of dressing—also it keeps well, and can be used on other salads.)

¼ cup white vinegar *or* lemon juice
1–2 tablespoons Dijon mustard
½ cup tightly packed fresh basil *or* 2 teaspoons dried basil leaves
¾ cup chopped parsley
1–3 cloves garlic, minced
2 tablespoons oil
1 cup plain nonfat yogurt
Pepper

SALAD INGREDIENTS

1 cup frozen peas, uncooked
1 cup broccoli (cut into small pieces)
2 cups halved cherry tomatoes
1 cup sliced mushrooms
1 cup sliced zucchini
6 green onions, chopped
2 cups fresh spinach leaves (torn into bite-size pieces)

On the day before: Cook pasta in unsalted water. Drain and cool. Combine ingredients for marinade and mix with shrimp and cooked pasta. Refrigerate overnight. Place *Green Sauce* ingredients in food processor or blender and mix until smooth. Refrigerate for several hours; it will thicken.

Just before serving: Combine marinated pasta and shrimp with salad ingredients and toss. Add a small amount of the *Green Sauce* to the salad when you toss it and serve the rest on the side or toss the salad with the sauce as for other salads.

Makes 10 servings as a main dish (about 20 cups).

PER cup:
CALORIES 154   FIBER 2 gm
CSI <1   SODIUM 53 mg
FAT 3 gm

FRUIT AND RICE SALAD

The sweet taste of dates gives this cold salad a lovely flavor.

3 cups cooked brown rice
2 tablespoons freshly squeezed lemon juice
1 tablespoon olive oil
¼ teaspoon cinnamon
½ cup chopped parsley
2 tablespoons dried mint *or* ¼ cup fresh
¼ cup chopped green onions
⅓ cup pitted dates
2 large oranges, sliced *or* 2 cans (11 ounces each) mandarin oranges, drained

Put cooked rice into mixing bowl. Add lemon juice, olive oil, cinnamon, parsley, mint, and onions. Add dates and orange slices and gently toss. Cover and chill.
    Makes 7 cups.

PER cup:
CALORIES 169   FIBER 4 gm
CSI trace   SODIUM 4 mg
FAT 3 gm

MONTANA PASTA SALAD

A very pretty salad—the pineapple gives it a little sweetness.

1 can (15 ounces) chunk pineapple, unsweetened
2 cups broccoli or asparagus tips
4 cups cooked pasta, shaped like a corkscrew
1 cup frozen peas, uncooked
1 cup sliced celery
½ cup chopped parsley
⅓ cup chopped green onion
⅓ cup diced pimiento *or* sweet red bell pepper

Drain pineapple, reserving 2 tablespoons juice for dressing. Wash broccoli or asparagus and cut in bite-size pieces. Combine all ingredients and toss with *Spring Dressing.* Chill at least 1 hour.

SPRING DRESSING

2 tablespoons juice from canned pineapple
1 clove garlic, crushed
2 tablespoons olive oil
⅓ cup white wine vinegar
2 tablespoons freshly squeezed lemon juice
2 tablespoons Dijon mustard
2 teaspoons basil leaves
½ teaspoon Lite Salt or less

Combine ingredients in jar and shake well.
    Makes 6 servings (1½ cups each).

PER cup:
CALORIES 169   FIBER 3 gm
CSI <1   SODIUM 121 mg
FAT 4 gm

MOROCCAN SALAD

A beautiful, unusual salad that is definitely worth the effort!

SALAD

> 1 cup uncooked orzo*
> 2 quarts boiling water
> ½ cup diced red bell pepper (½ medium)
> ½ cup diced green or yellow bell pepper (½ medium)
> ½ cup minced red onion (¼ medium)
> ½ cup chopped dates
> ½ cup chopped dried apricots (½ of 6-ounce bag)
> ¼ cup currants
> 2 tablespoons unsalted sunflower seeds *or* chopped pistachio nuts
> 2–4 tablespoons chopped cilantro (¼ bunch)
> Zest of ½ orange† (1 tablespoon), saving fruit for dressing
> Zest of ½ lemon (1 tablespoon), saving fruit for dressing

HONEY DRESSING

> 2 tablespoons freshly squeezed lemon juice (from ½ lemon)
> 3 tablespoons freshly squeezed orange juice (from ½ orange)
> ½ teaspoon ground cumin
> ¼ teaspoon ground cardamom
> ¼ teaspoon cinnamon
> ½ tablespoon honey
> ¼ teaspoon turmeric
> 1 teaspoon grated fresh ginger root
> 1 tablespoon olive oil

Add orzo to boiling water and continue boiling until tender (about 10 minutes). Drain well. Mix all salad ingredients with cooked orzo. Combine all dressing ingredients and blend well. Pour dressing over salad and mix well. Chill and serve.

Makes 6 cups.

PER cup:
CALORIES 229   FIBER 4 gm
CSI <1   SODIUM 9 mg
FAT 4 gm

*Orzo is a rice-shaped macaroni product found in the macaroni/noodle section of most supermarkets.

†Zest of orange and lemon is the outer peel without any of the white layer. It is obtained by using a vegetable peeler or "zester."

ORANGE BULGUR SALAD

These unusual combinations make a delicious salad. This would be a nice dish for a backyard barbecue.

> 1 cup uncooked bulgur
> 3 cups boiling water
> ⅔ cup grated carrots
> ½ cup chopped green onions, including green part
> ⅓ cup raisins
> ¼ cup frozen orange juice concentrate, thawed
> 2 tablespoons vinegar
> ½ teaspoon cinnamon
> Dash allspice
> Dash cayenne

Put bulgur in bowl and pour boiling water over it; let sit for about 20 minutes. Drain thoroughly. Add carrots, green onions, and raisins. In separate bowl combine orange juice concentrate, vinegar, cinnamon, allspice, and cayenne to make dressing. Add to bulgur mixture and toss lightly. Serve at room temperature.

Makes 4 cups.

PER cup:
CALORIES 252   FIBER 7 gm
CSI trace   SODIUM 15 mg
FAT 1 gm

POTATO SALAD

This tastes like the all-American favorite and is much lower in fat. Remember, low-fat dressings need to be added just before serving or the salad will be dry.

> 6 medium potatoes
> 3 hard-cooked egg whites
> ½ cup finely chopped sweet pickles
> ¼ cup finely chopped onion
> ⅛ teaspoon pepper

Cook unpeeled potatoes until tender (about 45 minutes). Drain and peel while hot. Stir with fork to break up into very small pieces. Add chopped egg whites, pickles, onion, and pepper. Refrigerate in covered container until serving time.

DRESSING

> 1 cup plain nonfat yogurt
> ¼ cup light mayonnaise
> 6 tablespoons sweet pickle juice
> 1 tablespoon prepared mustard

Mix together and refrigerate.

Just before serving: Mix dressing with potato mixture. Garnish with paprika. Leftover salad will become dry and need more dressing before it is served.

Makes 4–6 servings (about 1 cup each).

PER cup:
CALORIES 206   FIBER 4 gm
CSI 1   SODIUM 306 mg
FAT 4 gm

TABOULI

This salad keeps very well and can be made ahead of time.

> 1 cup uncooked bulgur
> 2 cups boiling water
> 2 tomatoes, finely diced
> 1 bunch green onions with tops, sliced
> 3 tablespoons chopped fresh mint *or* 2 teaspoons dried mint
> 1 cup finely chopped parsley
> 3 tablespoons olive oil
> ½ cup freshly squeezed lemon juice
> Pepper to taste

Three to 4 hours before serving time, place uncooked bulgur in a large bowl. Pour boiling water over the bulgur and let soak for 1 hour. Stir occasionally. Drain well in fine strainer. Return bulgur to bowl and stir in other ingredients. Chill for about 2 hours.

Makes 6 cups.

PER cup:
CALORIES 178   FIBER 4 gm
CSI 1   SODIUM 72 mg
FAT 8 gm

BEAN SALADS

CALIFORNIA BEANS—*EASY*

This colorful salad is high in fiber and iron. It makes a great filling for pocket bread for lunch or serve as a hearty salad with a favorite fish.

1 can (16 ounces) kidney beans,* drained and rinsed under cold water
3 cups broccoli flowerets
1½ cups chopped celery
1¼ cups chopped green onions
⅓ cup raisins
Freshly ground black pepper
2 tablespoons light mayonnaise
¼ cup wine vinegar

Combine beans, vegetables, raisins, and pepper. Mix light mayonnaise and vinegar until smooth. Add to rest of ingredients and chill.
Makes 6 cups.

*Use low-sodium beans if available.

PER cup:
CALORIES 126   FIBER 7 gm
CSI trace   SODIUM 182 mg
FAT 2 gm

CHILI BEAN SALAD

A colorful and unusual salad. This is a great main dish sandwich when served in pocket bread. Try it for a brown bag lunch (assemble at eating time).

1 can (16 ounces) kidney beans*
1 can (16 ounces) pinto beans*
1 can (16 ounces) garbanzo beans*
1 can (16 ounces) unsalted whole kernel corn
½ cup chopped green onions
¼ cup chopped parsley
1 cup sliced celery
1 can (4 ounces) diced green chiles, drained

Drain and rinse beans and corn. Combine all ingredients.

DRESSING

2 tablespoons oil
¼ cup vinegar
1–2 cloves garlic, minced
1 teaspoon chili powder
1 teaspoon oregano leaves
¼ teaspoon ground cumin
⅛–½ teaspoon pepper *or* taco sauce (to taste)

Mix all ingredients together. Pour dressing over salad, mix well, and chill 6 hours or overnight (stirring several times).
Makes 10 servings (1 cup each).

*Use low-sodium beans if available.

PER cup:
CALORIES 255   FIBER 9 gm
CSI <1   SODIUM 353 mg
FAT 5 gm

SPICY BLACK BEAN SALAD—*EASY*

A delicious salad we originally found in a deli. Be creative and use as a filling for pita bread or roll up in a flour tortilla. Several companies are marketing canned black beans, which greatly speeds up the preparation time.

1 can (15 ounces) black beans,* drained and rinsed *or* 1⅓ cups cooked dry beans
½ cup chopped celery
⅓ cup chopped green onion
1 cup chopped tomato
1 tablespoon chopped fresh cilantro
1 tablespoon wine vinegar
1 tablespoon olive oil
½ teaspoon Tabasco sauce
¼ teaspoon pepper
1 cup cooked rice (white or brown)

Combine black beans, celery, green onion, tomato, and cilantro. Mix together vinegar, oil, Tabasco sauce, and pepper; pour over bean mixture and mix. Add cooked rice and mix well. Serve cold.

Makes 4 cups.

*Use low-sodium beans if available.

PER cup:
CALORIES 228   FIBER 11 gm
CSI <1   SODIUM 245 mg
FAT 4 gm

SUMMER BEAN SALAD

A very colorful salad that is easy to prepare.

1 can (15 ounces) black beans,* drained
1 can (15 ounces) white beans,* drained
½ cup sliced green onions
1 cup diced red bell pepper
1 cup diced green bell pepper
1½ cups chopped tomatoes
3 tablespoons red wine vinegar
2 tablespoons olive oil
½ teaspoon Lite Salt or less
1 clove garlic, minced
½ teaspoon freshly ground black pepper

Combine beans, onions, bell peppers, and tomato in a salad bowl. Mix vinegar, oil, Lite Salt, garlic, and black pepper until well blended. Pour over bean mixture, toss gently. Cover and marinate in refrigerator for at least 4 hours.

Makes 7 cups.

*Use low-sodium beans if available.

PER cup:
CALORIES 199   FIBER 12 gm
CSI <1   SODIUM 329 gm
FAT 4 gm

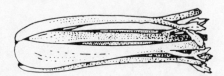

SALAD DRESSINGS

A variety of salad dressings can add a great deal to greens. You will see how we use nonfat plain yogurt to dilute the fat of even light mayonnaise or Miracle Whip Light. If you find the proportion of yogurt to mayonnaise too much for your tastes, alter it and then gradually increase the yogurt and decrease the mayonnaise until you reach the amounts given in the recipes.

Fresh Ginger Salad Dressing
Hearty Ranch Salad Dressing
Red French Salad Dressing
Russian Salad Dressing
Tangy Salad Dressing

Thousand Island Salad Dressing
Vinaigrette Salad Dressing with Greens
    (see page 294 in "Salads" section)
Western Salad Dressing and Mix

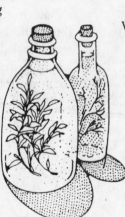

FRESH GINGER SALAD DRESSING

Serve over fresh greens with any Oriental dish.

6 tablespoons rice vinegar
3 tablespoons lower-sodium soy sauce
2 tablespoons sugar
1 tablespoon sesame oil
1½ tablespoons minced ginger root
1 clove garlic, minced

Combine all ingredients and stir or shake in jar with a tight lid, until sugar is dissolved.

Makes 14 tablespoons (enough for 10 cups of greens).

PER tablespoon:
CALORIES 19　　　　FIBER trace
CSI trace　　　　　SODIUM 129 mg
FAT 1 gm

HEARTY RANCH SALAD DRESSING

This dressing is thinner than the commercial version, but the flavor is great.

1 package (1 ounce) Ranch Salad
　Dressing Mix
1 cup buttermilk
¾ cup nonfat plain yogurt
¼ cup light mayonnaise

Combine all ingredients and mix well with wire whisk. Store in covered container in refrigerator. (Keeps fresh for 3 to 4 weeks.)

Makes 2 cups.

PER tablespoon:
CALORIES 13　　　　FIBER 0 gm
CSI trace　　　　　SODIUM 85 mg
FAT <1 gm

RED FRENCH SALAD DRESSING

The secret is to have this prepared and ready to use.

1 cup ketchup
½ cup sugar
⅓ cup oil
½ cup vinegar
Onion powder
Freshly ground black pepper

Combine all ingredients and mix well.
Makes about 2⅓ cups.

PER tablespoon:
CALORIES 37　　　　FIBER trace
CSI trace　　　　　SODIUM 79 mg
FAT 2 gm

RUSSIAN SALAD DRESSING

A delicious low-salt and low-fat version.

1 can (10½ ounces) low-sodium tomato soup
¼ cup oil
Peel of ½ lemon, grated
2 tablespoons freshly squeezed lemon juice
2 tablespoons chopped green onion
1 teaspoon prepared horseradish
Dash ground cinnamon (optional)
1 clove garlic, crushed (optional)

Blend tomato soup. Combine all ingredients in jar with lid. Chill. Shake well before serving.
Makes about 1¾ cups.

PER tablespoon:
CALORIES 25   FIBER trace
CSI trace   SODIUM 1 mg
FAT 2 gm

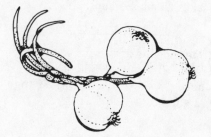

TANGY SALAD DRESSING

We've found this combination to be creamy enough in taste for mayonnaise lovers, yet low enough in fat to be a real improvement over commercial "imitation" salad dressings, which still contain considerable fat.

1 cup nonfat yogurt
¼ cup light mayonnaise

Blend well.
Makes 1¼ cups.

NOTE: This makes an excellent homemade creamy salad dressing. Use it for cole-slaw, potato salad, or in recipes where large amounts of mayonnaise are required. It is somewhat tarter than mayonnaise alone, so you may want to reduce the vinegar or lemon juice in your tried-and-true recipes.

PER tablespoon:
CALORIES 14   FIBER 0 gm
CSI trace   SODIUM 22 mg
FAT <1 gm

THOUSAND ISLAND SALAD DRESSING

A low-fat version of an all-time favorite.

½ cup low-fat cottage cheese
2 tablespoons plain nonfat yogurt
2 tablespoons light mayonnaise
2 tablespoons ketchup
Dash cayenne pepper
1 tablespoon skim milk (or more for desired thickness)

Combine ingredients and blend thoroughly. Add:

1 tablespoon chopped dill pickles
1 tablespoon finely chopped onion

Makes 1 cup.

PER tablespoon:
CALORIES 17   FIBER trace
CSI trace   SODIUM 70 mg
FAT <1 gm

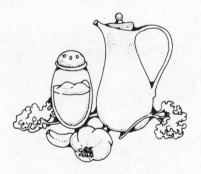

WESTERN SALAD DRESSING AND MIX

This is a ranch-type salad dressing that is much lower in salt than the commercial versions.

WESTERN DRESSING

1 teaspoon Dry Mix, (see below)
¼ cup light mayonnaise
¾ cup plain nonfat yogurt
1 cup buttermilk

Prepare Dry Mix. Carefully measure 1 teaspoon of the mix and add to mayonnaise, yogurt, and buttermilk. Blend well (a wire whisk is handy for this). Store in an airtight container in the refrigerator. (Flavor is best when made 24 hours before using.)
Makes 2 cups salad dressing.

DRY MIX

2 teaspoons Lite Salt or less
2 teaspoons dried parsley flakes
1 teaspoon garlic powder
½ teaspoon pepper
½ teaspoon onion powder

Put all ingredients in a small jar and shake well to mix. Store in airtight container. Shake before measuring out to use.
Makes 6 teaspoons (enough for 12 cups of prepared dressing).

PER tablespoon of prepared dressing:
CALORIES 13   FIBER trace
CSI trace   SODIUM 35 mg
FAT <1 gm

SOUPS

One can never have enough soup recipes. Not all recipes that could be categorized as "soups" are in this section. A recipe for a chili made from black beans is in our section of main dishes featuring vegetables, grains, and beans. Recipes for soups that contain small bits of fish, poultry, or lean red meats can be found in those sections. As always, all soups taste better if allowed to simmer two to three hours and are even better if refrigerated overnight and served the next day.

Lighter Soups
  French Onion Soup
  Gazpacho (a cold soup)
  Hot and Sour Soup
  Tomato Soup

Hearty Soups
  Creamy Chicken Noodle Soup
  Fish and Leek Chowder (see page 374 in "Fish and Shellfish" section)
  Greek Lentil Soup—*Easy*
  Greek-Style Garbanzo Soup—*Quick*
  Hungarian Mushroom Soup

  Lentil Soup
  Minestrone Soup
  Navy Bean Soup
  Potato Leek Soup
  Split Pea Soup
  Turkey-Vegetable Chowder (see page 396 in "Chicken and Turkey" section)
  Vegetable Beef Soup (see page 405 in "Beef and Pork" section)

Specialty Soup
  Homemade "Cream" Soup Mix

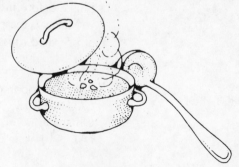

LIGHTER SOUPS

FRENCH ONION SOUP

An elegant soup for onion lovers.

SOUP

>   1 tablespoon oil
>   6 cups sliced onions
>   ¼ teaspoon sugar or less
>   2 tablespoons flour
>   3 cups water
>   1 can (10½ ounces) beef broth
>   ½ cup dry white wine *or* vermouth
>   Pepper

Heat oil in 3-quart pan. Add onions and sugar and sauté slowly until golden brown. Use medium-low heat and stir often (takes 30 minutes or more). Stir in flour and cook 2 minutes longer. Remove from heat and stir in water, broth, and wine. Simmer partially covered for 15 minutes. Season to taste with pepper. Can be refrigerated at this point to serve later, if desired. The flavor is enhanced by refrigerating overnight and reheating.

BREAD

>   6 slices French bread (with small diameter), cut ½ inch thick
>   3 tablespoons grated part-skim mozzarella cheese
>   3 tablespoons grated Parmesan cheese

Toast bread in 325° oven for 20 minutes. Save cheese to add at serving time. Store bread in an airtight container to keep bread crisp until ready to serve.

To serve:

Heat soup slowly until very hot. Sprinkle cheese on toasted bread and brown under broiler. Float 1 piece bread in each bowl of soup.

Makes 6 servings (1⅓ cups each).

PER cup:
CALORIES 109   FIBER 2 gm
CSI 2   SODIUM 203 mg
FAT 4 gm

GAZPACHO (A COLD SOUP)

This is a cold tomato soup made with small chunks of your favorite vegetables. Prepare early on a hot day so it will be nicely chilled. This soup travels very well to concerts in the park.

>   2 cans (16 ounces each) unsalted tomatoes
>   ¼ cup wine vinegar
>   ½ teaspoon garlic powder or less
>   Cayenne pepper to taste
>   1 can (14½ ounces) lower-salt chicken broth
>   1 small avocado, cut in half, peeled, and sliced
>   1 tomato, chopped
>   12 ripe olives, cut into wedges
>   ½ cup thinly sliced and chopped cucumber
>   2 tablespoons sliced green onions
>   2 limes, cut into wedges (optional)

(continued)

Mix first 4 ingredients in a blender. Add chicken broth, vegetables, and olives. Chill at least 4 hours. Serve very cold and with lime wedges, if desired.

Makes 7 cups.

PER cup:
CALORIES 99
CSI 1
FAT 6 gm
FIBER 4 gm
SODIUM 264 mg

HOT AND SOUR SOUP

3 or 4 dried black mushrooms
1 cup boiling water
12 ounces tofu (bean curd)
2 tablespoons cornstarch
¼ cup water
5 cups lower-salt chicken broth
1 tablespoon sherry
2 tablespoons white vinegar
1 teaspoon lower-sodium soy sauce
¼ teaspoon white pepper
2 tablespoons egg substitute, beaten (commercial *or Homemade Egg Substitute,* page 283)
½ cup frozen peas
Few drops sesame oil
1 green onion, minced

Soak dried mushrooms in 1 cup boiling water for 30 minutes, reserving soaking liquid for later use. Sliver mushrooms and bean curd. Blend cornstarch and ¼ cup water to a paste. Bring broth and mushroom-soaking liquid to a boil. Add mushrooms and simmer, covered, 10 minutes. Stir in sherry, white vinegar, soy sauce, and pepper. Thicken with cornstarch paste. Slowly add egg substitute, stirring gently once or twice. This may be prepared in advance and refrigerated until serving time. When ready to serve, heat the soup, add the bean curd and frozen peas, and heat for 1 minute or until peas are thawed. Remove from heat. Sprinkle with sesame oil and green onion.

VARIATIONS

In place of white vinegar, substitute wine vinegar or lemon juice. For the sesame oil, substitute Tabasco sauce. Omit vinegar and pepper—it's then called "Mandarin Soup."

Makes 9 cups.

PER cup:
CALORIES 68
CSI <1
FAT 3 gm
FIBER <1 gm
SODIUM 468 mg

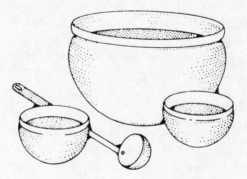

TOMATO SOUP

A homemade version of an old standby.

- 1 carrot, chopped
- 2 stalks celery, chopped
- ¼ cup water
- 3 cups unsalted canned *or* fresh tomatoes, peeled
- ½ teaspoon basil leaves
- ¼ teaspoon oregano leaves
- 1 cup powdered nonfat milk
- 2 bouillon cubes
- 1 quart water
- Pepper to taste

Steam carrots and celery in ¼ cup water until tender. Add tomatoes, basil and oregano. Simmer gently for 5 minutes. Puree tomato mixture in blender or food mill. Blend in powdered milk. Pour back into pan. Dissolve bouillon cubes in 1 quart of water and add to other ingredients. Heat thoroughly but do not boil. Add pepper to taste.

Makes 8 cups.

OPTIONAL
A little wine *or* brandy makes this a very fancy soup.

PER cup:
CALORIES 55   FIBER 1 gm
CSI trace   SODIUM 299 mg
FAT trace

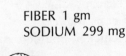
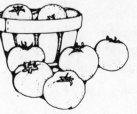

HEARTY SOUPS

CREAMY CHICKEN NOODLE SOUP

- 2 teaspoons oil
- 1¼ cups chopped onion (1 large)
- 1 can (14½ ounces) *or* 2 cups lower-salt chicken broth
- 6 cups water
- 3 cloves garlic, minced
- 1 teaspoon thyme leaves
- ¼ teaspoon pepper
- ¼ teaspoon dill weed
- 1 teaspoon Lite Salt or less
- 4 or 5 sprigs parsley
- 1 cup sliced carrots (3 small)
- 6 ounces wide eggless noodles (about 2 cups)
- 1¼ cups cubed, cooked chicken (2 chicken breasts)
- 2 cups nonfat plain yogurt
- 1 tablespoon cornstarch
- ½ teaspoon sugar
- 6 green onions, chopped (including green tops)

Heat oil in 6-quart kettle; add onion and cook until limp, about 5 minutes. Add broth, water, garlic, thyme, pepper, dill, Lite Salt, parsley, and carrots. Bring to a boil; reduce heat, cover, and simmer for about 30 minutes or until carrots are partially cooked.

Remove parsley sprigs and discard. Stir in noodles and cook, uncovered until ten-

(continued)

der, about 8–10 minutes. Add cooked chicken.

In separate bowl, blend yogurt and cornstarch until smooth. Add to soup, stirring and increase heat to high until soup boils and thickens slightly. Add sugar to offset tartness of yogurt. Serve hot and garnish each serving with green onions.

Makes 8 cups.

PER cup:
CALORIES 185   FIBER 2 gm
CSI 3   SODIUM 366 mg
FAT 3 gm

GREEK LENTIL SOUP—*EASY*

Lentil soup and baked potatoes are a natural combination. Serve the potatoes with *Mock Sour Cream* (page 451) or nonfat yogurt.

    2 cups uncooked lentils
    8 cups water
    ½ cup chopped onions
    ¾ cup chopped carrots
    1 cup chopped celery
    1 cup chopped potatoes
    2 bay leaves
    ½ teaspoon ground cumin
    ½ teaspoon Lite Salt or less
    2 teaspoons freshly squeezed lemon
      juice

Cook all ingredients except lemon juice in a large pot until lentils are soft, about 45 minutes. Add lemon juice and serve.

Makes about 10 cups.

PER cup:
CALORIES 149   FIBER 7 gm
CSI trace   SODIUM 67 mg
FAT 1 gm

GREEK-STYLE GARBANZO SOUP—*QUICK*

Very quick to prepare and delicious! Serve with whole wheat rolls.

    2 tablespoons olive oil
    2 medium onions, chopped
    1 clove garlic, minced
    2 stalks celery, chopped
    1 or 2 carrots, sliced
    1 large potato, diced
    1 sprig parsley, finely chopped
    1 green bell pepper, chopped
    1 can (6 ounces) unsalted tomato paste
    ¼ teaspoon black pepper
    2 cans (16 ounces each) garbanzo
      beans, drained*
    5 cups water
    1 chicken bouillon cube

Heat oil in a kettle and sauté onions, garlic, and celery for about 5 minutes. Add the remaining vegetables, tomato paste, and pepper. Add garbanzo beans, water,

*Use low-sodium beans if available.

(continued)

and bouillon cube. Bring to boil and simmer for 10 minutes. Stir well before serving.

Makes 14 cups.

PER cup:
CALORIES 156   FIBER 4 gm
CSI trace   SODIUM 240 mg
FAT 4 gm

HUNGARIAN MUSHROOM SOUP

Nice to make a day ahead so the flavors can develop.

2 cups chopped onions
1 tablespoon olive oil
3 cups sliced mushrooms
½ teaspoon Lite Salt or less
1 teaspoon dill weed
½ cup water
1 tablespoon lower-sodium soy sauce
¼ cup chopped parsley
⅛ teaspoon black pepper
1 tablespoon Hungarian sweet paprika
1½ cups water
1 cup skim milk
2 tablespoons cornstarch (for a thinner soup, reduce cornstarch)
¼ cup cold water
¾ cup plain nonfat yogurt
2 teaspoons freshly squeezed lemon juice
¼ cup chopped parsley, to garnish

Sauté onions in oil. Add mushrooms, Lite Salt, dill weed, ½ cup water, soy sauce,

parsley, pepper, and paprika. Cover and simmer 30 minutes. Add 1½ cups water, and the skim milk. Dissolve cornstarch in ¼ cup water. Bring soup to a boil and while stirring, add cornstarch/water mixture. Cook 1–2 minutes. Soup can be made ahead to this point and chilled.

Just before serving, add yogurt and lemon juice and heat through. If serving immediately, do not add cold yogurt to hot soup or it will curdle. Rather, while stirring yogurt, add a cup of hot soup to yogurt. Then stir mixture into hot soup, add lemon juice, and serve. Chopped parsley makes a nice garnish.

Makes 5 cups (4 servings).

PER cup:
CALORIES 116   FIBER 2 gm
CSI <1   SODIUM 277 mg
FAT 3 gm

LENTIL SOUP

An old standby—nice to serve with *Cereal Bran Muffins* (page 271).

½ pound lentils
2 tablespoons olive oil
2 medium onions, finely chopped
1 clove garlic, minced
2 stalks celery, finely chopped
1 carrot, thinly sliced
¼ cup chopped parsley
½ teaspoon Lite Salt or less
¼ teaspoon black pepper
6 cups water
2 beef bouillon cubes
1 tablespoon freshly squeezed lemon juice

(continued)

Wash lentils well. Cover with water. Bring to a boil and cook gently for 10 minutes. Drain and set aside. Heat oil in a skillet. Sauté onions and garlic for five minutes. Add chopped vegetables and sauté for 15 minutes. Place lentils, sautéed vegetables, water, Lite Salt, and pepper in kettle. Bring to a boil and cook slowly for 2 hours. Add bouillon cubes and stir to dissolve. Before serving add lemon juice.

Makes 8 cups.

PER cup:

CALORIES 145	FIBER 5 gm
CSI <1	SODIUM 317 mg
FAT 4 gm	

MINESTRONE SOUP

This hearty soup needs only some crusty French bread and fruit to make a fine meal.

- ½ cup uncooked navy beans
- 1 can (14½ ounces) lower-salt chicken broth
- 1 quart water
- 2 medium carrots, cut in small strips
- ½ small head cabbage, shredded
- 1 medium potato, diced
- 1 can (16 ounces) unsalted tomatoes
- 1 medium onion, sliced
- 1½ tablespoons olive oil
- 1 stalk celery, sliced diagonally
- 1 zucchini, sliced
- 2 cloves garlic, minced

- ⅛ teaspoon pepper
- ¼ teaspoon Lite Salt or less
- ½ teaspoon basil leaves
- ¼ teaspoon marjoram leaves *or* ⅛ teaspoon ground marjoram
- 2 tablespoons chopped parsley
- 1 can (8 ounces) unsalted tomato sauce (optional)
- ½ cup broken uncooked spaghetti*

In a very large kettle (6–8 quart) add navy beans to chicken broth and water. Cover and cook together for 1 hour. Add carrots, cabbage, potatoes, and tomatoes. Cook another 30 minutes. Sauté onions in oil until translucent. Add celery, zucchini, garlic, pepper, Lite Salt, basil, and marjoram. Continue to sauté until tender. Add to beans and vegetable mixture. Add parsley and tomato sauce. Cook 20 minutes. Add more water if too thick. Add spaghetti and cook for 10 additional minutes.

Makes 14 cups.

*If you are going to freeze leftover soup, do not add spaghetti as it does not freeze well.

PER cup:

CALORIES 81	FIBER 4 gm
CSI trace	SODIUM 102 mg
FAT 2 gm	

NAVY BEAN SOUP

The Senate's famous bean soup without the meat! The ground cloves add an unusual flavor.

2 cups uncooked white beans
8 cups water
½ teaspoon Lite Salt or less
⅛ teaspoon pepper
1 bay leaf
2 cups chopped celery
1 cup chopped carrots
1 cup chopped onion
1 can (8 ounces) unsalted tomato sauce
¼ cup chopped parsley
Dash of ground cloves

Soak beans at least 3 hours in cold water. Drain. Add 8 cups water, Lite Salt, pepper, and bay leaf. Bring to a boil, then simmer for 2 hours or until beans are tender. Add celery, carrots, onions, tomato sauce, parsley, and cloves. Mash some of the beans to thicken the soup. Simmer for 2 hours.

Makes 16 cups.

———————

PER cup:
CALORIES 79   FIBER 6 gm
CSI trace   SODIUM 49 mg
FAT <1 gm

POTATO LEEK SOUP

Chunky potatoes and savory leeks make this soup very tasty. Serve with bread and a tossed green salad.

4 leeks
1 tablespoon margarine
4 cups potatoes, peeled and chopped (3 large or 4 medium)
5 cups water
1 cup skim milk
½ teaspoon Lite Salt or less
¼ teaspoon pepper

Wash leeks thoroughly and cut up into small rounds. Use both the white and green parts. Melt the margarine in a large pot. Add cut-up leeks and cook for 5 minutes over medium heat, until leeks are limp. Add potatoes and water and bring to a boil. Boil uncovered for 30 minutes until potatoes are thoroughly cooked. (They should fall apart when prodded with a folk.) Add the skim milk, Lite Salt, and pepper. The soup should be thick, creamy, and green from the color of the leeks. Mash some of the potato chunks to thicken the soup or puree in blender if smooth creamy soup is desired.

Makes 10 cups.

———————

PER cup:
CALORIES 61   FIBER 1 gm
CSI trace   SODIUM 68 mg
FAT 1 gm

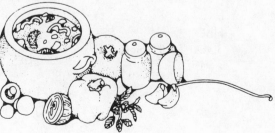

Exc!

SPLIT PEA SOUP

Hearty enough for a meal—try this with *Onion Squares* (page 338).

- 2 cups uncooked split peas
- 5 cups water or more
- 1 bay leaf
- ¾ teaspoon Lite Salt or less
- 2 cups chopped carrots
- 1 cup chopped celery
- 1 cup chopped onion
- ½ teaspoon thyme leaves
- ½ teaspoon pepper
- ½ teaspoon garlic powder
- 2 tablespoons vinegar *or* freshly squeezed lemon juice

Combine dried split peas, water, bay leaf, and Lite Salt in a large kettle. Bring to a boil and then reduce heat and simmer for 2 hours. Stir occasionally and check to make sure there is enough water and that the split peas do not stick. Add more water if it becomes too dry. Add carrots, celery, onions, and herbs. Continue to simmer for 30 minutes or longer (overcooking cannot hurt this soup, as long as it is stirred to prevent sticking). Just before serving add the vinegar or lemon juice and more pepper, if desired.

Makes about 12 cups.

PER cup:
CALORIES 106   FIBER 5 gm
CSI trace   SODIUM 91 mg
FAT 1 gm

SPECIALTY SOUP

HOMEMADE ''CREAM'' SOUP MIX

Use this in place of canned cream soups in casseroles or as a base for your own soups. Much lower in fat and salt than the canned versions. The trick is to have it made up ready to use!

- 2 cups powdered nonfat milk
- ¾ cups cornstarch
- ¼ cup (or less) instant chicken bouillon
- 2 tablespoons dried onion flakes
- 1 teaspoon basil leaves
- 1 teaspoon thyme leaves
- ½ teaspoon pepper

Combine all ingredients, mixing well. Store in an airtight container until ready to use.

To substitute for one can of condensed soup: Combine ⅓ cup of dry mix with 1¼ cups of cold water in a saucepan. Cook and stir until thickened. Add to casserole as you would the canned product.

Makes equivalent of 9 cans of soup.

PER ⅑ recipe:
CALORIES 131   FIBER trace
CSI <1   SODIUM 728 mg
FAT 1 gm

SANDWICHES

Recipes for sandwiches with low CSIs are not easy to come by. This section should help. We are promoting bean burritos, meatless pizzas, and there are ideas for lean hamburgers.

Sandwich Spreads
    "Egg" Salad Sandwich Spread
    Fruit-Nut Sandwich Spread
    Tofu "Egg" Salad Sandwich
    Tuna Salad Sandwich Spread—*Quick*
    Veggie Pockets with Creamy Dressing
    Vegetable–Cottage Cheese Sandwich
       Spread

Sandwiches
    Baked Bean Special Sandwich
    Burritos with Black Beans
    Falafel—*Quick*
       Tahini Dressing
       Yogurt Dressing
    Pita Pizza—*Quick*
    Skinny Burgers—*Quick*
    Very Skinny Burgers—*Quick*
    Your Basic Bean Burrito—*Quick*

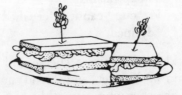

SANDWICH SPREADS

"EGG" SALAD SANDWICH SPREAD

Use as a sandwich filling or as a salad on crisp lettuce leaves.

1 cup egg substitute (commercial *or* *Homemade Egg Substitute,* page 283)
2 hard-boiled egg whites, chopped
2 tablespoons finely chopped celery
2 tablespoons finely chopped green bell pepper
2 tablespoons finely chopped onion
¼ cup Miracle Whip Light *or* light mayonnaise
Dash pepper
½ teaspoon prepared mustard

Pour egg substitute into an 8-inch nonstick skillet. Cover tightly. Cook over very low heat until just firm to the touch, about 10 minutes. Remove from skillet in large pieces. Cut into small cubes.

Combine cooked egg substitute, egg whites, celery, green peppers, and onions in a mixing bowl. In a separate bowl combine mayonnaise, pepper, and mustard; blend well. Lightly toss with egg substitute mixture. Chill before serving.

Makes filling for 4 sandwiches (2 cups spread).

PER ½ cup:
CALORIES 110
CSI <1
FAT 5 gm
FIBER trace
SODIUM 274 mg

FRUIT-NUT SANDWICH SPREAD

Looking for variety in lunches? Use wheatberry rolls or graham crackers with this filling.

1½ cups low-fat cottage cheese
1 teaspoon freshly squeezed lemon juice
⅓ cup chopped pecans *or* walnuts
⅓ cup raisins
⅓ cup canned crushed pineapple, drained

Place the cottage cheese and lemon juice in a blender and blend until smooth. Scrape mixture out of the blender and into bowl. Stir in pecans *or* walnuts, raisins, and pineapple. Spread ½ cup of mixture on 2 slices of bread to make a sandwich.

Makes filling for 5 sandwiches (2½ cups spread).

PER ½ cup:
CALORIES 162
CSI 2
FAT 7 gm
FIBER 1 gm
SODIUM 279 mg

TOFU "EGG" SALAD SANDWICH

Some say this sandwich spread is even better than the real thing!

4 ounces firm tofu, drained
1½ teaspoons tahini*
1 dill pickle, chopped (about two tablespoons)
¼ teaspoon minced onion
½ teaspoon prepared mustard
½ teaspoon oil
¼ teaspoon turmeric
Pinch basil and celery seed

Crumble tofu into small pieces with a fork. Combine with other ingredients.

Makes 1 cup spread (filling for 2 sandwiches).

*Tahini is sometimes labeled "sesame seed butter" and is usually available in supermarkets in the specialty food section.

PER ½ cup:
CALORIES 66   FIBER 1 gm
CSI <1   SODIUM 168 mg
FAT 5 gm

TUNA SALAD SANDWICH SPREAD—*QUICK*

Yogurt and a small amount of imitation mayonnaise with tuna makes a nice sandwich filling.

1 can (6½ ounces) water-packed tuna
¼ cup diced celery
¼ cup chopped onion
¼ cup plain nonfat yogurt
1 tablespoon light mayonnaise

Drain tuna. Combine with celery, onions, yogurt, and mayonnaise and stir to blend well.

Makes 1½ cups spread.

VARIATION
For a hot sandwich—spread on English muffin halves and place under broiler 2–3 minutes.

PER ½ cup:
CALORIES 111   FIBER trace
CSI 3   SODIUM 285 mg
FAT 2 gm

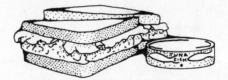

VEGGIE POCKETS WITH CREAMY DRESSING

A meatless lunch idea—fill pockets at serving time and enjoy a light, low-calorie sandwich. This is the day to include a fa-

(continued)

vorite low-fat dessert and fruit for additional calories.

1 cup plain nonfat yogurt
2 tablespoons light mayonnaise
1 tablespoon finely chopped cilantro
1 clove garlic, minced
½ teaspoon sugar
¼ teaspoon Lite Salt or less
¼ teaspoon pepper
2 large tomatoes, chopped (about 2 cups)
1 cup peeled and chopped cucumber
½ cup chopped red onion
10 small or 5 large whole wheat pita breads
4 cups alfalfa sprouts *or* finely chopped lettuce

Combine yogurt, mayonnaise, cilantro, garlic, sugar, ⅛ teaspoon Lite Salt, and ⅛ teaspoon pepper in bowl. In a second bowl, combine tomatoes, cucumber, onion, and remaining Lite Salt and pepper.

When ready to eat, split each pita in half. Line each with about ⅓ cup sprouts or lettuce. Fill with ¼–⅓ cup veggie mixture. Top each with 2 tablespoons dressing.

Makes 10 small pocket sandwiches or 5 large pockets.

PER two small pockets or one large pocket:
CALORIES 234   FIBER 7 gm
CSI <1   SODIUM 448 mg
FAT 3 gm

VEGETABLE-COTTAGE CHEESE SANDWICH SPREAD

Who says sandwiches must have meat?

1½ cups low-fat cottage cheese
½ teaspoon sugar
1 teaspoon freshly squeezed lemon juice
1 tablespoon chopped onion
⅓ cup chopped carrot
¼ cup chopped celery
Dash of Worcestershire sauce

Place the cottage cheese, sugar, and lemon juice in a blender and blend until smooth. Scrape mixture out of the blender and into bowl. Stir in vegetables and Worcestershire sauce.

Makes 2½ cups of spread.

SERVING IDEAS
Serve on whole wheat, pumpernickel, Vienna, rye, or French bread. For a sack lunch, make a poor-boy sandwich of the vegetable spread, lettuce, and tomato slices.

PER ½ cup:
CALORIES 68   FIBER trace
CSI 1   SODIUM 287 mg
FAT 1 gm

slice rye bread, half of an English muffin, or half of a hamburger bun. Top with tomato or pineapple slice. Broil for a few minutes, if desired. Garnish with parsley.

Makes 4 servings.

PER serving:
CALORIES 374   FIBER 11 gm
CSI <1   SODIUM 698 mg
FAT 3 gm

SANDWICHES

BAKED BEAN SPECIAL SANDWICH

An open-faced sandwich that is served warm.

1 can (16-ounces) vegetarian-style baked beans in tomato sauce*
½ cup chopped onion
¼ cup chopped green bell pepper
3 tablespoons brown sugar
1 tablespoon molasses
2 teaspoons Worcestershire sauce
¼ teaspoon dry mustard
¼ teaspoon pepper

8 slices rye bread, English muffin halves, or hamburger buns
8 slices tomato *or* canned pineapple
Parsley (for garnish)

Preheat oven to 400°. Mix first 8 ingredients together well. Place in ovenproof dish, cover, and bake for approximately 45 minutes, stirring occasionally.

Spread ¼ cup of bean mixture on one

*Use low-sodium beans if available.

BURRITOS WITH BLACK BEANS

2 cups *Black Beans With 1000 Uses* (page 357)
4 flour tortillas (8-inch diameter)
1 cup shredded lettuce
¼ cup salsa
½ cup plain nonfat yogurt

Heat black bean filling in saucepan. Soften tortillas by warming in oven or microwave, *or* by placing in an unoiled heated skillet for 1 minute on each side.

Place ½ cup of the hot black beans on a warm tortilla. Add lettuce, salsa, and yogurt. Fold tortilla over and serve.

Makes 4 burritos.

PER burrito:
CALORIES 242   FIBER 5 gm
CSI 2   SODIUM 415 mg
FAT 4 gm

FALAFEL—*QUICK*

Traditional filling for pocket or pita bread in the Middle East.

To make a falafel "sandwich," all you need to do is cut a pita bread in half and put 2 or 3 cooked falafel balls or patties into the open half. Add lettuce, alfalfa sprouts, sliced tomatoes, chopped green onions, and *Yogurt Dressing* or *Tahini Dressing* (see recipes below).

Falafel is not difficult to make, particularly if you use falafel mix found in many supermarkets or delicatessens. Most mixes list the traditional garbanzo beans and yellow peas, wheat germ, onion, parsley, herbs, spices, salt, and baking soda as ingredients.

Instructions on preparation and serving are on the back of the package. We edited them as follows:

1 cup falafel mix
¾ cup water

Mix instant falafel and water. Let stand for 10 minutes. Make into tablespoon-sized patties or balls. Preheat oven to 350°. Place on nonstick cookie sheets and bake for 10 minutes on each side for patties or for 20 minutes if shaped into balls.

Makes 4 servings (one 10-ounce package contains 2 cups dry mix).

Falafel per serving:
CALORIES 124   FIBER 3 gm
CSI trace   SODIUM 39 mg
FAT 2 gm

FALAFEL DRESSINGS

TAHINI DRESSING

¼ cup tahini*
½ cup water or more
1 tablespoon freshly squeezed lemon juice
⅛ teaspoon Lite Salt or less
1 clove garlic (optional)

Mix and serve. Should be the consistency of a creamy salad dressing. Add more water if necessary. Use about 2 tablespoons as a sauce for a falafel sandwich.

Makes ¾ cup.

*Tahini is sometimes labeled "sesame seed butter" and is usually available in supermarkets in the specialty food section.

Tahini Dressing per ¼ cup:
CALORIES 67   FIBER 2 gm
CSI <1   SODIUM 77 mg
FAT 6 gm

YOGURT DRESSING

1 cup plain nonfat yogurt
1 tablespoon freshly squeezed lemon juice
¼ teaspoon Lite Salt or less
1 tablespoon chopped parsley

Combine and serve.
Makes 1 cup.

Yogurt Dressing per ¼ cup:
CALORIES 37   FIBER trace
CSI <1   SODIUM 90 mg
FAT <1 gm

PITA PIZZA—QUICK

A quickie! The amounts listed make one pita pizza.

   1 whole wheat pita bread
   2 tablespoons no-salt-added spaghetti
     sauce
   2 tablespoons finely chopped green bell
     pepper
   2 tablespoons finely chopped mush-
     rooms
   2 tablespoons finely chopped onion
   2 black olives, sliced (optional)
   2 tablespoons shredded imitation moz-
     zarella cheese

Preheat oven to 425°. Spread sauce on one side of unsliced pita bread. Sprinkle green peppers, mushrooms, onions, and black olives over sauce. Sprinkle cheese over vegetables. Place on ungreased pizza pan or cookie sheet. Bake 5–10 minutes or until done.

   Makes 1 pita pizza.

PER pizza:
CALORIES 255   FIBER 1 gm
CSI 3   SODIUM 458 mg
FAT 5 gm

SKINNY BURGERS—QUICK

A hamburger made with a small amount of very lean ground beef can fit into a beginning low-fat eating style. Be sure to include other dishes that are very low in fat (baked beans, a hearty salad, fruit, and a dessert, etc.).

   1 pound ground beef (10 percent fat)
   4 hamburger buns
   ¼ cup ketchup *or* mustard
   12 slices dill pickle
   ¼ cup light mayonnaise
   4 lettuce leaves
   4 tomato slices
   4 onion slices

Make 4 patties of equal size and grill over charcoal or broil. Toast buns and assemble with remaining ingredients.

   Makes 4 hamburgers.

PER serving:
CALORIES 375   FIBER 1 gm
CSI 8   SODIUM 708 mg
FAT 15 gm

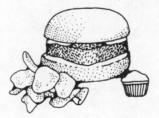

VERY SKINNY BURGERS—QUICK

A small burger naturally means fewer calories. For a filling meal, add corn on the cob, a large salad, and dessert.

> ¾ pound ground beef (10 percent fat)
> 4 hamburger buns *or* English muffins
> ¼ cup ketchup *or* mustard
> 2 tablespoons light mayonnaise
> 4 lettuce leaves
> 4 tomato slices
> 4 onion slices

Make 4 patties and grill over charcoal or broil. Toast buns and assemble with remaining ingredients.

Makes 4 hamburgers.

PER serving:

CALORIES 288	FIBER 1 gm
CSI 5	SODIUM 471 mg
FAT 10 gm	

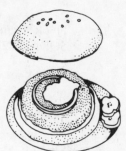

YOUR BASIC BEAN BURRITO—QUICK

Perfect for a quick meal. This recipe is for 1 burrito and is very low-fat.

> ½ cup *Refried Beans* (page 331) *or* ½ cup canned vegetarian refried beans*
> 1 tablespoon canned, chopped green chiles (optional)
> 1 flour tortilla (8-inch diameter)
> 2 tablespoons chopped tomato
> 1 tablespoon chopped green onion
> ¼ cup shredded lettuce
> 2 tablespoons plain nonfat yogurt

Heat refried beans in a small saucepan. Add green chiles if used. Soften tortilla by warming in oven or microwave *or* by placing in an unoiled heated skillet for 1 minute on each side. Place hot beans on warm tortilla and sprinkle chopped tomatoes, onions, lettuce, and yogurt over beans. Fold tortilla over and eat quickly—before it cools.

Makes 1 serving.

*Use low-sodium beans if available.

PER burrito:

CALORIES 269	FIBER 9 gm
CSI 2	SODIUM 221 mg
FAT 5 gm	

SIDE DISHES

We always debate whether these recipes should go into the section on main dishes featuring vegetables, grains, and beans—because many of us serve these recipes as main dishes. However, we elected to place them in the side dish section because we feel most people would serve them as accompaniments for fish, poultry, or lean red meat entrées. Plan to have leftovers of these dishes—they make for great lunches.

Grain Dishes
   Bulgur Pilaf—*Easy*
   Calico Pasta
   Fettuccine, at Last!
   Gourmet Curried Rice—*Easy*
   Green Rice
   Lemon Rice—*Easy*
   Mushroom Barley Pilaf
   Pine Needle Rice
   Pulihora (Tamarind Rice)
   Spanish Rice
   Spicy Peanut Noodles
   Spinach and Rice Casserole

Bean Dishes
   Classic Baked Beans
   Rancher's Beans—*Quick*
   Refried Beans

Potato Dishes
   Holiday Yams
   Homemade Tatertots
   Italian Potatoes
   Mashed Potatoes

Plank Potatoes—*Easy*
Potato Puff
Scalloped Potatoes
Skinny "French Fries"
Skinny Hash Browns (see page 284 in "Breakfasts and Brunches" section)
Spuds and Onions
Super Stuffed Potatoes

Vegetable Dishes
Acorn Squash with Roasted Onions
Cheesy Cauliflower—*Quick*
Corn Bake—*Easy*
Easy Acorn Squash
Eggplant Parmesan
Grilled Zucchini—*Quick*
Onion Squares
Oriental Broccoli
Ratatouille Provençale
Stir-Fried Mushrooms and Broccoli
Stuffed Zucchini Boats
Tomatoes "Provençale"
Zucchini Puff—*Easy*

GRAIN DISHES

BULGUR PILAF—*EASY*

1 teaspoon margarine
1 cup uncooked bulgur
1 teaspoon minced onion
1 cup lower-salt chicken broth
1 cup water
¼ teaspoon oregano leaves
Few grains pepper

Melt margarine in skillet. Add bulgur and onion. Stir and cook until golden. Add broth, water, and seasonings. Cover and bring to boil. Reduce heat and simmer for 15 minutes.

Makes 4 servings.

PER serving:
CALORIES 156   FIBER 4 gm
CSI trace   SODIUM 208 mg
FAT 2 gm

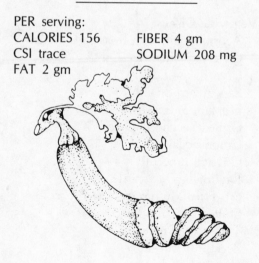

CALICO PASTA

An excellent pasta and vegetable side dish for *Juicy Flank Steak* (page 407) or any fish entrée. Use couscous for something unusual.

1 cup uncooked acini* *or* couscous
1 tablespoon olive oil
2 cloves garlic, minced
1 sweet green or red bell pepper, cut into ½-inch squares (red makes it look very nice)
1½ cups chopped zucchini
2 green onions, sliced
1 teaspoon Lite Salt or less
1 teaspoon basil leaves
¼ teaspoon white pepper

Boil acini or couscous until tender, 4–6 minutes. Drain and rinse with cold water. Drain again.

Heat olive oil in a large nonstick skillet. Add garlic, pepper, zucchini, green onion, Lite Salt, basil, and pepper. Sauté 1 minute. Add cooked acini or couscous and cook until vegetables are heated through, about another 3 to 4 minutes. Serve immediately.

Makes 5 cups.

*Spaghetti that has been cut very short.

PER cup:
CALORIES 142   FIBER 1 gm
CSI trace   SODIUM 198 mg
FAT 3 gm

FETTUCCINE, AT LAST!

An easy-to-make, low-fat version of Fettuccine Alfredo. Make immediately before serving for best results.

- 8 ounces fettuccine or linguini, eggless if possible
- 2 teaspoons olive oil
- 1 can (12 ounces) evaporated skim milk
- 4 tablespoons freshly grated Parmesan cheese, divided
- ¼ cup sliced green onion
- 2 tablespoons snipped fresh basil *or* ½ teaspoon dried basil leaves, crushed
- ¼ teaspoon finely shredded lemon peel
- 2 cloves garlic, crushed
- ⅛ teaspoon pepper
- **Fresh basil sprigs (for garnish)**

Cook pasta in unsalted water. Drain; immediately return to pan. Add olive oil; toss to coat.

Add milk, 3 tablespoons Parmesan cheese, onion, basil, lemon peel, garlic, and pepper. Cook over medium heat until bubbly, stirring constantly. Top with 1 tablespoon Parmesan cheese and decorate with fresh basil. Serve immediately.

Makes 4 servings (1 cup each).

PER cup:
CALORIES 358   FIBER 2 gm
CSI 2   SODIUM 206 mg
FAT 5 gm

GOURMET CURRIED RICE—*EASY*

Treat your family like company with this delicious dish.

- 1 tablespoon oil
- ½ teaspoon finely chopped garlic
- ½ cup finely chopped onion
- 1 cup uncooked rice
- 2 tablespoons black or golden raisins
- 1 tablespoon curry powder
- 1½ cups water
- 1 bay leaf
- ½ teaspoon thyme leaves
- 1 teaspoon Lite Salt or less
- ¼ teaspoon pepper

Heat the oil and garlic in a saucepan. Add onion and cook until wilted. Add the remaining ingredients and bring to a boil, stirring. Cover tightly and simmer for 15 minutes. Remove the bay leaf. Mix well and serve hot.

Makes 4 servings.

PER serving:
CALORIES 212   FIBER 2 gm
CSI 1   SODIUM 247 mg
FAT 4 gm

GREEN RICE

If you have leftover rice, this is a great way to use it.

1 cup chopped onion
1 tablespoon margarine
2 cups cooked rice
1 package (10 ounces) frozen chopped spinach, thawed
1 tablespoon chopped parsley
1 teaspoon garlic powder
½ teaspoon Lite Salt or less
½ teaspoon white pepper
1 tablespoon freshly squeezed lemon juice
¾ cup egg substitute (commercial or Homemade Egg Substitute, page 283)
½ cup grated Parmesan cheese

Preheat oven to 375°. Melt margarine in a nonstick skillet. Sauté onion. Add rice, spinach, parsley, garlic powder, Lite Salt, pepper, lemon juice, and egg substitute. Immediately pour into lightly oiled casserole. Sprinkle with Parmesan cheese. Bake for 20 minutes.

Makes 6 servings (1 cup each).

PER cup:
CALORIES 169   FIBER 3 gm
CSI 3   SODIUM 375 mg
FAT 5 gm

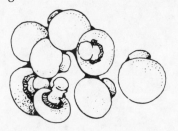

LEMON RICE—*EASY*

A "dress-up" rice—very tasty and simple to make.

2 cups lower-salt chicken broth
2 cups water
2 cloves garlic, crushed
¼ teaspoon Lite Salt or less
2 cups uncooked white rice
2 tablespoons finely grated lemon rind (yellow part only)
1 tablespoon finely minced fresh dill or 1 teaspoon dried
¼ teaspoon white pepper

Bring chicken broth and water to boil. Add garlic, Lite Salt, and rice. Reduce heat to low, cover, and cook for 15 minutes. Remove from heat. Add lemon rind, dill, and white pepper. Stir only to mix. Cover and let stand 10 minutes. Fluff and serve.

Makes 6 servings (1 cup each).

PER cup:
CALORIES 221   FIBER 1 gm
CSI trace   SODIUM 273 mg
FAT <1 gm

MUSHROOM BARLEY PILAF

A hearty casserole that is especially good when served with chicken or fish.

1 pound fresh mushrooms
1 cup chopped onion
1 tablespoon margarine
1½ cups uncooked pearl barley
1 jar (4 ounces) pimiento, chopped (optional)
2 cups lower-salt chicken broth
¼ teaspoon pepper

Preheat oven to 350°. Wash, dry, and slice mushrooms. Sauté onions and mushrooms in the margarine in a large skillet for 4 or 5 minutes. Transfer to a large casserole. Add barley and pimiento, if used, to the casserole dish. Stir in broth and pepper. Cover and bake for 50–60 minutes or until barley is tender and liquid is absorbed. Additional water may be needed during cooking if mixture seems dry.

This pilaf can also be cooked on stove top in a large kettle. Cook on low heat for 45 minutes.

Makes 8 servings.

PER serving:
CALORIES 196   FIBER 4 gm
CSI trace   SODIUM 223 mg
FAT 2 gm

PINE NEEDLE RICE

Pine nuts, orange juice, and wild rice combine flavors for this very popular side dish. It can be mostly prepared ahead of time and is delicious either at room temperature or heated.

4 cups water
1 cup uncooked wild rice
1 cup uncooked white rice (basmati works well, also)
3 tablespoons pine nuts
1 cup dried currants
¼ cup chopped fresh parsley
2 tablespoons grated orange zest*
¼ cup freshly squeezed orange juice (1 orange)
2 teaspoons olive oil
½ teaspoon Lite Salt or less
Freshly ground black pepper

Bring 4 cups water to boil and add wild rice. Return to boil and cover tightly. Reduce heat to simmer for 15 minutes. Add white or basmati rice, stir well, return cover, and continue on simmer for another 25 minutes or until rice is done. Remove rice from heat and let stand covered 10 minutes.

Toast pine nuts in nonstick skillet over medium heat until brown. Remove from heat and set aside. At serving time combine cooked rice with rest of ingredients and mix well. Serve at room temperature or cover tightly and heat through for 20 minutes in 350° oven.

Makes 6 cups.

*Zest of orange is the outer peel without any of the white layer. It is obtained by using a vegetable peeler or "zester."

PER cup:
CALORIES 318   FIBER 5 gm
CSI <1   SODIUM 96 mg
FAT 5 gm

PULIHORA (TAMARIND RICE)

A spicy, crunchy Indian rice dish that we have found very popular. It's worth the effort to find the special ingredients.

4 cups water
2 cups uncooked rice (basmati is best)
1 tablespoon oil
¼ teaspoon turmeric
¼ cup chana dal* or yellow lentils
2 teaspoons mustard seed
2 jalapeño peppers, seeded and finely minced (thinner ones are hotter, fatter ones are milder)
1 tablespoon finely minced fresh ginger root
8 whole dried red chiles
¼ cup unsalted peanuts
½ cup water
1½ teaspoons Lite Salt or less
1 tablespoon tamarind paste* (a very thick black paste)

Bring 4 cups water to boil. Add rice and bring to boil. Reduce heat to low and stir rice. Cover and cook 15 minutes. Remove from heat and cool (works best if made the day before and refrigerated).

In a small skillet heat oil and turmeric. Add uncooked chana dal or yellow lentils and sauté for a few minutes. Add mustard seeds and sauté for 1 minute. Add jalapeño peppers, ginger, red chiles, and peanuts and sauté. Mix Lite Salt and tamarind paste in ½ cup water and stir until paste is dis-

*Available in specialty stores (can be ordered by mail from Gulmohar Spices and Foods, 10195 SW Beaverton-Hillsdale Highway, Beaverton, Oregon 97005).

solved completely. Add to skillet and cook until mixture is slightly thickened. Add more water if necessary. Remove from heat. Put cooked rice in a large bowl; add sauce and mix thoroughly. Serve warm or at room temperature. It also works well to refrigerate and reheat in the microwave oven.

Makes 8 cups.

PER cup:
CALORIES 264   FIBER 2 gm
CSI 1   SODIUM 186 mg
FAT 5 gm

SPANISH RICE

This rice dish is a natural with Mexican food. Try it with *Acapulco Enchiladas* (page 397) and *Chocolate Zucchini Cake* (page 431) for a feast.

1 cup uncooked, long-grain white rice
1 clove garlic, minced
1 tablespoon oil
1 medium onion, sliced
1 green bell pepper, chopped
1 can (16 ounces) unsalted tomatoes, drained (use liquid as part of the 2 cups of water)
2 cups water
¾ teaspoon chili powder
¼ teaspoon marjoram leaves
½ teaspoon Lite Salt or less

Brown the rice and garlic in the oil in a 10-inch skillet. Add all the other ingredients and bring to a boil. Reduce heat to low, cover, and continue cooking for about 15 minutes or until rice has absorbed all the liquid. Remove from heat. Let stand covered 10 minutes before serving.

Makes 6 servings (1 cup each).

PER cup:
CALORIES 149   FIBER 2 gm
CSI trace   SODIUM 75 mg
FAT 3 gm

SPICY PEANUT NOODLES

A popular cold pasta side dish—you be the judge for the heat you add from the red pepper flakes! Pasta of any shape works well.

  1 tablespoon sesame oil
  ½–1 teaspoon crushed dried red pepper flakes (this adds the "spice")
  2 tablespoons honey
  2 tablespoons lower-sodium soy sauce
  ½ teaspoon Lite Salt or less
  8 ounces vermicelli, rotini, or other pasta
  2 tablespoons chopped cilantro
  2 tablespoons chopped peanuts
  ¼ cup minced green onions
  1 teaspoon toasted sesame seeds
  Cilantro leaves for garnish

Early in the day or the day before serving: Heat oil in saucepan. Stir in crushed pepper flakes and heat to bring out flavor. Add honey, soy sauce, and Lite Salt. Stir to combine and set aside. Cook vermicelli in boiling, unsalted water until tender. Drain well and combine with honey/soy sauce mixture. Cover and refrigerate for at least four hours or overnight.

When ready to serve: Add chopped cilantro, peanuts, and green onions to noodles, toss together and sprinkle with sesame seeds. Garnish with whole cilantro leaves.

Makes 6 cups.

PER cup:
CALORIES 223   FIBER 1 gm
CSI <1   SODIUM 284 mg
FAT 4 gm

SPINACH AND RICE CASSEROLE

  1 pound fresh spinach *or* 1 package (10 ounces) frozen chopped spinach
  ½ cup chopped onion
  ¼ cup sliced mushrooms
  1 tablespoon oil
  3 tablespoons whole wheat flour
  2 cups low-fat cottage cheese
  2 egg whites
  ¼ cup egg substitute (commercial *or Homemade Egg Substitute,* page 283)
  3 cups cooked brown rice
  ¼ teaspoon pepper
  ½ teaspoon thyme leaves or more
  ½ teaspoon garlic powder
  ½ teaspoon Lite Salt or less
  1 tablespoon sesame seeds
  1 tablespoon grated Parmesan cheese

(continued)

Preheat oven to 350°. Wash and tear up fresh spinach or defrost frozen spinach, if used.

Sauté onions and mushrooms in the oil. Combine with flour, cottage cheese, egg whites, egg substitute, uncooked spinach, cooked brown rice, and seasonings. Pat into a shallow 9-by-13-inch baking dish and top with sesame seeds and Parmesan cheese. Bake for 40–50 minutes until bubbling hot.

Makes 8 servings.

PER serving:
CALORIES 174   FIBER 3 gm
CSI 2   SODIUM 343 mg
FAT 4 gm

BEAN DISHES

CLASSIC BAKED BEANS

Dark, sweet and flavorful—these beans have the aroma of a country picnic. Let them bake for several hours.

  1 pound uncooked navy beans
  3 tablespoons brown sugar
  ¾ teaspoon Lite Salt or less
  1 teaspoon dry mustard
  ⅓ cup dark molasses
  ½ cup ketchup
  2 onions, cut in quarters

Wash the beans and soak overnight in enough water to cover them. Drain. Place in a saucepan and cover with water. Simmer, covered, 1–2 hours.

Mix with beans and remaining liquid the brown sugar, Lite Salt, mustard, molasses, and ketchup. Preheat oven to 325°. Place onion quarters in the bottom of a 2-quart casserole. Pour in the beans. Add enough boiling water to cover beans. Cover casserole; place in oven, and bake for 5–6 hours, adding more water, if needed.

Makes 8 cups.

PER cup:
CALORIES 230   FIBER 14 gm
CSI trace   SODIUM 283 mg
FAT 2 gm

RANCHER'S BEANS—QUICK

Almost too easy to believe. This delicious dish can increase your bean consumption by 500 percent!

  2 cans (16 ounces each) vegetarian beans in tomato sauce*
  2 tablespoons molasses
  1 teaspoon dry mustard
  ¼ teaspoon onion powder

Mix all ingredients in a medium saucepan. Simmer, uncovered, 10 minutes, or until thoroughly heated.

Makes 8 servings (½ cup each).

*Use low-sodium beans if available.

PER ½ cup:
CALORIES 171   FIBER 11 gm
CSI trace   SODIUM 276 mg
FAT trace

REFRIED BEANS

Make your own! Contains less salt than the canned ones. If this is below your salt threshold, add a little Lite Salt.

> 1½ cups uncooked pinto beans
> ¼ cup chopped onion
> 2 cloves garlic, minced
> 1 tablespoon oil
> 1 teaspoon ground cumin

Soak beans overnight in water. The next day boil beans in 6 cups fresh water until tender (2–3 hours). Drain and save some liquid.

Sauté onions and garlic in oil until clear. Add a little water if vegetables stick. Mash half of the beans, and add to onion and garlic. Continue to sauté for 10 minutes, stirring frequently. Allow some of the mashed beans to brown. Add cumin. Add remaining beans and continue cooking until they are warmed through. Water or liquid from beans may be added to keep the beans soft and mushy.

Makes 4 cups.

PER cup:
CALORIES 225   FIBER 16 gm
CSI 1   SODIUM 12 mg
FAT 6 gm

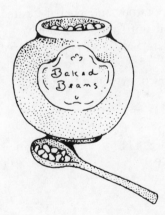

POTATO DISHES

HOLIDAY YAMS

This is so good, you won't want to wait for a holiday!

> 1 cup brown sugar
> 1 tablespoon melted margarine
> ⅓ cup water
> 2 cups fresh cranberries
> 6 medium yams, cooked, peeled, and quartered, *or* 3 cans (16 ounces each) yams, drained

Preheat oven to 350°. Combine all ingredients except yams in a 2-quart shallow baking dish. Bake about 5 minutes. Remove from oven and add yams; stir gently to mix. Return to oven; bake 25 minutes or until mixture bubbles at edges and yams are warm.

Makes 6 servings.

PER serving:
CALORIES 287   FIBER 6 gm
CSI trace   SODIUM 48 mg
FAT 2 gm

HOMEMADE TATERTOTS

A good way to use leftover mashed potatoes and cooked rice.

⅓ cup chopped onion
1 tablespoon margarine
½ cup cooked mashed potatoes
1 cup cooked brown rice
1 tablespoon unsalted tomato paste
½ teaspoon Lite Salt or less
½ cup whole-grain bread crumbs
3 tablespoons grated Parmesan cheese

Preheat oven to 350°. Sauté onions in margarine. Combine all ingredients and form into 1½-inch balls. Bake until delicately browned, approximately 15–20 minutes.
Makes 2½ cups.

PER cup:
CALORIES 192   FIBER 3 gm
CSI 2   SODIUM 390 mg
FAT 7 gm

ITALIAN POTATOES

This dish can be made ahead of time and reheated just before serving.

5 medium potatoes
2 cloves garlic, minced
¼ cup finely chopped fresh parsley
⅛ teaspoon Lite Salt or less
¼ teaspoon freshly ground pepper
1 tablespoon olive oil

Boil potatoes with their skins on until fork tender. While the potatoes are cooking combine garlic, parsley, Lite Salt, pepper, and oil. Put topping aside.

When potatoes are done, drain and slice into ¼-inch rounds. Arrange on a serving platter or dish. Spread topping evenly over the potatoes.
Makes 4 servings.

PER serving:
CALORIES 200   FIBER 4 gm
CSI <1   SODIUM 44 mg
FAT 4 gm

MASHED POTATOES

Simple and always good.

6 medium potatoes
⅓–½ cup skim milk
½ teaspoon Lite Salt or less
Pepper

Scrub potatoes and peel if desired. Cube and boil until tender. Mash well, adding milk, Lite Salt, and pepper. Serve piping hot.
Makes 6 servings (1 cup each).

PER cup:
CALORIES 111   FIBER 3 gm
CSI trace   SODIUM 79 mg
FAT trace

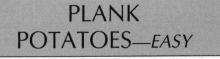

PLANK POTATOES—*EASY*

Homemade jumbo French fries without the deep-fat frying . . .

4 large baking potatoes, sliced lengthwise into ¼-inch-thick pieces
1 tablespoon oil

Preheat oven to 400°. Spray baking sheets with nonstick spray. Place sliced potatoes close together on prepared baking sheets and brush lightly with oil. Turn potatoes over and brush lightly with remainder of oil. Bake for 20 minutes, turn potatoes with spatula, and continue baking another 25 minutes or until brown.

Makes 4 servings.

PER serving:
CALORIES 231   FIBER 5 gm
CSI <1   SODIUM 15 mg
FAT 4 gm

POTATO PUFF

An easy, fancy mashed potato dish. It looks very pretty.

6 potatoes, cooked and drained
¾ cup skim milk
¾ teaspoon Lite Salt or less
⅓ cup grated low-fat cheese
2 teaspoons Dijon mustard
¼ cup chopped green onions
2 egg whites

Add the skim milk and Lite Salt to potatoes and mash until smooth. Add cheese, mustard, and green onions to the mashed potatoes. Mix well. Place in a lightly oiled 1½-quart baking dish. May be prepared ahead to this point and refrigerated.

Just prior to baking, preheat oven to 375°. Beat egg whites until very stiff and spread over potatoes. Bake 50–60 minutes and serve immediately.

Makes 4–6 servings.

PER ⅙ recipe:
CALORIES 142   FIBER 3 gm
CSI 1   SODIUM 223 mg
FAT 2 gm

SCALLOPED POTATOES

The secret of these scalloped potatoes is long, slow cooking—well worth the time and effort.

6 medium potatoes
¼ cup finely chopped onion
3 tablespoons flour
½ teaspoon Lite Salt or less
¼ teaspoon pepper
1 tablespoon margarine
2½ cups skim milk

Heat oven to 350°. Wash potatoes and remove eyes. Cut potatoes into thin slices—no need to peel them.

In a lightly oiled 2-quart casserole, arrange potatoes in 4 layers, sprinkling each of the first 3 layers with 1 tablespoon on-

(continued)

ion, 1 tablespoon flour, ⅛ teaspoon Lite Salt, and a dash pepper. Dot each layer with 1 teaspoon margarine. Sprinkle top with remaining onion, Lite Salt, and pepper. Heat milk just to scalding (bubbles around edge) and pour over potatoes. Cover and bake 30 minutes. Uncover and bake 60–70 minutes until potatoes are tender. Let stand 5–10 minutes before serving.

Makes 4–6 servings.

PER ⅙ recipe:

CALORIES 219	FIBER 5 gm
CSI <1	SODIUM 150 mg
FAT 2 gm	

SKINNY "FRENCH FRIES"

The taste and texture of French fries—without the fat!

4 medium potatoes, cut in strips or lengthwise, about ½ inch thick
1 tablespoon oil
Paprika
½ teaspoon Lite Salt or less

Preheat oven to 450°. While cutting potatoes, keep strips in bowl of ice water to crisp. Drain and pat dry on paper towels. Return to bowl and sprinkle with oil. Mix with hands to distribute oil evenly over potatoes. Bake on a baking pan coated with nonstick spray until golden brown and tender, about 30–40 minutes, turning fre-

quently. Sprinkle generously with paprika, and sparingly with Lite Salt.

Makes 4 servings.

PER serving:

CALORIES 134	FIBER 3 gm
CSI <1	SODIUM 101 mg
FAT 4 gm	

SPUDS AND ONIONS

An easy baked potato dish that will fill your kitchen with a wonderful aroma.

4 large baking potatoes, unpeeled (about 2 pounds)
1 large onion
1 tablespoon olive oil
¼ teaspoon Lite Salt or less
⅛ teaspoon pepper
1 teaspoon thyme leaves

Preheat oven to 425°. Cut potatoes and onions into 1-inch chunks. Place in a single layer on a nonstick cookie sheet. Sprinkle on olive oil, Lite Salt, pepper, and thyme. Toss to coat. Bake for 30 minutes or until potatoes are tender. Turn vegetables with a spatula several times while baking.

Makes 6 cups (about 4 servings).

PER cup:

CALORIES 185	FIBER 4 gm
CSI trace	SODIUM 53 mg
FAT 2 gm	

SUPER STUFFED POTATOES

Very versatile! These stuffed potatoes can be made ahead since they freeze very well. The "stuffing" can be served in a casserole dish when time is limited.

- **6 medium potatoes**
- **1½ cups broccoli**
- **¾ cup grated low-fat cheese, divided**
- **1 tablespoon margarine**
- **¼ cup skim milk**
- **⅛ teaspoon pepper**
- **½ teaspoon Lite Salt or less**

Preheat oven to 400°. Scrub potatoes. Make shallow slits around the middle as if you were cutting the potatoes in half lengthwise. Bake until done, 30–60 minutes.

Steam broccoli until just tender and finely chop.

Carefully slice the potatoes in half and scoop the insides into a bowl with the broccoli. Add ½ cup of the cheese and the margarine, milk, Lite Salt, and pepper. Mash all together until mixture is pale green with dark flecks. Heap into the potato jackets and sprinkle with remaining cheese. Return to the oven to heat through.

Makes 12 servings (½ potato each).

PER ½ potato:
CALORIES 113 FIBER 3 gm
CSI 1 SODIUM 94 mg
FAT 3 gm

VEGETABLE DISHES

ACORN SQUASH WITH ROASTED ONIONS

The roasting onions fill the house with a wonderful aroma. For a holiday treat, use 8 mini-pumpkins in place of the acorn squash. Rinse the pumpkins, then place slightly apart on a 10-by-15-inch baking pan. Bake uncovered at 375° until soft when pressed, about 40 minutes. Let cool. Cut off tops to make a lid; scoop seeds from pumpkin and discard. Fill with baked onions, set lid on top, and continue as directed.

- **4 small acorn squash**
- **2 packages (16 ounces each) frozen tiny onions**
- **½ cup balsamic vinegar* _or_ red wine vinegar**
- **1 tablespoon sugar**
- **4 teaspoons melted margarine**

Preheat oven to 375°. Cut squash in half lengthwise, remove seeds, and put cut side down in a pan. Add 1 cup water and bake covered until tender when pierced, 45–60 minutes. Let cool.

At the same time, put onions in a 9-by-13-inch baking pan. Add vinegar. Bake uncovered, stirring every 10 minutes, until

*Available in deli or food specialty shops.

(continued)

vinegar is almost gone (45 minutes). Mix sugar into onions and continue to bake until lightly glazed, about 10 minutes.

Brush inside of squash with melted margarine. Spoon onions into squash. Place close together in a shallow 9-by-13-inch baking dish. Return to oven. Heat through and serve.

If made ahead, cover and chill until next day. Bake covered in a 375° oven until hot, 15–25 minutes. Or cover loosely with plastic wrap and heat in microwave at full power, about 12 minutes.

Makes 8 servings.

PER serving:
CALORIES 135   FIBER 7 gm
CSI <1   SODIUM 30 mg
FAT 3 gm

CHEESY CAULIFLOWER—QUICK

A microwave "find."

1 head cauliflower (1½ pounds, cleaned)
½ cup grated low-fat cheese
2 teaspoons Dijon mustard
¼ teaspoon Worcestershire sauce

Place cauliflower in bowl containing ½ inch water. Cover with plastic and microwave on high until just tender (about 7–10 minutes). Drain water from cauliflower.

Combine cheese, mustard, and Worcestershire sauce. Pat cheese mixture over top of hot cauliflower. Cover with plastic wrap and microwave just until cheese is melted (about 1 minute).

Makes 4 servings.

PER serving:
CALORIES 76   FIBER 4 gm
CSI 2   SODIUM 131 mg
FAT 3 gm

CORN BAKE—EASY

A nice dish to serve with enchiladas for a Mexican dinner, and it's so easy to prepare!

1 small onion, finely chopped
1 small green bell pepper, finely chopped
1 can (16 ounces) unsalted cream-style corn
½ teaspoon Lite Salt or less
Pepper to taste
½ cup bread crumbs

Preheat oven to 350°. Mix chopped onions and green peppers with corn, Lite Salt, and pepper. Place in baking dish. Sprinkle with bread crumbs. Bake for 45 minutes.

Makes 4 servings.

PER serving:
CALORIES 118   FIBER 7 gm
CSI trace   SODIUM 139 mg
FAT <1 gm

EASY ACORN SQUASH

This is also a delicious way to serve spaghetti squash. Use either leftover *Marinara Sauce* or a commercial tomato sauce.

1 cup *Marinara Sauce* (page 450), heated
2 acorn squash, cut in half and seeds removed

Preheat oven to 350°. Place squash cut side down in baking dish. Add water to one-inch depth. Bake 40 minutes or until squash is tender. Turn squash over and fill each center with ¼ cup warm *Marinara Sauce*.

Makes 4 servings.

_____

PER serving:
CALORIES 101   FIBER 6 gm
CSI trace   SODIUM 19 mg
FAT 2 gm

EGGPLANT PARMESAN

Simple, elegant, and delicious.

3 cups *Marinara Sauce* (page 450)
1 eggplant, sliced ½ inch thick
½ cup grated Parmesan cheese

Preheat oven to 350°. Steam eggplant slices *or* roll in flour and broil for 3 minutes on each side. Place in a casserole dish and cover with *Marinara Sauce*. Sprinkle with Parmesan cheese. Heat in oven for about 20 minutes until bubbly.

Makes 6 servings.

_____

PER serving:
CALORIES 124   FIBER 4 gm
CSI 2   SODIUM 146 mg
FAT 6 gm

GRILLED ZUCCHINI—*QUICK*

Garden-fresh small Japanese eggplants are also great prepared this way.

2 tablespoons chopped fresh basil *or* 2 teaspoons dried basil
1 tablespoon low-calorie Italian salad dressing
4 medium zucchini, cut in half lengthwise (about 1½ pounds)

Combine basil and salad dressing. Brush cut surfaces of sliced squash or eggplants with one-half the mixture; set aside. Coat charcoal grill with nonstick cooking spray. Place vegetables cut side down on rack and cook 3 minutes. Turn vegetables over; brush with remaining basil mixture and cook an additional 5 minutes or until vegetables are tender.

Makes 4 servings.

_____

PER serving:
CALORIES 32   FIBER 2 gm
CSI trace   SODIUM 35 mg
FAT 1 gm

ONION SQUARES

We can't decide if this is a side dish or a cornbread—it came to us from Eastern Oregon and goes very well with chili or a bean soup. If cut in small squares it makes a great appetizer.

1 onion, sliced
½ cup nonfat yogurt
¼ teaspoon dill weed
¼ teaspoon Lite Salt or less
½ cup flour
½ cup cornmeal
1 teaspoon sugar
1½ teaspoons baking powder
3 tablespoons oil
½ cup skim milk
1 egg white
1 package (10 ounces) frozen corn, thawed
2 drops Tabasco sauce
2 tablespoons grated Parmesan cheese

Preheat oven to 450°. Sauté onion slices in nonstick skillet until soft and slightly browned. Add yogurt, dill weed, and Lite Salt. In a separate bowl combine flour, cornmeal, sugar, baking powder, oil, skim milk, and egg white. Mix well. Add corn and Tabasco sauce. Pour batter into lightly oiled 9-inch-square pan. Spread onion mixture over batter. Sprinkle Parmesan cheese over onions. Bake for 25–30 minutes. Cut into squares to serve.

Makes 9 servings.

PER serving (3 by 3 inches):
CALORIES 140   FIBER 3 gm
CSI 1   SODIUM 121 mg
FAT 5 gm

ORIENTAL BROCCOLI

This is a delicious way to serve broccoli. The sweet red pepper makes the dish look beautiful, but it can be left out when red peppers are out of season or outrageously priced.

1 head fresh broccoli (about 1½ pounds) cut into small flowerets
½ red bell pepper, cut into thin strips

SAUCE

1 tablespoon lower-sodium soy sauce
1 teaspoon sesame oil
1 teaspoon sugar
1 teaspoon sesame seeds

Combine sauce ingredients in a small bowl. Steam broccoli until tender crisp. Stir-fry broccoli, red pepper, and sauce ingredients in nonstick pan over medium-high heat just until red pepper is crisp tender (about 1 minute).

Makes 4 cups.

PER cup:
CALORIES 70   FIBER 7 gm
CSI trace   SODIUM 191 mg
FAT 2 gm

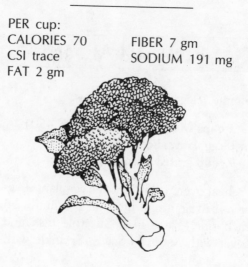

RATATOUILLE PROVENÇALE

2½ cups diced eggplant
¾ cup thinly sliced onion
2 cloves garlic, minced
1 tablespoon olive oil
4 green bell peppers, sliced
2 cups quartered tomatoes
3 cups sliced zucchini (½ inch thick)
1 teaspoon oregano leaves
Pepper to taste
1 cup plain nonfat yogurt *or Mock Sour Cream* (page 451)

Dice eggplant in ½-inch cubes. Sauté onions and garlic in olive oil. Add green peppers, tomatoes and zucchini; sauté until heated. Add eggplant, oregano, and pepper. Cook very slowly in covered dish for about an hour. Uncover and cook about 15 minutes longer. Serve with dollop of plain yogurt *or Mock Sour Cream;* may be served hot or cold in small bowls.

Makes 8 servings.

PER serving:
CALORIES 72   FIBER 3 gm
CSI <1   SODIUM 30 mg
FAT 2 gm

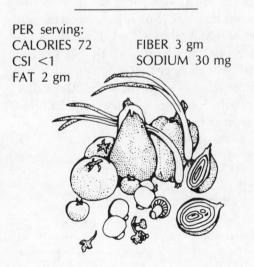

STIR-FRIED MUSHROOMS AND BROCCOLI

Great over fresh pasta, too.

1 tablespoon margarine
½ cup chopped onion
½ pound fresh mushrooms, sliced
1 tablespoon oil
1 bunch broccoli, cut into flowerets
1 clove garlic, minced
1 can (8 ounces) sliced water chestnuts, drained
1 tablespoon cornstarch
1 teaspoon sugar
¼ teaspoon ground ginger
1 teaspoon lower-sodium soy sauce
½ bouillon cube
¾ cup boiling water

Melt margarine and add onions. Sauté 2 minutes. Add mushrooms and stir for 5 minutes. Remove and set aside. Heat oil. Add broccoli and garlic, cooking for 3 minutes. Add water chestnuts and cook 2 minutes longer. Blend cornstarch, sugar, and ginger with soy sauce. Dissolve bouillon in water and pour into pan. Add cornstarch mixture. Cook and stir until thickened. Reduce heat and simmer, covered, 5 minutes, or until broccoli is just crisp-tender. Add mushrooms. Serve over rice, if desired.

Makes 8 servings.

PER serving:
CALORIES 69   FIBER 2 gm
CSI <1   SODIUM 120 mg
FAT 3 gm

STUFFED ZUCCHINI BOATS

This recipe is excellent with Italian dishes.

2 medium zucchini (8 inches long)
2 teaspoons olive oil
1 clove garlic, minced
¼ cup minced onion
¼ cup chopped green bell pepper
4 large fresh mushrooms, chopped
1 tomato, chopped
½ teaspoon oregano leaves (see variations)
3 tablespoons grated Parmesan cheese

Preheat oven to 350°. Cut zucchini in half. Scoop out pulp and dice. Place scooped-out zucchini shells cut side down in a baking dish with a small amount of water. Bake or heat in a microwave oven until crisp-tender. Heat olive oil in a skillet and stir-fry garlic, onion, green pepper, and mushrooms until crisp-tender. Add a little water if vegetables stick. Add diced zucchini and stir-fry for 1 minute. Add tomato and oregano. Cool slightly. Add 1 tablespoon Parmesan cheese. Mix well. Spoon mixture into zucchini boats. Top with remaining Parmesan cheese. Broil for a few minutes to brown cheese or cover and heat in a microwave oven. Do not overcook.

Makes 4 servings.

VARIATIONS

Substitute ¼ to ½ teaspoon turmeric for the oregano as an accompaniment for Indian food *or* use ¼ to ½ teaspoon ground cumin instead of oregano when serving Mexican food.

PER serving:
CALORIES 66   FIBER 3 gm
CSI 1   SODIUM 74 mg
FAT 4 gm

TOMATOES "PROVENÇALE"

Stuffed tomatoes can be easily served at home, too—not just in restaurants.

6 firm tomatoes
¼ teaspoon thyme leaves
¼ teaspoon rosemary leaves
¼ teaspoon ground coriander
¼ teaspoon garlic powder
Pepper
½ cup soft bread crumbs
¼ cup chopped onion
1 tablespoon oil

Preheat oven to 400°. Cut tomatoes in half crosswise. Press out juice and seeds. Turn upside down on a paper towel to remove excess moisture. Mix spices, bread crumbs, onions, and oil in a bowl. Place the tomatoes side by side in a lightly oiled baking dish. Fill each with spice mixture. Place in upper third of oven. Bake for 20 minutes, until the tomatoes are tender and the filling browned.

Makes 6 servings.

PER serving:
CALORIES 73   FIBER 2 gm
CSI trace   SODIUM 31 mg
FAT 3 gm

ZUCCHINI PUFF—*EASY*

2 cups grated zucchini
½ cup grated low-fat cheese
3 egg whites *or* ½ cup egg substitute
  (commercial *or Homemade Egg Substitute,* page 283)
1 tablespoon dried onion flakes
¼ cup *Baking Mix* (page 275)

Preheat oven to 350°. Coat 1½-quart baking dish with nonstick spray. Combine ingredients and pour into dish. Bake uncovered for 45 minutes.

Makes 4 servings.

PER serving:
CALORIES 93
CSI 3
FAT 4 gm
FIBER 1 gm
SODIUM 202 mg

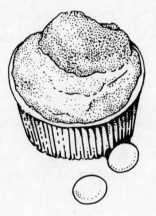

MAIN DISHES FEATURING VEGETABLES, GRAINS, AND BEANS

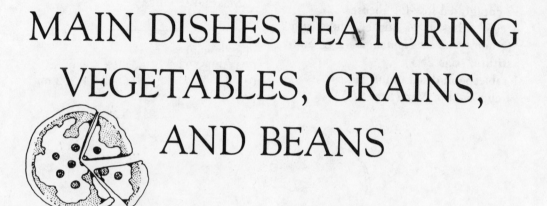

If you are trying to double your complex carbohydrate and fiber intakes, this is the section for you. You'll notice that many of these dishes are ethnic—because other cultures often have main dishes that use lots of whole grains and beans. You will not miss the meat because there never was any in the original recipes—and they taste great just as they are. We like these recipes very much.

Featuring Vegetables
Baguette with Vegetable Filling
Baked Burrito Squares
Broccoli Quiche
Lasagna Primavera
Moroccan Vegetable Stew—*Easy*
Quick-and-Easy Pan Bread Pizza
Spicy Cheese Pizza
Spinach Lasagna
Vegetable Calzone
Zucchini Pie

Featuring Grains
Baked Spaghetti Pie
Broccoli with Rice
Cabbage Rolls
Cheese-Stuffed Manicotti

Chinese Noodles
Creamy Enchiladas—*Easy*
Macaroni Bake
Pasta with Fresh Tomato Sauce—*Easy*
Vegetable Pulav

Featuring Beans
Acapulco Bean Casserole—*Easy*
Bean Lasagna
Black Bean Chili
Black Beans with 1000 Uses
Chile Relleno Casserole
Garbanzo Goulash—*Quick*
No-Meat Enchiladas
Pinto Bean Chow Mein—*Quick*
Rick's Chili—*Easy*
Spicy Lentils

san cheese. Baked uncovered about 15 minutes.

Makes 2 servings.

PER serving:
CALORIES 500   FIBER 6 gm
CSI 2   SODIUM 827 mg
FAT 10 gm

FEATURING VEGETABLES

BAGUETTE WITH VEGETABLE FILLING

Our favorite Friday night casual dinner! Just pick it up with your hands and eat it.

1 loaf (16 ounces) baguette bread (3 by 20 inches)
2 teaspoons margarine
2 cloves garlic, minced, divided
1 cup thinly sliced green or red bell pepper
1 cup thinly sliced onion
1 cup thinly sliced mushrooms
½ cup *Marinara Sauce* (page 450) *or* use commercial marinara sauce
½ teaspoon olive oil
2 teaspoons grated Parmesan cheese

Preheat oven to 375°. Cut baguette crosswise into two pieces. Slice ½ inch from top of each piece and use for something else. Hollow the loaf out. Mix together margarine and 1 clove garlic and scrape onto cut edges of bread. Toast under broiler or over grill. Heat oil and 1 clove garlic until bubbly. Add vegetables and stir-fry until crisp tender. Add *Marinara Sauce* and spoon mixture into bread. Sprinkle with Parme-

BAKED BURRITO SQUARES

Tortillas are filled with vegetables and rice, crisped in the oven, and served with salsa.

4 flour tortillas (8-inch diameter)
1 teaspoon oil
1 medium onion, chopped
1 small red bell pepper, chopped
1 cup chopped jicama
1 teaspoon cumin
1 cup cooked brown rice
⅓ cup chopped cilantro
½ cup shredded part-skim mozzarella cheese

½ cup salsa

Preheat oven to 400°. Wrap tortillas in foil and heat until warm, about 10 minutes.

Meanwhile, in a skillet, heat oil and cook onion, green pepper, jicama, and cumin about 10 minutes. Remove from heat and stir in cooked rice, cilantro, and cheese.

Place ¼ of vegetable/rice mixture in center of each warm tortilla. Fold over tortilla sides and ends to enclose filling and

(continued)

form a square-shaped bundle. Place seam side down in a baking dish. Bake until crisp, about 30 minutes. Serve with salsa to spoon over top.

Makes 4 servings.

_____

PER serving:
CALORIES 298   FIBER 4 gm
CSI 4   SODIUM 586 mg
FAT 8 gm

BROCCOLI QUICHE

A crisp potato crust with a delicious creamy broccoli filling.

MASHED POTATO CRUST

2 large potatoes
2 tablespoons margarine
¼ teaspoon Lite Salt or less
Freshly ground black pepper
½ cup finely minced onion

BROCCOLI FILLING

1 cup evaporated skim milk
2 egg whites
6 tablespoons egg substitute (commercial or *Homemade Egg Substitute*, page 283)
1 teaspoon tarragon leaves
¼ teaspoon nutmeg
¼ teaspoon Lite Salt or less
⅛ teaspoon pepper
½ cup shredded low-fat cheese
1 package (10 ounces) frozen chopped broccoli, thawed

Preheat oven to 375°. Scrub unpeeled potatoes; cut into chunks and boil them until soft. Drain well and mash. Add margarine, Lite Salt, pepper, and minced onion. Mix well and spoon into 9-inch pie plate that has been sprayed with nonstick spray. Bake for 45 minutes.

While crust is baking, prepare filling. In a small bowl beat together milk, egg whites, egg substitute, tarragon, nutmeg, Lite Salt, and pepper.

Remove crust from oven. Lower oven temperature to 350°. Put thawed broccoli in warm crust. Sprinkle with shredded cheese. Pour over milk/egg mixture. Return to oven and bake for 30 minutes or until custard is set. Wait a few minutes before serving.

Makes 6 servings.

_____

PER serving:
CALORIES 189   FIBER 3 gm
CSI 2   SODIUM 292 mg
FAT 6 gm

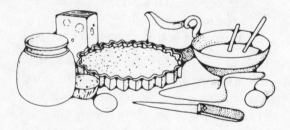

LASAGNA PRIMAVERA

A colorful and delicious meatless dish.

10 lasagna noodles
1 tablespoon olive oil
1 small clove garlic, minced
1 medium onion, chopped
1 pound carrots, shredded
1 pound mushrooms, sliced
¾ cup sliced black olives
1 can (15 ounces) unsalted tomato sauce
1 can (6 ounces) unsalted tomato paste
1½ teaspoons oregano leaves
⅛ teaspoon black pepper
2 cups low-fat cottage cheese, drained
1 package (10 ounces) frozen chopped spinach, thawed and squeezed dry
8 ounces imitation or part-skim mozzarella, grated
3 tablespoons grated Parmesan cheese

Preheat oven to 350°. In a large kettle, bring water to a boil. Add the lasagna noodles and cook 8–10 minutes. Drain and return to the cooking pot, adding a little warm water to keep them from sticking.

Heat oil in a large skillet. Add garlic and onion and sauté, stirring continuously, for 2 minutes. Add mushrooms and cook, stirring occasionally, until the moisture evaporates—about 15 minutes. Add carrots and cook 3–5 minutes. Add tomato sauce and paste, olives, oregano, and black pepper. Stir well and remove from heat.

Spray a 13-by-9-inch baking pan with nonstick spray. Spread 1 cup of tomato mixture in bottom of pan. Line the bottom with 5 drained lasagna noodles. Spread on top of them half the drained cottage cheese, then half the spinach. Cover with half of the remaining tomato mixture. Repeat the layering and bake for 30 minutes. Top with cheese and continue baking another 15 minutes. Let sit for a few minutes before serving.

Makes 12 servings.

PER serving:
CALORIES 240   FIBER 4 gm
CSI 4   SODIUM 529 mg
FAT 7 gm

MOROCCAN VEGETABLE STEW—EASY

1 medium onion, chopped
2 tablespoons water
1 tablespoon oil
2 cups chopped potatoes, in 1-inch-square pieces
2 cups carrots, chopped into large chunks
1 can (16 ounces) unsalted tomatoes or 2 cups fresh tomatoes
¾ teaspoon ground cumin
½–1 cup unsalted tomato juice
2 cups fresh green beans, sliced into 2-inch pieces
¼ teaspoon black pepper or cayenne, to taste

Simmer onions in oil and water until transparent. Add potatoes and carrots and simmer for 15 minutes, stirring occasionally. Add chopped tomatoes and cumin. Cover

(continued)

and simmer for about 1 hour, checking to see if the stew needs more liquid. If so, add tomato juice. Add green beans and cook for 15 minutes more. Check seasoning— add ¼ teaspoon or more black pepper and more cumin, if desired.

Makes 4 servings (about 8 cups).

PER cup:
CALORIES 81   FIBER 4 gm
CSI trace   SODIUM 14 mg
FAT 2 gm

QUICK-AND-EASY PAN BREAD PIZZA

The brown-and-serve bread is a quick premade crust. The rest is easy.

1 loaf (15–16 ounces) round brown-and-serve pan bread (focaccia, fugasa, etc.)
1½ cups *Marinara Sauce* (page 450) *or* commercial pizza sauce
½ cup chopped onion
½ cup chopped green bell pepper
1 cup sliced mushrooms
¼ cup sliced ripe olives
1 cup grated imitation mozzarella cheese

Preheat oven to 425°. Slice unbaked bread horizontally and place cut sides up on baking sheet. Spread *Marinara Sauce* or pizza sauce over bread. Top with chopped vegetables and grated cheese. Bake for 15–20 minutes. Remove from oven, cut into wedges, and serve.

Makes 6 servings.

PER serving:
CALORIES 339   FIBER 3 gm
CSI 2   SODIUM 742 mg
FAT 11 gm

SPICY CHEESE PIZZA

Choose a thick or thin crust (see *Pizza Crusts*, page 276) and add the following toppings:

1 can (6 ounces) unsalted tomato paste
2 cans (8 ounces each) unsalted tomato sauce
2 teaspoons ground anise seed
¼ teaspoon pepper
¼ teaspoon garlic powder
1 teaspoon oregano leaves
1 teaspoon Italian seasonings
1 teaspoon chopped parsley
½ cup fresh mushrooms, sliced, *or* 1 can (4 ounces) sliced mushrooms, drained
1 green bell pepper, chopped
1 medium onion, chopped
6 ounces part-skim or imitation mozzarella cheese, grated

Preheat oven to 425°. Combine tomato paste, tomato sauce, and seasonings. Spread sauce over the dough. Sprinkle pizza with the remaining ingredients. Bake 25–30 minutes.

Makes enough for 1 pizza.

PER ⅛ recipe (topping only):
CALORIES 101   FIBER 2 gm
CSI 3   SODIUM 128 mg
FAT 4 gm

SPINACH LASAGNA

This is a low-fat version of an old favorite. Other vegetables such as zucchini or eggplant may be added for extra appeal.

SAUCE

1 large onion, chopped
3 cloves garlic, minced
1 tablespoon oil
2 cans (16 ounces each) unsalted tomatoes, chopped
1 can (6 ounces) unsalted tomato paste
Pinch of basil, oregano, rosemary leaves

NOODLES AND VEGETABLE

12 ounces lasagna noodles
1 pound fresh spinach, lightly steamed and chopped, *or* 1 package (10 ounces) frozen chopped spinach, thawed

FILLING

½ cup chopped tofu
½ cup part-skim ricotta cheese
2 tablespoons grated Parmesan cheese
½ cup low-fat cottage cheese
½ cup sliced mushrooms (optional)

TOPPING

6 ounces part-skim mozzarella cheese

Make sauce: Sauté onions and garlic in oil. Add tomatoes, tomato paste, and herbs. Simmer for ½ hour or longer.

Prepare noodles and vegetables: Cook noodles according to package directions in un-

salted water until tender. Drain. Steam spinach and drain, if using fresh, or thaw and drain, if using frozen.

Prepare filling: Mix tofu, ricotta, Parmesan cheese, cottage cheese, and mushrooms. Blend well so tofu is thoroughly mixed in.

Complete casserole: Preheat oven to 350°. Assemble ingredients in a 9-by-13-inch baking dish in the following order:

Small amount of tomato sauce
Cooked noodles
⅓ of cheese/tofu mixture
⅓ of drained spinach
Tomato sauce
Repeat as above ending with noodles and tomato sauce

Place thinly sliced mozzarella cheese on top of casserole and bake for about 40 minutes until bubbly. Let stand about 15 minutes before serving.

Makes 12 servings (about 3 by 3 inches).

PER serving:
CALORIES 223   FIBER 3 gm
CSI 3   SODIUM 172 mg
FAT 6 gm

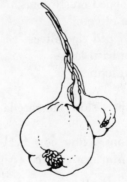

VEGETABLE CALZONE

Some restaurants have built a reputation around this entrée. You can do the same thing. . . .

DOUGH

> 1 package yeast
> ½ cup warm water
> 2–2½ cups flour
> 1 teaspoon sugar
> ½ teaspoon Lite Salt or less
> 1 egg white
> 1½ teaspoons oil

Dissolve yeast in warm water. Stir in 1 cup flour, sugar, and Lite Salt. Add egg white and oil; beat until smooth and glossy. Stir in 1 to 1½ cups flour—until dough is no longer sticky. Knead 10 minutes. Place in lightly oiled bowl and cover. Let rise 1 hour in warm place or until double in volume.

FILLING

> 2 green bell peppers, chopped
> 2 medium onions, chopped
> 2 cups chopped mushrooms
> 1 teaspoon olive oil
> ¼ cup chopped ripe olives
> 1 teaspoon basil leaves
> 1 teaspoon fennel
>
> 4 ounces part-skim mozzarella cheese, grated
> 2 tablespoons yellow cornmeal
> 1⅓ cups *Marinara Sauce* (page 450)

Prepare filling while dough is rising: Sauté green peppers, onions, and mushrooms in oil until limp. Add olives, basil, and fen-

nel. On lightly floured board, roll dough into 2 large circles about ¼ inch thick. Spread cooked vegetables on half of each circle, cover with grated cheese. Fold ½ of circle over and pinch edges tightly to close and seal. (Prongs of a fork work well for this.)

Preheat oven to 425°. Cover a nonstick baking sheet with a light coat of cornmeal. Place two prepared calzones onto it and bake 15–20 minutes or until slightly browned. Remove from oven and cut into wedges. Serve warm with *Marinara Sauce* over top.

Makes 4 servings.

PER serving including ⅓ cup sauce:

CALORIES 437	FIBER 6 gm
CSI 5	SODIUM 378 mg
FAT 11 gm	

ZUCCHINI PIE

Our version of a vegetable quiche.

CRUST

> 1 tablespoon yeast
> ½ cup warm water
> ½ cup whole wheat flour
> ¾ cup white flour
> ½ teaspoon Lite Salt

FILLING

> 4 cups zucchini, unpeeled, thinly sliced
> 1 cup coarsely chopped onion
> 1 tablespoon margarine
> 2 tablespoons chopped parsley

½ teaspoon Lite Salt or less
½ teaspoon pepper
¼ teaspoon garlic powder
¼ teaspoon basil leaves
¼ teaspoon oregano leaves
3 egg whites
2 cups grated, part-skim mozzarella cheese

2 teaspoons Dijon-style or prepared mustard

Dissolve yeast in water. Stir in flours and Lite Salt. Knead dough on floured board for 5 minutes or until smooth and elastic. Let rise for 45 minutes.

Preheat oven to 375°. In large skillet, cook zucchini and onions in margarine until tender, about 10 minutes. Stir in parsley and seasonings. In large bowl, blend egg whites and cheese. Stir into vegetable mixture.

Transfer raised dough to an ungreased 11-inch quiche pan, 10-inch pie pan, or 9-by-13-inch baking dish. Press over bottom and up sides to form crust. Spread crust with mustard. Pour vegetable mixture evenly over crust.

Bake for 25–35 minutes or until knife inserted near center comes out clean. If crust becomes too brown, cover with foil during last 10 minutes of baking. Let stand 10 minutes before serving.

Makes 8 servings.

PER serving:
CALORIES 188   FIBER 3 gm
CSI 5   SODIUM 317 mg
FAT 7 gm

FEATURING GRAINS

BAKED SPAGHETTI PIE

These pie-shaped spaghetti wedges are especially good covered with *Marinara Sauce* (page 450) or *Light Mushroom Sauce for Pasta* (page 450).

7 ounces spaghetti
1 cup low-fat cottage cheese
½ cup commercial egg substitute *or* *Homemade Egg Substitute* (page 283)
¼ teaspoon Lite Salt or less
⅛ teaspoon pepper
½ cup grated low-fat cheese
1 tablespoon grated Parmesan cheese

Preheat oven to 350°. Cook spaghetti according to package directions in unsalted water. Drain well and mix hot spaghetti with cottage cheese, egg substitute, Lite Salt, pepper, and ½ cup grated cheese. Place in 9-inch pie plate that has been sprayed with nonstick spray. Sprinkle with Parmesan cheese and bake 45–50 minutes or until knife inserted in center comes out clean. Cut into wedges and serve warm garnished with parsley or covered with sauces suggested above.

Makes 6 servings.

PER serving:
CALORIES 213   FIBER <1 gm
CSI 2   SODIUM 305 mg
FAT 3 gm

BROCCOLI WITH RICE

A true favorite. Very popular for potluck dinners.

2 onions, chopped
2 stalks celery, chopped
1 tablespoon margarine
3 cups chopped fresh broccoli *or* 2 packages (10 ounces each) chopped frozen broccoli
2 cans (10¾ ounces each) cream of celery soup *or* use *Homemade "Cream" Soup Mix* (page 314)
¼ cup grated Parmesan cheese
5 cups cooked brown rice
4 drops Tabasco sauce
1 can (8 ounces) sliced water chestnuts, drained
¼ cup soft bread crumbs

Preheat oven to 350°. In large skillet, sauté the onions and celery in margarine until clear. Cook broccoli until barely tender and drain well. Mix broccoli with soup and cheese. Add to celery and onions. Stir in rice, Tabasco sauce, and water chestnuts and mix well. Pour into a lightly oiled casserole dish and top with bread crumbs. Bake for about 20–30 minutes, until bubbly and heated through.

Makes 6 servings as a main dish, 12 servings as a side dish (about 12 cups total).

PER cup:
CALORIES 157   FIBER 3 gm
CSI 2   SODIUM 495 mg
FAT 5 gm

CABBAGE ROLLS

These are very popular as a main dish, but can also be a delicious side dish with a fish entrée. They are easily made when cooked rice is on hand.

2 small heads cabbage

SAUCE

1 onion, chopped
3 cans (8 ounces each) unsalted tomato sauce
1 bay leaf
½ teaspoon ground ginger
¼ cup honey
¼ cup vinegar
¼ teaspoon thyme leaves
½ teaspoon Lite Salt or less
Pepper to taste

FILLING

1 large onion, chopped
8 ounces tofu, cubed
½ cup chopped fresh parsley
½ cup unsalted tomato paste
2 cups cooked brown rice
½ teaspoon Lite Salt or less
¼ teaspoon garlic powder

Steam cabbage 20 minutes. Cool, then carefully separate leaves from the head.

Prepare sauce: Steam onion until transparent; add remaining ingredients and gently simmer for about 30 minutes.
Preheat oven to 350°.

Prepare filling: Steam the chopped onion, add the tofu, and stir to crumble. Add remaining ingredients and heat thoroughly. Place about 1 tablespoon on each cabbage leaf, roll up tightly, and secure with a wooden pick.

Assemble dish: Place a small amount of sauce in shallow baking pan and add cabbage rolls. Pour remaining sauce over. Cover pan and bake for 45 minutes to 1 hour, until cabbage is soft.

Makes 16 cabbage rolls, about 4 servings.

PER roll:
CALORIES 80   FIBER 2 gm
CSI trace   SODIUM 70 mg
FAT <1 gm

CHEESE-STUFFED MANICOTTI

Simple to fix—the manicotti shells do not need to be precooked!

TOMATO SAUCE

1 clove garlic, minced
1 tablespoon olive oil
2 cans (8 ounces each) unsalted tomato sauce
2 cans (16 ounces each) unsalted tomatoes
1½ teaspoons oregano leaves
1 tablespoon chopped parsley

FILLING

2 cups low-fat cottage cheese
1 cup part-skim ricotta cheese
3 tablespoons grated Parmesan cheese
2 egg whites
¼ cup chopped parsley
Dash pepper
8 ounces uncooked manicotti shells (15 pieces)
1 cup water

Preheat oven to 375°.

To prepare sauce: Sauté garlic in olive oil; add tomato sauce and tomatoes slowly. Stir in oregano and parsley. Bring to boil and simmer covered for 20 minutes to 2 hours, stirring occasionally. Makes 5 cups.

Next combine filling ingredients and stuff *uncooked* manicotti shells using small butter knife. Fill bottom of 9-by-13-inch casserole dish with 2 cups tomato sauce. Arrange stuffed manicotti shells in a single layer over sauce side by side. Cover shells with remaining 3 cups sauce and pour *1 cup water* over sauce.

Cover dish with foil and bake for 50 minutes. Remove foil and bake another 10 minutes.

Makes 5–6 servings.

PER manicotti:
CALORIES 135   FIBER 1 gm
CSI 2   SODIUM 216 mg
FAT 4 gm

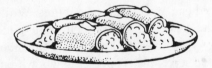

CHINESE NOODLES (HOMEMADE TOP RAAMEN)

An excellent idea for a weekend lunch dish.

SOUP

1 can (14½ ounces) lower-salt chicken broth
1 can water
1 teaspoon lower-sodium soy sauce
1 teaspoon white vinegar
½ teaspoon sesame oil
½–1 teaspoon black bean sauce with chili* (optional)
1 tablespoon fresh chopped cilantro

1 package (8 ounces) chuka soba noodles* or 3 cups cooked spaghetti

VEGETABLES

1 teaspoon oil
1 onion, cut in half and thinly sliced
2 cups sliced mushrooms
4 cups chopped Chinese cabbage
1 teaspoon lower-sodium soy sauce

Combine ingredients for soup and heat to boiling. Add noodles or cooked spaghetti, reduce heat, and cook for 2 minutes. While noodles are cooking, heat oil in skillet, and stir-fry vegetables; add soy sauce. Stir noodles. To serve, place noodles in a bowl, put vegetables on top, and spoon broth over the vegetables and noodles.
Makes 9 cups (about 4 servings).

*Available in Oriental grocery stores or some large supermarkets.

PER serving:
CALORIES 192   FIBER 3 gm
CSI trace   SODIUM 496 mg
FAT 3 gm

CREAMY ENCHILADAS—EASY

This is quick to assemble as it calls for canned enchilada and tomato sauces.

2 cups nonfat yogurt
2 cups low-fat cottage cheese
5–8 green onions, finely chopped
1 can (16 ounces) enchilada sauce
2 cans (8 ounces each) unsalted tomato sauce
12 corn tortillas
4 ounces low-fat cheese, grated

Preheat oven to 350°. Mix yogurt, cottage cheese, and green onions (including tops). Set aside.
Mix enchilada sauce and tomato sauce in saucepan and heat. To make enchiladas, dip corn tortillas into warm sauce in pan to soften or warm for a few seconds in a microwave oven. Spoon generous amount of yogurt mixture into center. Roll up tortillas and place in baking dish. Pour remaining enchilada sauce over the top. Sprinkle with the grated cheese. Bake uncovered for 30 minutes. Let set for 5 minutes before serving.
Makes 6 servings (2 enchiladas each).

PER enchilada:
CALORIES 179   FIBER 2 gm
CSI 3   SODIUM 687 mg
FAT 4 gm

MACARONI BAKE

A light version of macaroni and cheese. It is very low in calories so serve with generous portions of vegetables, salad, and bread, or try it as a side dish with baked chicken.

2 cups uncooked elbow macaroni
1 onion, chopped
2 tablespoons margarine
¼ cup flour
2 cups skim milk
2 teaspoons dill weed
2 teaspoons parsley flakes
⅛ teaspoon garlic powder
½ teaspoon pepper
½ teaspoon Lite Salt or less
2 cups low-fat cottage cheese
⅓ cup bread crumbs
Paprika

Preheat oven to 350°. Cook and drain elbow macaroni. Sauté onions in margarine until tender. Stir in flour. Cook 1 minute, stirring constantly. Blend in milk. Cook and stir over medium heat until thick. Add spices, cottage cheese, and cooked macaroni to the sauce. Pour into shallow, 2-quart baking dish. Top with crumbs and paprika. Bake for 45 minutes or until bubbly.

Makes 4 servings (2 cups each).

PER cup:
CALORIES 246   FIBER 1 gm
CSI 2   SODIUM 381 mg
FAT 5 gm

PASTA WITH FRESH TOMATO SAUCE—*EASY*

Hot pasta mixed with a cold sauce makes a delicious dish. Great with fresh corn, lots of French bread, and a fruit dessert.

1 clove garlic, minced
2 tablespoons red wine vinegar
4 teaspoons olive oil
1 teaspoon Dijon mustard (optional)
¼ teaspoon pepper
½ cup fresh basil, chopped *or* 1 tablespoon dried basil leaves, crumbled
4 cups diced ripe tomatoes
⅓ cup diced red onion
¼ cup sliced black olives
1 pound linguini, fresh if possible (but look for eggless)
¼ cup grated Parmesan cheese

Early in the day or a few hours before dinner (the longer this marinates, the better): Mash garlic in a medium-size bowl. Stir in vinegar, oil, mustard, pepper, and basil. Add the diced tomatoes, onions, and olives and toss to mix.

When nearly ready to eat: Cook pasta in boiling water with no fat added. Drain and return to kettle. Add cheese and toss until heat of pasta begins to melt cheese. Add tomato mixture and toss again to blend. Serve.

Makes 6 servings as a main dish *or* 8 servings as a side dish.

PER ⅙ recipe:
CALORIES 397   FIBER 4 gm
CSI 2   SODIUM 157 mg
FAT 6 gm

VEGETABLE PULAV

Our friend, Anu, brought this from India—

PULAV TOPPING

1 teaspoon oil
1 jalapeño pepper, seeded and finely minced (thinner peppers are hotter; fatter are milder)
1 cup minced onion
1½ cups finely chopped tomato
½ teaspoon Lite Salt or less
¾ cup plain nonfat yogurt

Heat oil in skillet. Add jalapeño pepper and cook 1 minute. Add onions and brown lightly. Add tomatoes and Lite Salt. Cook until mixture is soft. Remove from heat and cool. Stir in yogurt before serving.

MASALA

8 whole cloves
Cardamom seeds from 8 cardamom pods *or* 1 teaspoon cardamom powder
1 jalapeño pepper, seeded
2-inch piece stick cinnamon
3 cloves garlic
1-inch piece fresh ginger root, peeled
¼ cup water

1 tablespoon oil
1½ cups sliced onions (finger-sized pieces)
2 cups sliced potatoes (finger-sized pieces)
1¾ cups (½ of a 16-ounce bag) frozen mixed vegetables
1 cup uncooked rice (basmati is best)
1 teaspoon Lite Salt or less
1 tablespoon freshly squeezed lemon juice
2 cups water

Puree cloves, cardamom, jalapeño pepper, cinnamon, garlic, ginger, and ¼ cup water in blender to make *Masala.* Heat oil in skillet. Add onions and brown lightly. Add potatoes and cook 2 minutes. Add frozen mixed vegetables and cook for 1 minute. Add *Masala* and cook 5 minutes. Add uncooked rice and stir and cook 2 minutes. Add Lite Salt, lemon juice, and 2 cups water. Bring to boil, reduce heat, cover and cook 15 minutes.

Serve warm rice in large bowl with cool pulav topping in a side dish to spoon over top.

Makes 4 servings.

PER serving:
CALORIES 389   FIBER 8 gm
CSI 1   SODIUM 470 mg
FAT 6 gm

FEATURING BEANS

ACAPULCO BEAN CASSEROLE—*EASY*

Tortillas and beans combined for a great dish! The use of canned products makes it very quick to prepare.

1 cup chopped onion
1 cup chopped celery
2 teaspoons margarine
2 cans (16 ounces each) chili with beans*
1 can (16 ounces) refried beans*
1 can (16 ounces) unsalted whole kernel corn, drained
½ cup taco sauce
8 corn tortillas, torn up
1 cup grated low-fat cheese
Fresh whole chile peppers (optional for garnish)

Preheat oven to 350°. In a skillet sauté onions and celery in margarine until tender but not brown, about 10 minutes. Stir in chili, refried beans, corn, and taco sauce. Arrange half the tortilla pieces in a 10-inch-square baking dish; top with half the chili mixture. Repeat layer. Bake, covered, for 45–50 minutes. Sprinkle cheese atop. Bake, uncovered, 2–3 minutes more or until cheese is melted. Garnish with fresh whole chile peppers, if desired.

Makes 8 servings (1½ cups each).

*Use low-sodium beans if available.

PER cup:
CALORIES 236   FIBER 9 gm
CSI 5   SODIUM 626 mg
FAT 9 gm

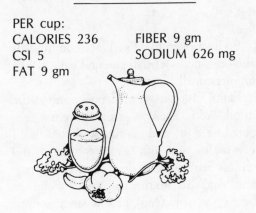

BEAN LASAGNA

A great meatless dish! Make a double batch and freeze one to use later.

2 medium onions, chopped
4 cloves garlic, minced
½–¾ pound mushrooms, sliced
2 teaspoons oil
2 teaspoons oregano leaves
1 teaspoon basil leaves
¼ cup chopped fresh parsley
½ teaspoon Lite Salt or less
1 can (16 ounces) kidney or pinto beans*
½ cup liquid from beans
1 can (16 ounces) unsalted tomatoes

8 ounces uncooked lasagna noodles

3 cups low-fat cottage cheese
4 ounces part-skim mozzarella cheese, grated
2 tablespoons grated Parmesan cheese

Prepare the sauce: Sauté onions, garlic, and mushrooms in oil with oregano, basil, parsley, and Lite Salt, stirring constantly. Drain beans and reserve the liquid. Add this liquid to the sautéed vegetables and herbs; simmer for 5–10 minutes. When onions look clear, stir in beans and tomatoes. Cover pan and simmer sauce for about ½ hour, until slightly thickened. Break up the tomatoes with a fork and stir sauce occasionally while simmering.

Cook lasagna noodles in large pot of boiling water until tender. Rinse in cold

*Use low-sodium beans if available.

(continued)

water to prevent sticking together. Drain well.

Preheat oven to 375°.

Assemble lasagna in a 9-by-13-inch baking dish using a third of each ingredient to layer in this order:

Noodles
Tomato-bean sauce
Cottage cheese
Mozzarella cheese
(Repeat above sequence twice more)

Top with grated Parmesan cheese. Bake 20–30 minutes.

Makes 12 servings (about 3 by 3 inches).

PER serving:

CALORIES 220	FIBER 3 gm
CSI 3	SODIUM 420 mg
FAT 5 gm	

BLACK BEAN CHILI

Very popular! Canned black beans make this chili very quick to prepare.

2 cups dried black beans *or* 3 cans (15 ounces each) black beans*
1 tablespoon whole cumin seed
1 tablespoon oregano leaves
1 cup finely chopped onion (1 small)
2 cups finely chopped green bell pepper (1 large)

*Use low-sodium beans if available.

1 clove garlic, minced
1 tablespoon olive oil
1 teaspoon Tabasco sauce *or* ½ teaspoon cayenne pepper (if you like it hot, use the cayenne)
1 teaspoon Lite Salt or less, omit if using canned beans
1 tablespoon paprika
1 can (16 ounces) unsalted tomatoes, chopped
2 jalapeño chiles, finely chopped (if you like it milder, remove seeds)
1 tablespoon chopped cilantro

GARNISH

⅔ cup nonfat plain yogurt
6 sprigs cilantro

To cook dried beans: Place them in a 3-quart kettle. Cover with water to several inches above top of beans. Cover pot and bring to a boil. Reduce heat and cook for 1¾ hours or until tender. Add more water as needed. When done, strain and reserve ½ cup liquid. Add the liquid back to the beans.

To use canned beans: Pour beans undrained into a 3-quart kettle and heat until simmering.

Preheat oven to 325°. Place cumin seeds and oregano in a small pan and bake 10–12 minutes until toasted.

Sauté onions, green pepper, and garlic in oil. Add Tabasco sauce or cayenne pepper, Lite Salt, and paprika and cook until vegetables are soft. Add tomatoes and chiles. Stir in the toasted cumin and oregano. Add this mixture to cooked or canned beans and stir. Cook at low simmer until heated through.

To serve, top with a dollop of yogurt and a sprig of cilantro.

Makes 6 cups.

PER cup:

CALORIES 277	FIBER 16 gm
CSI <1	SODIUM 237 mg
FAT 4 gm	

BLACK BEANS WITH 1000 USES

We chose the name because, once made, these beans can be used in many ways; in a burrito, as a side dish with chicken fajitas, or—for the daring—served over rice and topped with red salsa. In a hurry? Several companies now have canned black beans available, which greatly reduces the cooking time.

1¼ cups uncooked black beans *or* 2 cans (15 ounces each) black beans*

4 cups water when using uncooked beans *or* 1 cup water when using canned beans

2 cups chopped onion (1 large)

1 cup diced red or green bell pepper (1 large)

2–3 cloves garlic, minced

1 tablespoon ground cumin

1 teaspoon oregano leaves

¼ teaspoon ground black pepper

2 bay leaves

*Use low-sodium beans if available.

6 tablespoons coarsely chopped cilantro *or* parsley, divided

2 tablespoons dry sherry

1 tablespoon brown sugar

¼ cup freshly squeezed lemon juice

2–3 drops Tabasco sauce

¼ teaspoon Lite Salt or less

When using uncooked black beans: Soak beans overnight in enough water to cover entirely. In the morning drain beans and add 4 cups water. Cook one-half hour over moderate heat and proceed as for canned beans.

When using canned black beans: Rinse beans under cold water and drain. Add onion, red or green pepper, garlic, spices, and 3 tablespoons cilantro or parsley to beans. Add 1 cup water and cook for 20 minutes or until beans are soft. Add remaining parsley, sherry, brown sugar, lemon juice, Tabasco sauce, and Lite Salt. Simmer until ready to serve.

Makes 4 cups.

PER ½ cup:

CALORIES 63	FIBER 3 gm
CSI trace	SODIUM 38 mg
FAT trace	

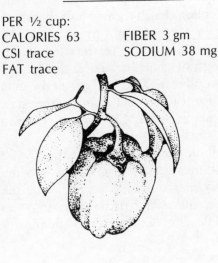

CHILE RELLENO CASSEROLE

A spicy, hearty casserole—serve with a crisp salad and *Baked Corn Chips* (page 262).

⅔ cup uncooked brown rice
2 cups *Refried Beans* (page 331) *or* 1 can (16 ounces) refried beans*
1 can (7 ounces) whole green chiles *or* 8 fresh chiles
4 ounces low-fat cheese
1 can (8 ounces) unsalted tomato sauce
1 teaspoon oregano leaves
¼ teaspoon Lite Salt or less
½ teaspoon garlic powder
2 tablespoons minced chives *or* green onions

Cook rice. Lightly oil a large, deep casserole dish. Mix beans and rice. Place half of this mixture on the bottom of the dish and set aside.

Prepare chile peppers. If you are using fresh chiles, blanch them or hold them over an open gas flame until the skin crackles and burns all around; peel the skins off. Slit the fresh or canned chiles lengthwise and remove all of the seeds and cut off the stem ends. Rinse under cold water if you prefer a less spicy casserole. Cut peppers crosswise into 1-inch-long sections.

Preheat oven to 350°. Cut the low-fat cheese into chunks that will fit into the chiles. Stuff the chile peppers with the cheese chunks and nestle them into the casserole dish. Cover them with the re-

maining rice-bean mixture. Mix tomato sauce, spices, and chives *or* green onions. Pour over top. Bake for 30 minutes.
Makes 4 servings.

PER serving:
CALORIES 310   FIBER 10 gm
CSI 4   SODIUM 217 mg
FAT 8 gm

GARBANZO GOULASH—*QUICK*

A quick macaroni dish. Nice to serve with *Old-Style Wheat Biscuits* (page 276).

1½ cups uncooked small shell macaroni *or* 2 cups uncooked large-sized macaroni
1 medium onion, chopped
2 teaspoons oil
1 can (16 ounces) garbanzo beans, drained*
1 can (16 ounces) unsalted tomatoes
2 tablespoons chopped fresh parsley
1 teaspoon ground cumin

Cook macaroni in unsalted boiling water according to package directions. In the meantime, sauté onions in oil until tender. Add drained beans and canned tomatoes with juice. Cut up canned tomatoes with spatula. Let simmer until macaroni is ready.

Drain macaroni. Add to bean-tomato mixture and mix. Add seasonings. For best

---

*Use low-sodium beans if available.

*Use low-sodium beans if available.

flavor, let mixture simmer or boil for a few minutes until macaroni has been slightly colored by the tomato juice.

Makes 3 to 4 servings (about 8 cups).

PER cup:
CALORIES 208   FIBER 4 gm
CSI trace   SODIUM 135 mg
FAT 3 gm

NO-MEAT ENCHILADAS

Bean-filled corn tortillas.

SAUCE (very quickly prepared)

1 tablespoon oil
1 tablespoon chili powder
1½ tablespoons flour
1½ cups water
1 teaspoon vinegar
½ teaspoon garlic powder
½ teaspoon onion powder
½ teaspoon Lite Salt or less
¼ teaspoon oregano leaves

FILLING

½ cup low-fat cottage cheese
¾ cup *Refried Beans* (page 331) or ¾
    cup canned refried beans*
1 cup grated low-fat cheese, divided
1 medium onion, finely chopped

8 corn tortillas
1 cup *Mock Sour Cream* (page 451)
¼ cup chopped green onions

*Use low-sodium beans if available.

To make sauce: Heat oil, chili powder, and flour in a small saucepan to make a paste. Add water gradually to make a smooth sauce; add vinegar, garlic powder, onion powder, Lite Salt, and oregano. Bring to a boil. Lower heat; simmer uncovered for about 3 minutes.

To assemble dish: Preheat oven to 350°. Reserve a third of the grated cheese for topping. Mix refried beans, remaining cheese, cottage cheese, and onions in a bowl. Warm tortillas in the oven or microwave or dip in warm sauce. Place ¼ cup of the bean filling down center of each tortilla. Roll up; place seam side down in shallow baking dish. Pour sauce over filled enchiladas and sprinkle with reserved cheese. Bake for 20 minutes or until bubbly.

Top with *Mock Sour Cream* and chopped green onions before serving.

Makes 4 servings (2 enchiladas each).

PER enchilada:
CALORIES 202   FIBER 3 gm
CSI 4   SODIUM 371 mg
FAT 7 gm

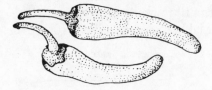

PINTO BEAN CHOW MEIN—*QUICK*

An Oriental stir-fry with beans. Fruit salad goes well with this.

        3 tablespoons cornstarch
        ¼ cup cold water
        ¼ cup lower-sodium soy sauce
        ½ bouillon cube
        1¼ cups boiling water
        3 cups diagonally sliced celery
        1 cup sliced onions
        ¾ cup sliced mushrooms
        1 tablespoon oil
        1 can (16 ounces) pinto beans, drained*
        1 can (16 ounces) bean sprouts, drained
        1 can (8 ounces) sliced water chestnuts, drained
        1 can (6 ounces) bamboo shoots (optional)

Blend cornstarch in ¼ cup cold water and soy sauce; dissolve ½ bouillon cube in 1¼ cups boiling water. Set aside. Stir-fry celery, onions, and mushrooms in oil until crisp-tender. Add cornstarch mixture and bouillon to vegetables.

Add pinto beans, bean sprouts, water chestnuts, and bamboo shoots. Cook and stir until thickened. Serve over rice.

Makes 6 servings (about 10 cups).

*Use low-sodium beans if available.

PER cup:
CALORIES 96   FIBER 4 gm
CSI trace   SODIUM 416 mg
FAT 2 gm

RICK'S CHILI—*EASY*

A meatless version that is simple and delicious. *Onion Squares* (page 338) are great with it.

        2 cloves garlic, minced
        1 medium onion, chopped
        2–3 stalks celery, chopped
        ½ pound mushrooms, sliced
        1½ green bell peppers, chopped
        1 tablespoon oil
        1 tablespoon water
        2 cans (16 ounces each) unsalted tomatoes, cut up
        2 cans (16 ounces each) kidney beans, drained*
        1–3 tablespoons chili powder, or to taste

Lightly sauté fresh vegetables in oil and water until onions are tender. Add tomatoes, beans, and chili powder. Cook covered for 1 hour or longer on low heat.

Makes 6 servings (about 10 cups).

*Use low-sodium beans if available.

PER cup:
CALORIES 126   FIBER 5 gm
CSI <1   SODIUM 189 mg
FAT 3 gm

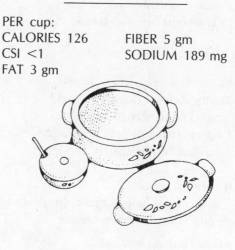

SPICY LENTILS

1½ cups lentils, rinsed under cold water
3 cups water
1 cup chopped onion
½ cup chopped red bell pepper
1 tablespoon oil
1 teaspoon Lite Salt or less
1 teaspoon ground cumin
¾ teaspoon turmeric
½ teaspoon ground coriander
¼ teaspoon cinnamon
⅛ teaspoon cayenne pepper, or to taste
⅛ teaspoon ground cloves

Nonfat yogurt, for garnish
Chutney, for garnish

In a saucepan combine the lentils with 3 cups water, bring the water to a boil, and cook the lentils over moderately low heat for 15–20 minutes, or until they are tender. Remove from heat and *do not drain.* In a large skillet cook onion and pepper in the oil, stirring until the vegetables are softened. Add Lite Salt, cumin, turmeric, coriander, cinnamon, cayenne pepper, and cloves; cook the mixture, stirring, for 1 minute. Add the cooked lentils with the cooking liquid and simmer the mixture, stirring occasionally, for 10 minutes. Transfer the lentils to a serving dish and garnish them with yogurt and chutney.

Makes 4 cups.

PER cup:
CALORIES 137   FIBER 5 gm
CSI <1   SODIUM 247 mg
FAT 4 gm

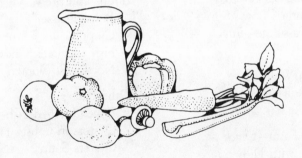

FISH AND SHELLFISH

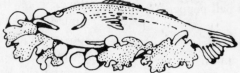

Fish and shellfish can add great variety to your eating style. The flavors and textures available are endless. There are two recipes for oysters that are not fried but are very tasty.

With Salmon
    Baked Salmon
    Peppered Salmon Steak—*Quick*
    Salmon Loaf—*Easy*

With Tuna
    Alphabet Seafood Salad—*Easy*
    Bean Sprout Tuna Chow Mein—*Quick*
    Tuna Noodle Casserole—*Easy*

Roll-Ups
    Fish Fillets with Walnuts
    Lively Lemon Roll-Ups

With Sauces
    Clam Sauce for Pasta—*Quick*
    Fish Almondine with Dilly Sauce
    Halibut Mexicana
    Peppers and Prawns
    Scallops in Creamy Sauce

Fancier
    Fancy Baked Scallops
    Fish à la Mistral—*Easy*
    Halibut and Vegetables
    Seafood Strudel

Soups and Stews
    Bouillabaisse
    Cioppino
    Fish and Leek Chowder
    Northwest Gumbo

Other Ideas
    Baked Herbed Fish—*Quick*
    Oysters in Crusty French Bread
    Oysters Sauté
    Seafood Pilaf
    Seafood Teriyaki and Kabobs
    Skinny Sole—*Quick*
    Sole with Spring Vegetables
    Wonderful Oriental Steamed Fish

WITH SALMON

BAKED SALMON

Fit for a picture—this whole salmon can be served warm or baked earlier, refrigerated, and served cold the next day. The skin is removed while the fish is still warm. The fish can be beautifully decorated just before serving.

> **One whole 6-to-8-pound salmon (including head and tail), cleaned**
> **4 teaspoons margarine**
> **1 lemon, sliced**
> **2 whole green onions**
> **1 stalk celery**
> **1 cup white wine**

GARNISH

> **1 bunch red leaf lettuce**
> **2 lemons *or* 1 cucumber, very thinly sliced**
> **1 bunch fresh parsley**

> **Lemon wedges**
> ***Cucumber-Dilly Sauce* (page 453)**

Heat oven to 350°. Wipe cleaned salmon inside and out with paper towels. Line baking sheet with large sheets of foil that can be wrapped around salmon. Lay salmon on foil. Rub margarine on both sides of salmon including the tail and head. This prevents foil from sticking to fish. Place lemon slices from one lemon, green onions, and celery inside salmon. Heat wine to boiling and pour carefully over salmon. Seal foil tightly. Bake for 25 minutes. Carefully turn unwrapped salmon over and bake for 15 minutes. Fish is done when a knife inserts easily into the thickest part and salmon is opaque in color all the way through.

When done, remove salmon from oven, open foil carefully, and immediately remove skin and dark meat from one side of salmon. Roll fish onto a large sheet of plastic wrap. Remove skin and dark meat from other side of salmon. Wrap salmon and juices tightly in the plastic wrap. Refrigerate salmon until serving time.

To serve, place salmon on a large platter or tray lined with red leaf lettuce. Decorate with lemon or cucumber slices and parsley. Serve with lemon wedges and *Cucumber-Dilly Sauce.*

Makes 24 servings (3 ounces each).

PER serving:

CALORIES 185	FIBER 0 gm
CSI 7	SODIUM 73 mg
FAT 11 gm	

PEPPERED SALMON STEAK—*QUICK*

This also works well with flank steak.

1 tablespoon coarsely ground pepper
1 teaspoon Italian seasoning
¼ teaspoon garlic powder
½ teaspoon dry mustard
2 pounds salmon steaks

Combine seasonings. Rinse fish in cold water and pat dry with paper towels. Rub seasoning mixture onto both sides of salmon steaks. Grill over charcoal or broil in oven about 5 minutes to a side.

Makes 4 servings.

PER serving:
CALORIES 251   FIBER trace
CSI 5   SODIUM 79 mg
FAT 10 gm

SALMON LOAF—*EASY*

Serve slices of this loaf with *Super Stuffed Potatoes* (page 335) and a favorite vegetable.

2 cups soft bread crumbs
1 onion, chopped
1 tablespoon melted margarine
¼ cup minced celery
1 cup skim milk
2 cups flaked canned salmon
1 tablespoon freshly squeezed lemon juice
Dash pepper
1 tablespoon minced parsley

3 egg whites
½ teaspoon Worcestershire sauce

Heat oven to 325°. Combine all ingredients and mix thoroughly. Place in lightly oiled 9-by-5-inch loaf pan. Bake for 45 minutes.

Makes 6 servings.

PER serving:
CALORIES 174   FIBER 1 gm
CSI 3   SODIUM 498 mg
FAT 7 gm

WITH TUNA

ALPHABET SEAFOOD SALAD—*EASY*

A popular cold pasta salad. Excellent for potlucks or picnics—children love this dish.

1 package (12 ounces) alphabet noodles
2 cans (6½ ounces each) water-packed tuna, drained and flaked
1 can (2.2 ounces) black olives, sliced
1 medium onion, finely chopped
¼ cup chopped parsley
¼ teaspoon paprika

DRESSING

1 cup plain nonfat yogurt
¼ cup light mayonnaise
1 teaspoon Dijon mustard
2 tablespoons sweet pickle juice

Cook alphabet noodles in unsalted water following package directions. Drain well and combine with tuna, drained olives, onions, parsley, and paprika. Cover and chill until serving time.

Meanwhile, mix dressing ingredients together and add to rest of salad *just before serving*. This is especially important in order to keep the salad creamy because the noodles absorb the yogurt dressing.

Makes 12 servings (1 cup each).

PER cup:

CALORIES 242	FIBER 1 gm
CSI 2	SODIUM 243 mg
FAT 3 gm	

BEAN SPROUT TUNA CHOW MEIN—*QUICK*

A tuna stir-fry dish that can be prepared in 20 minutes! Serve with rice, *Sunshine Spinach Salad* (page 294) and *Cocoa Cake* (page 431).

½ chicken bouillon cube
1 cup water
1 tablespoon lower-sodium soy sauce
2 tablespoons cornstarch
1 tablespoon oil
6 stalks celery, cut diagonally
2 medium onions, thinly sliced
1 can (6 ounces) bamboo shoots, drained
½ cup sliced fresh mushrooms *or* 1 can (4 ounces) mushrooms, drained
2 cups fresh bean sprouts *or* 1 can (15 ounces) bean sprouts
1 can (6½ ounces) water-packed tuna, drained

Dissolve bouillon in water. Add soy sauce. Stir in cornstarch until dissolved. Heat oil in skillet or wok over high heat. When hot, toss in celery and onions and stir-fry 1 minute. Add bamboo shoots, mushrooms, and bean sprouts. Stir bouillon mixture and add to vegetables. Stir and cook just until sauce is thickened. Add tuna and stir until hot and sauce is clear. Serve immediately over fluffy rice.

Makes 4 servings (1¾ cups each).

PER serving:

CALORIES 159	FIBER 3 gm
CSI 2	SODIUM 499 mg
FAT 5 gm	

TUNA NOODLE CASSEROLE—*EASY*

The unsalted canned soups and vegetables now readily available make this dish much lower in salt in addition to being lower in fat.

3 cups uncooked eggless noodles
½ small onion, chopped
¼ cup sliced mushrooms
1 can (6½ ounces) water-packed tuna, drained
1 can (10½ ounces) low-sodium cream of mushroom soup *or* use *Homemade "Cream" Soup Mix* (page 314)
½ teaspoon Lite Salt or less
Pepper to taste
1 can (16 ounces) unsalted green beans, drained
½ cup crushed Rice Krispies

(continued)

Preheat oven to 325°. Cook noodles in unsalted boiling water until tender. Drain well. Steam onions and mushrooms in a small amount of water until onions are transparent. Remove with slotted spoon and combine with the cooked noodles, tuna fish, soup, Lite Salt, pepper, and green beans in casserole dish. Bake uncovered for 15–20 minutes or until heated through. Sprinkle crushed cereal over top and serve.

Makes 4 servings (2 cups each).

PER serving:
CALORIES 292   FIBER 5 gm
CSI 2   SODIUM 328 mg
FAT 4 gm

ROLL-UPS

FISH FILLETS WITH WALNUTS

A very elegant and tasty dish. The walnuts make it special.

2 pounds sole fillets *or* other white fish
Freshly ground black pepper
1 tablespoon oil
1 tablespoon flour
1 cup clam juice
2 tablespoons prepared mustard
¼ cup chopped walnuts

Preheat oven to 400°. Season fish with pepper. Heat oil in a saucepan; blend in flour and cook over medium heat about 1 minute, stirring until smooth. Add clam juice and mustard. Cook until thickened, stirring constantly.

Roll fish fillets jelly-roll style and place seam side down in a shallow casserole. Spoon sauce over fish. Sprinkle with nuts. Bake 15–20 minutes, until fish flakes easily with a fork.

Makes 4 servings.

PER serving:
CALORIES 246   FIBER <1 gm
CSI 7   SODIUM 460 mg
FAT 11 gm

LIVELY LEMON ROLL-UPS

One of the favorite recipes in this book.

1 tablespoon margarine
½ cup freshly squeezed lemon juice
½ chicken bouillon cube
½–1 teaspoon Tabasco sauce
2 cups cooked brown rice
2 packages (10 ounces each) frozen chopped broccoli, thawed, *or* 1 head fresh broccoli, finely chopped
¾ cup chopped green onion
½ cup grated low-fat cheese
3 pounds sole (thin white fish works best)
Paprika

Preheat oven to 375°. In small saucepan, melt the margarine. Add lemon juice, bouillon cube, and Tabasco. Heat slowly until bouillon dissolves; set aside. In medium bowl combine cooked rice, broccoli, green onions, cheese, and half of the above sauce. Mix well and place half of rice mixture on bottom of shallow baking dish.

Cut fish into 6 fillets and spread flat on work surface. Divide remaining broccoli mixture equally among fillets. Roll fillets up around rice mixture (secure with wooden picks if necessary) and place seam side down on top of rice in baking dish. Pour remaining sauce over roll-ups. Bake 25 minutes or until fish flakes easily with a fork. Garnish with paprika.

Makes 6 servings.

PER serving:
CALORIES 281   FIBER 5 gm
CSI 7   SODIUM 351 mg
FAT 6 gm

WITH SAUCES

CLAM SAUCE FOR PASTA—*QUICK*

An elegant way to serve pasta—and easy to make as well!

3 cans (6½ ounces each) chopped *or* minced clams
2 cloves garlic, minced
4 teaspoons margarine
2 tablespoons flour

¼ **cup finely chopped fresh parsley**
¼ **teaspoon pepper**
¼ **teaspoon thyme leaves**
¼ **cup grated Parmesan cheese for topping**

Drain clams into a 2-cup measure and add water to make 2 cups. In a saucepan sauté garlic in margarine over medium heat. Add flour and mix well. It will be dry. Add clam juice/water mixture, stirring rapidly with wire whisk to smooth out lumps. Add parsley, pepper, and thyme. Stir and simmer for a few minutes. Add clams and heat through. Serve over warm pasta. Sprinkle with Parmesan cheese.

Makes about 4 cups sauce.

PER cup:
CALORIES 222   FIBER trace
CSI 8   SODIUM 274 mg
FAT 10 gm

FISH ALMONDINE WITH DILLY SAUCE

A meal fit for guests—the almonds add a great finishing touch.

2 pounds white fish
Juice of 2 lemons
2 teaspoons tarragon leaves
1 cup *Dilly Sauce* (see below)
¼ **cup sliced almonds, toasted**

Wash fish in cold water and pat dry. Place in a flat baking dish. Squeeze lemon juice

(continued)

over both sides of fish. Cover tightly and place in refrigerator until time to cook (no longer than 24 hours).

Twenty minutes before serving, preheat oven to 350°. Sprinkle tarragon over the fish. Cover the dish and bake for 15 minutes. Prepare *Dilly Sauce* while fish cooks. Remove the fish from the oven and pour off excess liquid. Spoon *Dilly Sauce* evenly over the fish. Place under the broiler until sauce starts to bubble, about 1 minute. Sprinkle the sliced almonds on top of each serving.

Makes 4 servings.

DILLY SAUCE

2 tablespoons light mayonnaise
1 cup plain nonfat yogurt
¾ teaspoon tarragon leaves
1½ teaspoons dill weed

Put the mayonnaise and yogurt in a mixing bowl. Mix thoroughly with a wire whisk. Add the other ingredients and blend well.

Makes about 1 cup.

PER serving:
CALORIES 248   FIBER 1 gm
CSI 7   SODIUM 255 mg
FAT 8 gm

HALIBUT MEXICANA

If you like the flavors of Mexican food and are learning to like fish, this dish is for you.

2 pounds halibut steaks or fillets

MARINADE

⅓ cup lime juice
3 cloves garlic, minced
1 tablespoon oil
¼ cup white wine, beer, *or* water
1 tablespoon chopped parsley
½ teaspoon ground cumin
2 teaspoons Dijon mustard
Freshly ground pepper to taste

SALSA (Makes about 1¼ cups salsa)

2 medium tomatoes, seeded and coarsely chopped
¼ cup chopped red onion
3 tablespoons diced green chiles
2 to 3 dashes Tabasco sauce

Place halibut in dish and set aside. Combine lime juice, garlic, oil, wine (or beer or water), parsley, cumin, mustard, and pepper; pour over halibut. Cover and marinate in refrigerator for 1 hour, turning once.

While halibut is marinating, make salsa. Combine tomatoes, onion, green chiles, and Tabasco sauce in blender and blend well. Let stand at room temperature or in refrigerator for at least 15–20 minutes to blend flavors.

Drain halibut, reserving marinade. Place on lightly oiled grill. Cook 4–5 minutes, baste with marinade, and turn. Cook an additional 4–5 minutes until fish flakes when tested with a fork. Can be broiled in oven 3–4 inches from broiler. Top with salsa to serve.

Makes 4 servings.

PER serving:
CALORIES 259   FIBER 1 gm
CSI 7   SODIUM 297 mg
FAT 6 gm

PEPPERS AND PRAWNS

The West Coast of the United States calls them prawns while on the East Coast they are labeled shrimp; all are the same delicious shellfish! This dish can be quite spicy depending upon the amount of Thai chili sauce you use.

½ cup ketchup
1–2 teaspoons Thai (sweet) chili sauce* (adjust to your taste)
1 tablespoon oil
1 clove garlic, minced
1 pound prawns, peeled and deveined (avoid the work of peeling by buying the ¾ pound rock shrimp, which are peeled when sold)
1 cup sliced onion (1 medium)
1 cup thinly sliced green bell pepper (1 medium)
1 cup thinly sliced red bell pepper (1 medium)
1 stalk celery, sliced diagonally
1 teaspoon freshly squeezed lemon juice (optional)

*Available in Oriental grocery stores.

Combine ketchup and Thai chili sauce; set aside. Heat oil in large skillet over medium heat. Add garlic and sauté until lightly golden. Add prawns and cook just until prawns turn pinkish-white. Remove prawns from skillet and cover to keep warm.

Add onion, red and green peppers, and celery to skillet and stir-fry until crisp-tender. Add prawns again and stir in ketchup–chili sauce mixture. Heat thoroughly. Sprinkle with lemon juice, if desired. Serve with steamed rice.

Makes 4 servings.

PER serving:
CALORIES 174   FIBER 2 gm
CSI 9   SODIUM 578 mg
FAT 5 gm

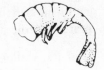
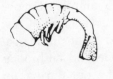

SCALLOPS IN CREAMY SAUCE

PER serving:
CALORIES 218   FIBER 1 gm
CSI 4   SODIUM 318 mg
FAT 6 gm

A low-fat version of the famous Coquilles St. Jacques. Lovely when baked in individual scallop shells. *Baba au Rhum* (page 429) for dessert would complete this elegant menu.

1 pound bay scallops (small ones)
½ cup dry sherry
¼ cup water
1 bay leaf
½ pound mushrooms, sliced
1 small onion, chopped
1½ tablespoons margarine
1½ tablespoons flour
1 tablespoon freshly squeezed lemon juice
⅛ teaspoon paprika
Dash ground pepper
1 tablespoon dry bread crumbs
1 tablespoon grated Parmesan cheese

Preheat oven to 325°. Put scallops, sherry, water, and bay leaf in skillet. Cover and simmer on stovetop for 5 minutes. Remove scallops, drain, and reserve broth. Cook and stir mushrooms and onions in margarine until onions are tender and mushrooms brown. Stir in flour and cook, stirring, for 1 minute or until bubbling. Stir in reserved broth, lemon juice, paprika, and pepper. Heat, stirring constantly, until mixture thickens. Add scallops. Pour into casserole dish or divide among individual scallop shells. Sprinkle bread crumbs and cheese on top. Garnish with a sprinkling of paprika for color. Bake until golden brown and heated through, 5–15 minutes.

Makes 4 servings.

FANCIER

FANCY BAKED SCALLOPS

This is a treat fit for royalty; *Gourmet Curried Rice* (page 325) makes it twice as good.

1 pound fresh scallops
1 tablespoon olive oil
2 teapoons finely chopped garlic
1 red bell pepper, cut into thin strips about 1½ inches long
2 green bell peppers, cut into thin strips about 1½ inches long
¾ cup sliced onions
1½ cups ripe plum tomatoes, cut into 1½-inch cubes
¼ cup sliced black olives
1 teaspoon oregano leaves
½ teaspoon fennel *or* anise seed
½ cup dry white wine
⅛ teaspoon dried hot red pepper flakes *or* ⅛ teaspoon Tabasco sauce
⅛ teaspoon freshly ground pepper
1 ounce crumbled feta cheese

Preheat oven to 375°. Spray 4 individual ovenproof serving dishes with nonstick spray. Divide the scallops evenly among the dishes.

Heat oil and garlic in a heavy skillet. Add peppers and onion. Cook and stir over medium-high heat until wilted. Add the tomatoes, olives, oregano, fennel, wine, pepper flakes, and pepper. Bring to a boil and simmer for 5 minutes. Add feta cheese and spoon the mixture evenly over the scallops. Bake 15–20 minutes or until lightly browned. Serve immediately.

Makes 4 servings.

PER serving:
CALORIES 226　　　FIBER 2 gm
CSI 5　　　SODIUM 464 mg
FAT 8 gm

FISH À LA MISTRAL—*EASY*

It's worth the effort to have fennel seeds on hand for this delicious dish.

1 onion, finely chopped
1 tablespoon oil
2 tomatoes, peeled and coarsely chopped
½ teaspoon Lite Salt or less
2 pounds fish steaks or fillets (white fish *or* salmon)
4 fresh lemon slices
1 tablespoon chopped parsley
⅛ teaspoon fennel seeds (optional)
½ cup dry white wine

Preheat oven to 350°. Sauté onions in oil in nonstick skillet until golden brown. Add tomatoes and Lite Salt; cook 3–5 minutes. Pour into baking dish large enough to hold fish. Lay fish on top of vegetable mixture.

Add 1 slice of lemon on top of each steak. Sprinkle with parsley, fennel seeds, and wine. Bake for 20–30 minutes or until fish flakes easily with a fork. (When serving, spoon vegetable mixture over fish.)

Makes 4 servings.

PER serving:
CALORIES 203　　　FIBER 1 gm
CSI 6　　　SODIUM 274 mg
FAT 5 gm

HALIBUT AND VEGETABLES

The fish and vegetables can be baked in the oven if you do not have parchment paper* on hand. This dish is very attractive.

1 cup asparagus spears *or* green beans
½ cup sliced red bell pepper
⅓ cup sliced red onion
1 tablespoon olive oil
¼ cup slivered almonds or hazelnuts†
½–1 teaspoon oregano leaves, crumbled
½ teaspoon Lite Salt or less
¼ teaspoon pepper
4 halibut steaks
Juice from 1 lemon

Sauté asparagus or beans, red pepper, and onion in olive oil for about 1 minute. Remove from heat; add nuts, oregano, Lite

---

*Cooking/baking paper that can be purchased in a food specialty store.

†To remove skins from hazelnuts, heat in 350° oven for 15 minutes; rub skins off with terry cloth towel.

(continued)

Salt, and pepper and toss gently. Cool slightly.

Preheat oven to 400°. Cut 4 sheets of parchment paper to measure 15 by 14 inches; fold in half and cut into heart shapes. Lightly spray paper with nonstick spray to within 1 inch of edges. Place halibut on one side of each heart. Season fish with pepper and sprinkle each with lemon juice.

Arrange ½ cup vegetable mixture around halibut. Fold other half of heart around halibut. Seal edges with tightly creased overlapping folds. Place on baking sheet. Bake for 10 minutes or until packets are puffed and lightly browned. Remove from oven; cut paper around halibut. Serve immediately.

As an alternative, bake fish surrounded by vegetables in covered casserole dish in 375° oven for 20–30 minutes or until fish flakes easily with a fork.

Makes 4 servings.

PER serving:

CALORIES 289 FIBER 2 gm
CSI 7 SODIUM 306 mg
FAT 10 gm

SEAFOOD STRUDEL

For ease in handling strudel, assemble phyllo* and the filling on plastic wrap. Then use the wrap like a sling to transfer to a baking sheet. Remove wrap before baking. It's important to have all the seafood fairly uniform in size.

1 teaspoon oil
1 carrot, sliced (½ cup)
½ cup chopped onion
1 package (10 ounces) frozen chopped spinach, thawed and squeezed dry
¼ teaspoon Lite Salt or less
¼ teaspoon dried sage
⅓ pound medium shrimp, shelled and deveined
⅓ pound scallops
⅓ pound boneless salmon, cut in 1-inch pieces
½ cup dry bread crumbs
6 sheets phyllo*
1½ tablespoons melted margarine
Carrot tops, if available
12 cherry tomatoes

Preheat oven to 375°. Heat oil in skillet over medium heat. Sauté carrots and onions. Add spinach, Lite Salt, and sage. Gently stir in seafood and ¼ cup bread crumbs, taking care not to break up the seafood. (The crumbs help prevent the bottom crust of strudel from getting soggy.) Remove from heat immediately (seafood will be cooked in oven).

On plastic wrap, place 1 sheet of phyllo. Brush the phyllo with small amount of melted margarine, using a pastry brush. Sprinkle with two teaspoons bread crumbs. Continue layering phyllo, brushing with margarine and sprinkling with crumbs. Starting with long side of phyllo, spoon seafood mixture to cover one-fourth of phyllo rectangle. Beginning with seafood

*A trick in handling phyllo pastry is to be sure to thaw it in the refrigerator and work with it while it is cold. If allowed to come to room temperature before unfolding, it is hard to handle. The remainder of the pastry keeps well in refrigerator if wrapped tightly.

mixture side, roll phyllo jelly-roll fashion. Tuck ends in to seal. Place roll, seam side down, on ungreased baking sheet. Brush with remaining margarine.

Bake strudel 20 minutes or until golden brown. Cool on baking sheet for 5 minutes for easier cutting.

To serve, cut strudel into 6 slices. Arrange on warm platter or individual plates and decorate with cherry tomatoes and carrot tops, if available.

Makes 6 servings.

PER serving:
CALORIES 232   FIBER 3 gm
CSI 4   SODIUM 369 mg
FAT 6 gm

SOUPS AND STEWS

BOUILLABAISSE

Serve with French bread to use for dipping in the soup, so all the sauce can be enjoyed! It's a great party dish.

2 large onions, thinly sliced
2 leeks, minced
1 tablespoon oil
4 cloves garlic, mashed
3 large tomatoes, peeled, seeded, and diced
5 cups water

3 cups clam juice (24 ounces)
2 tablespoons chopped parsley
1 bay leaf
⅛ teaspoon fennel seeds
½ teaspoon thyme or basil leaves
⅛ teaspoon saffron
2-inch-by-½-inch piece orange peel
½ teaspoon Lite Salt or less
½ teaspoon pepper
2 pounds lean fish bones, trimmings, etc. for stock
2 pounds assorted lean fish and shellfish (more than one kind—bass, snapper, halibut, turbot, cod, scallops, etc.), cut in large pieces

To prepare stock: In a large kettle cook onions and leeks slowly in oil until tender but not browned. Stir in the garlic and tomatoes. Cook 5 minutes. Add water, clam juice, herbs, and seasonings. Tie fish bones and trimmings together in a large piece of cheesecloth. Add this bundle to vegetables. Simmer covered for 30 minutes. Discard fish bones and trimmings, strain the stock or puree it through a food mill. Stock can be refrigerated or frozen at this point.

Twenty minutes before serving: Bring the fish stock to a boil. Add fresh fish and shellfish. Bring rapidly back to boiling and cook 5 minutes or until fish flakes easily with a fork. Do not overcook.

Makes 8 small servings (1½ cups each) or 4 larger servings (3 cups each).

PER serving (1½ cups):
CALORIES 123   FIBER 1 gm
CSI 3   SODIUM 422 mg
FAT 3 gm

CIOPPINO

A fine kettle of fish—serve with lots of crusty bread, salad, and a hearty fruit cobbler for dessert.

1 pound red snapper *or* halibut (*or* use ½ pound snapper *or* halibut, and ½ pound scallops *or* prawns)
1 tablespoon oil
1 cup chopped onion
2 cloves garlic, finely minced
1 can (8 ounces) unsalted tomato sauce
2 cans (16 ounces each) unsalted tomatoes
½ cup water *or* dry white wine
1 teaspoon basil leaves
1 teaspoon thyme leaves
1 teaspoon marjoram leaves
1 teaspoon oregano leaves
1 bay leaf
¼ teaspoon pepper
¼ cup chopped parsley *or* 1 tablespoon dried parsley flakes
1 dozen steamer clams (optional)
1 cup shrimp meat

Cut fish into ½-inch chunks and set aside. Heat oil in large kettle and sauté onions and garlic until onions are tender but not brown. Add tomato sauce, tomatoes, liquid, and all seasonings. Let simmer 20–30 minutes until as thick as desired, stirring occasionally. Soup base can be refrigerated at this point to serve at later time.

When ready to serve, reheat soup base and add fish chunks and scrubbed steamer clams (in shell). Cook until clams open, about 10 minutes. Just before serving, add shrimp meat. Serve warm in large soup bowls.

Makes 4 servings (2¼ cups each).

PER serving:
CALORIES 299   FIBER 4 gm
CSI 8   SODIUM 225 mg
FAT 7 gm

FISH AND LEEK CHOWDER

Prepare the chowder base ahead of time and add the fish just before serving for a convenient, quick meal.

1 tablespoon margarine
½ cup chopped onion (1 medium)
2 medium carrots, sliced
1½ cups chopped green bell pepper
2 cups chopped tomatoes (3 medium)
2 cups potatoes, peeled and cut into ½-inch cubes (4 medium)
1 cup clam juice
4 fresh leeks (use chopped white parts) *or* ½ envelope dry leek soup mix
1 bay leaf
1 teaspoon red pepper flakes (optional)
1 cup dry white wine *or* water
⅛ teaspoon freshly ground pepper
1 teaspoon thyme leaves
2 tablespoons chopped parsley
1 pound white fish fillets, cut into 1½-inch chunks
½ pound scallops
1 can (12 ounces) evaporated skim milk

Melt margarine in a large soup kettle. Add onion and cook over moderate heat until onion is soft. Add carrots, green pepper, tomatoes, potatoes, clam juice, leeks, bay leaf, red pepper flakes, wine *or* water, pepper, thyme, and parsley. Bring to boil, reduce heat and simmer, covered, 10 minutes or until potatoes are almost done. Add fish fillets and scallops and simmer covered, five to 10 minutes or until fish is just done (don't overcook). Add skim milk. Mix well. Heat just to serving temperature.

Makes 12 cups.

PER cup:
CALORIES 142   FIBER 3 gm
CSI 2   SODIUM 207 mg
FAT 2 gm

NORTHWEST GUMBO

A recent trip to New Orleans was the inspiration for this dish. Serve in large bowls over steamed rice.

1 tablespoon olive oil
8 ounces fresh okra, trimmed and cut into 1-inch lengths (optional)
1 cup coarsely chopped onion (1 large)
1 cup very finely chopped celery
1 large clove garlic, finely chopped
1 large shallot, finely chopped
3 tablespoons flour
2 teaspoons filé powder*
½ teaspoon Lite Salt or less
1 teaspoon sugar
1 teaspoon freshly ground black pepper

*Filé powder used to flavor and thicken Creole soups and stews is made from dried young sassafras leaves and is found in the spice department in most supermarkets.

1 teaspoon ground cumin
4 cups water or fish stock
1 cup coarsely chopped green bell pepper (½ large)
1 cup coarsely chopped red bell pepper (½ large)
1 pound tomatoes cored, and cut into thin wedges
⅓ cup chopped fresh parsley
2 tablespoons finely chopped cilantro
8 drops Tabasco sauce
½ pound halibut steaks, cut into 1-inch cubes
1 pound snapper or orange roughy fillets, cut into 1-inch pieces
½ pound medium shrimp, peeled and cleaned

6 cups steamed rice

Heat 1 tablespoon of oil in a heavy pot over medium-high heat. (If using okra, add now and sauté it, turning frequently, until it is evenly browned—about five minutes. Remove the okra and set it aside.)

Add onion and celery and cook them, covered, until the onion is translucent—about five minutes. Add the garlic and shallot and cook the mixture, stirring constantly for two minutes more. Sprinkle in the flour, filé powder, Lite Salt, sugar, black pepper, and cumin. Stir in water or fish stock and bring the liquid to a boil. Add the okra (if using), green and red peppers, and tomatoes. Partially cover the pot, then reduce the heat to simmer and cook, stirring occasionally, 8–10 minutes.

Stir in parsley, cilantro, and Tabasco sauce. Add the seafood and gently stir the gumbo to mix the fish and shrimp. Cover the pot, reduce the heat to low, and cook the gumbo for five minutes more.

(continued)

To serve: Spoon 1 cup warm steamed rice in large bowl and cover with gumbo.

Makes 6 servings (2½ cups each).

PER serving:
CALORIES 418
CSI 6
FAT 5 gm
FIBER 4 gm
SODIUM 246 mg

OTHER IDEAS

BAKED HERBED FISH—*QUICK*

Fresh fish is the secret ingredient!

2 pounds white fish fillets (red snapper, halibut, etc.)
1 tablespoon oil
½ teaspoon Lite Salt or less
½ teaspoon marjoram leaves
⅓ teaspoon thyme leaves
¼ teaspoon garlic powder
⅛ teaspoon white pepper
2 bay leaves
½ cup chopped onion
Paprika
½ cup white wine *or* skim milk
Lime wedges, for garnish

Preheat oven to 350°. Wash fish, pat dry, and put in dish. Combine oil with Lite Salt and herbs. Dribble over fish. Top with bay leaves and onions. Sprinkle with paprika. Pour wine *or* skim milk over all. Bake uncovered for 20–30 minutes or until fish flakes easily with a fork. Serve with lime wedges.

Makes 4 servings.

PER serving:
CALORIES 189
CSI 5
FAT 5 gm
FIBER trace
SODIUM 253 mg

OYSTERS IN CRUSTY FRENCH BREAD

A great way to fix oysters—after baking just pick up the sandwich and eat it for a very casual meal.

1 loaf (16 ounces) baguette bread (3 by 20 inches)
1 teaspoon margarine
2 cloves garlic, minced
1 jar (10 ounces) oysters
½ teaspoon olive oil
2 teaspoons grated Parmesan cheese

Preheat oven to 375°. Cut baguette crosswise into two pieces. Slice ½ inch from top of each piece and discard. Hollow out rest of loaf. Mix margarine with 1 clove garlic and scrape onto bread. Toast under broiler or over grill. Heat oil and 1 clove garlic until bubbly. Add oysters, including liquid, and cook slowly until heated through. Spoon oysters into bread and pour all liquid over oysters. Sprinkle with Parmesan cheese. Bake uncovered about 15 minutes or until golden brown.

Makes 2 servings.

PER serving:
CALORIES 527   FIBER 2 gm
CSI 9   SODIUM 1,024 mg
FAT 10 gm

OYSTERS SAUTÉ

Hot crusty French bread makes a great dipper for the juice.

1 tablespoon chopped onion
⅓ cup sliced fresh mushrooms
1 tablespoon chopped green bell pepper
1 teaspoon margarine
1 jar (10 ounces) oysters, drained
1 medium-size fresh tomato, cut into wedges
¼ cup dry white wine, vermouth, *or* water
2 teaspoons freshly squeezed lemon juice

Sauté onion, mushrooms, and green pepper in margarine until onion is transparent. Add oysters and heat through, turning occasionally. Add tomato wedges. Stir in wine and lemon juice. Heat and, because it is very juicy, serve in a bowl or over steamed rice.

Makes 2 servings.

PER serving:
CALORIES 173   FIBER 1 gm
CSI 7   SODIUM 253 mg
FAT 7 gm

SEAFOOD PILAF

The flavors of the seafood stand out in this delicious dish.

1 tablespoon margarine
¼ teaspoon turmeric (use more if you like it spicy) *or* ⅛ teaspoon saffron
1 cup uncooked white rice
1 cup chopped onion
1 clove garlic, chopped
1 can (14½ ounces) *or* 2 cups lower-salt chicken broth
¾ cup water
8 ounces small scallops
8 ounces shrimp, peeled and deveined
1 package (10 ounces) frozen peas

Melt margarine in large skillet over medium heat; stir in turmeric. Add rice, onion, and garlic. Stir often and cook about 3 minutes until onion is translucent. Pour in chicken broth and water; bring to a boil. Reduce heat, cover and simmer 15 minutes.

Add seafood and peas. Simmer, covered, 5 minutes longer or until scallops are opaque, shrimp turns pink, and peas are heated. Don't overcook; serve immediately.

Makes 7 cups (about 4 servings).

PER cup:
CALORIES 209   FIBER 2 gm
CSI 4   SODIUM 372 mg
FAT 3 gm

SEAFOOD TERIYAKI AND KABOBS

When you are in the barbecue mood, kabobs of green peppers and pineapple are great with fish steaks.

2 pounds fish steaks *or* 1½ pounds fillets (cod, halibut, snapper)
¾ cup pineapple chunks, juice packed
3 tablespoons juice from pineapple
2 tablespoons lower-sodium soy sauce
2 tablespoons sherry
1 tablespoon grated *or* minced ginger
½ teaspoon dry mustard
2 cloves garlic, crushed
1 teaspoon brown sugar
⅛ teaspoon black pepper
1 large green bell pepper, cut into large pieces

One hour before mealtime: Rinse fish with cold water; pat dry with paper towels. Place fish in single layer in baking dish; set aside. Make marinade by combining 3 tablespoons juice from pineapple, soy sauce, sherry, ginger, mustard, garlic, and brown sugar. Stir well and pour over fish. Cover and marinate in refrigerator for 1 hour, turning fish once.

Using bamboo or metal skewers, make kabobs by alternating pineapple chunks and green pepper; set aside. Drain fish, reserving marinade. Spray barbecue grill with nonstick cooking spray. Place steaks on grill and cook 4–5 minutes; baste with marinade and turn. Cook an additional 4–5 minutes or until fish flakes easily when tested with a fork. Baste fruit and vegetable kabobs and place on grill. Cook 1–2 minutes on each side, or until just brown. Makes 4 servings.

PER serving:
CALORIES 258   FIBER 1 gm
CSI 6   SODIUM 481 mg
FAT 3 gm

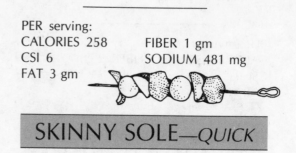

SKINNY SOLE—*QUICK*

Kids love this! It goes very well with *Classic Baked Beans* (page 330).

1½ pounds sole, cut into 4 pieces
½ cup cornmeal
2 tablespoons oil

Coat pieces of fish with cornmeal. Heat oil in skillet. Sauté fish quickly in oil, turning once.
Makes 4 servings.

PER serving:
CALORIES 227   FIBER 1 gm
CSI 5   SODIUM 128 mg
FAT 8 gm

SOLE WITH SPRING VEGETABLES

An easy-to-make microwave dish—the vegetables make it very attractive.

1½ pounds sole fillets, about ¼ inch thick (4 fillets)
½ teaspoon pepper

½ teaspoon paprika
2 tablespoons grated Parmesan cheese
1 cup julienne carrots
1 cup julienne zucchini
1 teaspoon grated lime peel
½ cup reconstituted Butter Buds or
  Molly McButter
Lime wedges for garnish

Sprinkle one side of each fillet with pepper, paprika, and Parmesan cheese. Roll up each fillet with seasoned side on the inside. Arrange in 9-inch round baking dish, seam side down. Set aside.

In small mixing bowl, combine carrot, zucchini, lime peel, and butter-flavor mix. Toss to coat. Cover. Microwave at high power for 2 minutes, stirring once. Spoon vegetable mixture over fish. Cover with wax paper. Microwave at high power for 5–9 minutes longer or until fish flakes easily with fork. Let stand, covered, for 5 minutes before serving. Serve with lime wedges.

Makes 4 servings.

PER serving:
CALORIES 184   FIBER 1 gm
CSI 5   SODIUM 242 mg
FAT 3 gm

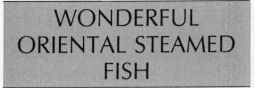

WONDERFUL ORIENTAL STEAMED FISH

A beautiful dish! A steamer makes this dish easier, but it can be prepared with a rack in a large covered pot. Add a small amount of water to cover bottom of pot.

SAUCE

2 tablespoons lower-sodium soy sauce
1 teaspoon sesame oil
¾ teaspoon finely minced or grated
  ginger
1 tablespoon white vinegar
6 tablespoons orange juice
¾ teaspoon grated orange rind

2 pounds fillets of red snapper, halibut, *or* other thick, firm-fleshed fish (approximately ¾ inch thick)
1½ cups sliced mushrooms
4 green onions, cut into 1-inch lengths
1½ cups asparagus (or green beans or snow peas) cut into 1-inch lengths
1½ cups sliced carrots

Combine all sauce ingredients and set aside for 30 minutes to blend flavors. Warm sauce as fish is cooking.

Rinse fish with cold water. Arrange on vegetable steamer tray. Place tray over ½ inch boiling water; cover and steam for 1–2 minutes. Top with vegetables and steam additional 5 minutes, or until fish flakes easily and vegetables are crisp-tender. Place in serving dish. Pour warm sauce over steamed fish and vegetables and serve.

Makes 4 servings.

PER serving:
CALORIES 268   FIBER 3 gm
CSI 7   SODIUM 498 mg
FAT 4 gm

CHICKEN AND TURKEY

People are always looking for new chicken recipes. Look no further, for there are some truly delicious recipes in this section. We have also provided some ideas for using ground turkey.

Stir-Fried
Cashew Chicken
Turkey Lettuce Stir-Fry
Zesty Stir-Fried Chicken

Baked
Chicken Parmesan—*Quick*
Curried Chicken Quickie—*Easy*
Oven-Fried Chicken—*Easy*
Portland Fried Chicken—*Easy*

With Sauce
Chicken Broccoli Roll-Ups
Chicken Cacciatore—*Easy*
Chicken Marbella
Chicken Paprika
Chicken with Apricot-Wine Glaze—*Easy*
Garlic Chicken with Balsamic Vinegar
Parmesan Yogurt Chicken—*Easy*

With Pasta
Easy Oven Lasagna
Homemade Raviolis
Poppyseed and Turkey Casserole

Sesame Linguini with Chicken
Texas Hash—*Easy*
Turkey-Mushroom Spaghetti Sauce—*Easy*
Turkey Tetrazzini

Salads
Chicken Salad with Yogurt-Chive Dressing
Curried Chicken and Peanut Salad
Simply Wonderful Turkey Salad

Stews and Chowders
Mulligatawny Stew
Rose Bowl Chili
Turkey-Vegetable Chowder

Other Ideas
Acapulco Enchiladas
Carmen's Curry
Chicken Fajitas Spicy-Style
Chicken Fajitas with Lime
Chicken in Pastry
Spicy Chicken with Peppers
Thai Barbecued Chicken—*Easy*

STIR-FRIED

CASHEW CHICKEN

Be sure to add the nuts as it makes this dish very special! With a small amount of chicken and lots of vegetables, this dish remains low-fat.

> 2 chicken breasts
> ½ pound pea pods *or* 1½ cups broccoli flowerets
> ½ pound mushrooms
> 4 green onions
> 1 can (8 ounces) bamboo shoots, drained
> 1 cup lower-salt chicken broth
> 1 tablespoon lower-sodium soy sauce
> 2 tablespoons cornstarch
> ½ teaspoon sugar
> 1 teaspoon oil
> ¼ cup cashew nuts, dry roasted

Bone chicken breasts and remove skin. Slice horizontally in ⅛-inch-thick slices, then cut in 1-inch squares. Arrange on a tray. Remove the ends and strings from pea pods or chop broccoli. Wash and slice mushrooms. Cut the green part of the onions into 1-inch lengths and then slash both ends several times making small fans; slice the white part ¼ inch thick. Slice bamboo shoots. Pour chicken broth into small pitcher. Mix together soy sauce, cornstarch, and sugar; pour into a small pitcher. Place oil and nuts in containers. Arrange at the table with electric skillet or wok.

Add oil to pan, add chicken and cook quickly, turning, until it turns opaque. Add peas and mushrooms; pour in broth, cover and simmer 2 minutes. Add bamboo shoots. Stir the soy sauce mixture into the pan juices and cook until sauce is thickened, stirring constantly; then simmer 2 minutes. Mix in the green onions, sprinkle with nuts. Serve with cooked rice.

Makes 4 servings.

PER serving:
CALORIES 242   FIBER 4 gm
CSI 4   SODIUM 391 mg
FAT 10 gm

TURKEY LETTUCE STIR-FRY

Do you have leftover turkey meat? This makes a cool summertime dish. Serve with rice and end the meal with fresh fruit or sherbet.

> 6 cups shredded iceberg lettuce
> 1 tablespoon oil
> 3½ cups carrots, cut into thin strips (approximately 6 carrots)
> 1 medium onion, sliced
> 1 clove garlic, crushed
> ½ chicken bouillon cube
> ⅔ cup water
> 2 tablespoons freshly squeezed lemon juice
> 1 teaspoon cornstarch
> 1 teaspoon basil leaves, crumbled
> ½ teaspoon brown sugar
> 1 cup cooked turkey, cut into strips (white meat)

(continued)

Shred lettuce and refrigerate in a plastic bag while preparing the remaining ingredients.

In a wok or large skillet, heat oil. Sauté the carrots with the onions and garlic for 3 minutes, stirring and tossing frequently. Combine bouillon cube, water, lemon juice, cornstarch, basil, and brown sugar. Add to the skillet. Add the cooked turkey and heat, stirring constantly, until the sauce boils and thickens. Toss with the crisp shredded lettuce and serve immediately over steamed rice.

Makes 4 servings.

PER serving:
CALORIES 147   FIBER 5 gm
CSI 2   SODIUM 191 mg
FAT 5 gm

ZESTY STIR-FRIED CHICKEN

A recent first-place winner in a cooking contest. You can increase the red pepper flakes if you wish a spicier flavor.

SAUCE

   3 tablespoons lower-sodium soy sauce
   ¼ cup water
   2 tablespoons dry sherry
   2 tablespoons orange marmalade
   1 tablespoon cornstarch
   2 teaspoons minced fresh ginger root
   ½ teaspoon crushed dried red pepper
      flakes (optional)

STIR-FRY

   3 stalks celery, sliced diagonally
   1 package (6 ounces) frozen pea pods, thawed and well drained
   4 teaspoons oil, divided
   4 chicken breast halves, skinned, boned, and cubed
   2 green onions, sliced thin on the diagonal

   2 teaspoons slivered almonds
   1 small orange, sliced into thin rounds

To make sauce, mix together soy sauce, water, dry sherry, orange marmalade, cornstarch, ginger, and red pepper, if desired. Set aside.

Stir-fry celery and pea pods in 2 teaspoons of the oil. Spoon these vegetables around the perimeter of a platter; keep warm. Add remaining 2 teaspoons of oil to the pan and stir-fry the chicken over medium high until done, but still tender. Add green onion and sauce mixture to the chicken and cook until sauce turns clear and thickens.

Spoon chicken and sauce into center of the warm platter, garnish with the sliced almonds and oranges. Serve with steamed rice.

Makes 4 servings.

PER serving:
CALORIES 266   FIBER 3 gm
CSI 5   SODIUM 540 mg
FAT 9 gm

BAKED

CHICKEN PARMESAN—*QUICK*

Quick, easy, and good! If you are really in a hurry, start with frozen chicken.

⅓ cup bread crumbs
¼ cup grated Parmesan cheese
½ tablespoon basil leaves
4 chicken breasts, skinned and boned
Vegetable cooking spray

Preheat oven to 350°. Combine bread crumbs, Parmesan cheese, and basil. Rinse chicken breasts in cold water and roll damp breasts in bread crumb mixture.

Spray shallow baking dish with nonstick cooking spray. Bake uncovered for 15–25 minutes until cooked through. Turn breasts once, about halfway through cooking.

Makes 4 servings.

PER serving:
CALORIES 205   FIBER trace
CSI 6   SODIUM 249 mg
FAT 6 gm

CURRIED CHICKEN QUICKIE—*EASY*

4 chicken breasts (boned, if desired)
1 can (10½ ounces) low-sodium cream of mushroom soup *or* use *Homemade "Cream" Soup Mix* (page 314)
2½ cups hot water
2 cups skim milk *or* lower-salt chicken broth
2½ cups uncooked white rice*
2 teaspoons curry powder
½ teaspoon Lite Salt or less

Heat oven to 350°. Skin chicken. Combine liquid ingredients in a saucepan. Bring to a boil. Add rice, curry powder, and Lite Salt and mix; heat to boiling again.

Lay chicken breasts in a 9-by-13-inch baking dish. Pour soup-rice mixture over the top. Cover tightly with foil and bake for 30 minutes. Remove from oven and let set for 10 minutes.

Makes 6 servings.

*When using brown rice, cook rice in hot soup mixture for 10 minutes before adding to chicken and putting into oven.

PER serving:
CALORIES 415   FIBER 1 gm
CSI 3   SODIUM 149 mg
FAT 4 gm

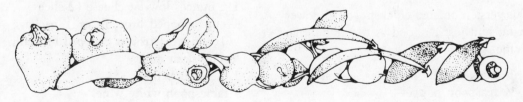

OVEN-FRIED CHICKEN—*EASY*

Crisp-coated chicken—an all-time favorite.

1 chicken, cut in pieces and skinned
1 cup crushed cornflakes *or* other flaked cereal
¼ teaspoon garlic powder
½ teaspoon onion powder
½ teaspoon paprika
½–1 teaspoon Italian seasoning *or* dried herb leaves of your choice

Preheat oven to 350°. Mix cereal and spices. Roll damp chicken in mix and place on nonstick baking sheet. Bake uncovered for 1 hour.
Makes 6 servings.

PER serving:
CALORIES 173   FIBER trace
CSI 5   SODIUM 110 mg
FAT 6 gm

PORTLAND FRIED CHICKEN—*EASY*

Our version of fried chicken—much lower in fat and just as good as the traditional recipe.

1 chicken, cut in pieces and skinned
¼ teaspoon pepper
1½ cups crushed Rice Krispies
¼ teaspoon paprika

Preheat oven to 350°. Roll damp chicken in crushed cereal. Place on nonstick baking sheet and sprinkle with pepper and paprika. Bake uncovered for 1 hour. If crispier chicken is preferred, begin baking at 400° for 20 minutes, then lower heat to 350°.
Makes 6 servings.

PER serving:
CALORIES 187   FIBER trace
CSI 5   SODIUM 154 mg
FAT 5 gm

WITH SAUCE

CHICKEN BROCCOLI ROLL-UPS

A microwave recipe, which makes this meal very speedy! The sauce is delicious over steamed rice.

4 chicken breasts, skinned and boned
1½ ounces low-fat cheese (2 slices)
1 cup chopped broccoli *or* 1 package (10 ounces) frozen chopped broccoli
½ cup skim milk
1 tablespoon flour
1 tablespoon white wine
1 tablespoon chopped fresh parsley
¼ teaspoon white pepper

Pound chicken breasts with mallet to flatten. Cut one slice cheese into 8 strips; place 2 strips lengthwise on each chicken piece. Place one fourth of broccoli over cheese in center of each piece. Fold ends of chicken over broccoli and secure with wooden picks or tie with string. Place rolls seam side down in baking dish. Cover with waxed paper. Microwave on high for 6–8 minutes, or until chicken is no longer pink, turning over once.

Meanwhile, blend milk with flour, wine, pepper, and parsley. Cook slowly over medium heat until thickened, stirring constantly—a wire whisk works well for this. Cut up remaining cheese slice and stir into sauce until melted.

Place chicken on serving dish or drain off liquid. Pour sauce over all.

Makes 4 servings.

PER serving:
CALORIES 195   FIBER 1 gm
CSI 6   SODIUM 139 mg
FAT 5 gm

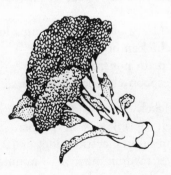

CHICKEN CACCIATORE—*EASY*

It tastes as good as it sounds—traditionally served with pasta, a salad, and French bread.

4 chicken breasts
2 tablespoons flour
1 tablespoon oil
2 tablespoons chopped onion
1 can (6 ounces) unsalted tomato paste
½ cup white wine
¼ teaspoon white pepper
¾ cup lower-salt chicken broth
½ bay leaf
⅛ teaspoon thyme leaves
½ teaspoon basil leaves
⅛ teaspoon marjoram leaves
1 cup sliced fresh mushrooms

Roll skinned chicken breasts in flour. Sauté in the oil until browned. Remove from skillet. Sauté onions in remaining trace of oil. Add remaining ingredients and stir together. Replace chicken breasts in skillet and spoon sauce over top. Simmer the chicken, covered, for 45 minutes or until tender.

Makes 4 servings.

PER serving:
CALORIES 222   FIBER 2 gm
CSI 4   SODIUM 212 mg
FAT 6 gm

CHICKEN MARBELLA

Especially for garlic lovers! Serve over cooked rice or pasta for an unusual and tasty dish. Dried prunes or apricots can be used in the sauce.

MARINADE

8 cloves garlic, minced
1–3 teaspoons oregano leaves
½ teaspoon pepper
½ cup red wine vinegar
2 tablespoons olive oil
1 cup pitted prunes, cut in half
⅓ cup Spanish green olives
½ cup capers with juice
6 bay leaves

6 chicken breasts, skinned and boned
2 tablespoons brown sugar
1 cup white wine

¼ cup chopped fresh parsley *or* cilantro

On the day before serving: Combine marinade (garlic, oregano, pepper, vinegar, oil, prunes, olives, capers, and bay leaves) with chicken breasts. Cover and marinate, refrigerated, overnight.
An hour before serving: Preheat oven to 350° and arrange chicken in a single layer in a shallow baking pan. Spoon marinade over all. Sprinkle chicken pieces with brown sugar and pour wine around them. Bake for 50 minutes to 1 hour, basting frequently with pan juices.

To serve: Transfer chicken, prunes, olives, and capers to a warm serving platter. Moisten with a few spoonfuls of pan juices and sprinkle generously with fresh parsley *or* cilantro. Pass remaining pan juices in a small bowl.
Makes 6 servings.

PER serving:
CALORIES 289   FIBER 4 gm
CSI 5   SODIUM 432 mg
FAT 9 gm

CHICKEN PAPRIKA

Do use Hungarian paprika, if it's available, for this delicious chicken.

1 chicken (2½–3 pounds), cut in serving pieces and skinned *or* 6 skinned and boned breasts
¼ teaspoon black pepper
1 tablespoon oil
1 cup chopped onion (1 small)
1 clove garlic, finely chopped
2 tablespoons unsalted tomato paste
1½ tablespoons sweet Hungarian paprika
1 can (14½ ounces) *or* 2 cups lower-salt chicken broth
1 cup plain nonfat yogurt
1 tablespoon chopped fresh parsley

Rinse chicken pieces and pat dry with paper towel. Sprinkle with pepper. Sauté chicken in oil in electric skillet or 10-inch skillet over medium heat, 6–8 minutes on each side. Remove chicken from skillet.

Sauté onion and garlic over medium heat until light brown, about 6 minutes. Stir in tomato paste and paprika until onion is evenly coated, then stir in chicken broth. Return chicken to skillet and reduce heat to low. Simmer, covered, until chicken is done, 10 minutes or so.

Remove chicken from skillet and keep warm. Boil liquid in pan, stirring constantly, until slightly reduced and thickened, about 5 minutes. In a separate bowl stir the yogurt and slowly add part of the hot sauce to it. This will prevent curdling. Return the sauce and chicken to skillet and heat just until chicken is hot. Transfer chicken to heated serving platter. Spoon thickened sauce from skillet over chicken and sprinkle with parsley. Serve immediately.

Makes 6 servings.

PER serving:
CALORIES 214   FIBER <1 gm
CSI 5   SODIUM 328 mg
FAT 6 gm

CHICKEN WITH APRICOT-WINE GLAZE—*EASY*

A true winner!

6 chicken breasts, skinned (and boned, if desired)
¼ teaspoon Lite Salt or less
¼ teaspoon pepper
1 tablespoon margarine
¾ cup apricot preserves
¼ teaspoon garlic powder
½ cup dry white wine *or* water

Preheat oven to 350°. Season the chicken with Lite Salt and pepper. Place into a roasting dish, making sure no two pieces

overlap. Top each piece of chicken with ½ teaspoon of margarine.

Place chicken in oven, uncovered, and bake for 15 minutes, if boned, or 30 minutes, if unboned. Combine preserves, garlic, and wine. Spoon this mixture over the chicken and bake for another 45–60 minutes, basting occasionally. Add more wine if sauce becomes too thick.

Makes 6 servings.

PER serving:
CALORIES 270   FIBER <1 gm
CSI 5   SODIUM 134 mg
FAT 5 gm

GARLIC CHICKEN WITH BALSAMIC VINEGAR

A dish that always gets rave reviews. *Lemon Rice* (page 326) is especially nice to serve with this dish.

4 chicken breasts, boned and skinned
¾ pound small to medium-sized mushrooms
2 tablespoons flour
⅛ teaspoon pepper
1 tablespoon olive oil
6 cloves garlic, peeled but left whole
¼ cup balsamic vinegar*
¾ cup lower-salt chicken broth
1 bay leaf
¼ teaspoon thyme leaves

*Available in deli or food specialty shops.

(continued)

Wash chicken breasts. Clean and quarter or halve mushrooms. Mix the flour and pepper and coat chicken breasts with mixture. Heat oil in a heavy skillet and cook chicken breasts until nicely browned on one side (about 3 minutes). Add the whole garlic cloves. Turn the chicken pieces and scatter mushrooms over all. Continue cooking, moving mushrooms and chicken so they cook evenly (about 3 minutes). Add balsamic vinegar, chicken broth, bay and thyme leaves. Cover and cook over moderately low heat (about 10 minutes). Move chicken and mushrooms around to keep from sticking.

Transfer chicken pieces to a warm serving platter. Remove bay leaf and garlic cloves. Cook until sauce is thickened. Spoon sauce and mushrooms over chicken and serve.

Makes 4 servings.

PER serving:
CALORIES 220   FIBER 2 gm
CSI 5   SODIUM 195 mg
FAT 7 gm

PARMESAN YOGURT CHICKEN—EASY

A quickly prepared baked chicken with a zippy sauce. For a company dinner, use thighs and breasts.

1 chicken, cut in pieces and skinned
2 tablespoons freshly squeezed lemon juice
Cayenne pepper or Tabasco sauce, to taste
1 cup plain nonfat yogurt
2 tablespoons flour
¼ cup light mayonnaise
2 tablespoons Dijon mustard
¼ teaspoon Worcestershire sauce
½ teaspoon thyme leaves
¼ cup minced green onions
Paprika
2 tablespoons grated Parmesan cheese

Preheat oven to 350°. Arrange chicken in lightly oiled baking dish. Drizzle with lemon juice. Sprinkle lightly with cayenne pepper or Tabasco sauce (use more if you like it hot!). In small bowl mix yogurt with flour and add mayonnaise, mustard, Worcestershire, and thyme. Spread over chicken. Top with green onions and sprinkle with paprika. Bake uncovered for 60 minutes or until fork tender. Sprinkle chicken evenly with Parmesan cheese. Broil 6 inches from heat until cheese is slightly brown. Serve warm. Sauce is good served over brown rice.

Makes 6 servings.

PER serving:
CALORIES 235   FIBER trace
CSI 7   SODIUM 212 mg
FAT 10 gm

WITH PASTA

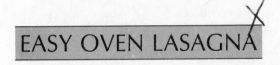

EASY OVEN LASAGNA

An old favorite, prepared an easier way—
with *uncooked noodles!*

- ¼ **pound ground turkey *or* ground beef (10 percent fat)**
- ¾ **cup water**
- 4 **cups *Marinara Sauce* (page 450)**
- 8 **ounces uncooked lasagna noodles**
- 1 **cup low-fat cottage cheese** /ricotta
- ¾ **cup sliced part-skim mozzarella** egg **cheese**
- ¼ **cup grated Parmesan cheese**

Preheat oven to 375°. Brown ground turkey in nonstick skillet and drain well. Add water and *Marinara Sauce*; bring to boil. Remove from heat. In 2-quart (9-by-13-inch) dish, layer sauce, uncooked lasagna noodles, cottage cheese, mozzarella cheese; repeat layers, ending with sauce and Parmesan cheese. The sauce will be runny. Cover dish with foil and bake for 1 hour. Let stand 5–10 minutes before cutting into squares.

Makes 12 servings (about 3 by 3 inches).

PER serving:
CALORIES 185　　FIBER 2 gm
CSI 3　　　　　　SODIUM 172 mg
FAT 6 gm

HOMEMADE RAVIOLIS

Have a party and make these with a group of friends! This recipe is for 12 servings, but it can be easily increased if you wish to put some in the freezer.

SAUCE

12 **cups *Marinara Sauce* (page 450)**

Prepare sauce and set aside to warm up at serving time.

FILLING

- 1½ **cups cooked chicken (white meat)**
- 1 **carrot, chopped**
- 1 **stalk celery, chopped**
- 1 **small onion, chopped**
- ⅓ **package frozen chopped spinach**
- ⅓ **cup chopped parsley**
- 2 **teaspoons garlic powder**
- 1 **teaspoon oregano leaves**
- 1 **teaspoon basil leaves**
- ¼ **teaspoon pepper**
- ¼ **teaspoon Lite Salt or less**

Bone and cube chicken. Steam carrots, celery, onions and frozen spinach together in a small amount of water until done. Drain well. Put chicken and vegetables through meat grinder using coarse grind or use a

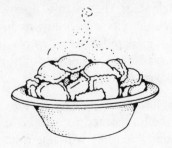

(continued)

food processor. Add spices to meat/vegetable paste and mix well together. Chill until pasta is prepared. (Unused filling may be frozen.)

Makes filling for 12 dozen raviolis.

PASTA
(These are easier to make if you have a ravioli rolling pin.)

4 cups flour
8 egg whites
4 tablespoons oil
Water

Measure 2 cups of flour into a large bowl; shape deep well in center. Place egg whites and oil in well. Beat egg white/oil mixture with fork until smooth; stir flour from well gradually into egg mixture to make a stiff sticky dough. Knead remaining 2 cups of flour into dough until smooth and elastic on a floured bread board. Sprinkle with water if more moisture is needed. Cover with towel; let stand for 10 minutes.

Roll the dough into a large rectangle on a large flat surface (the kitchen table works well). The dough should be about ⅛ inch thick. Spread ½ of dough with a thin layer of filling (about ⅛ inch thick also). Bring the unfilled half of dough over filled half to cover filling and roll a ravioli rolling pin over it, or mark in squares with a wooden yardstick. Cut the raviolis apart with a pastry cutter. Cook according to directions below or prepare for freezer by placing ravioli in plastic container, separating layers with waxed paper.

Cooking and serving: Place raviolis in unsalted boiling water for 10–12 minutes. Boil gently so they will not split. Drain carefully and arrange on a serving dish. Cover with hot *Marinara Sauce* and serve with grated Parmesan cheese.

Makes 12 servings (1 dozen raviolis each).

PER serving:
CALORIES 366   FIBER 5 gm
CSI 2   SODIUM 119 mg
FAT 10 gm

POPPYSEED AND TURKEY CASSEROLE

This is a great dish and a wonderful way to use ground turkey. The sauce can be made ahead and frozen to speed up preparation time.

½ pound ground turkey
3 tablespoons chopped onion
3 tablespoons chopped green bell pepper
1 can (8 ounces) unsalted tomato sauce
½ teaspoon Lite Salt or less
⅛ teaspoon pepper
½ package (5 ounces) wide eggless noodles
½ cup low-fat ricotta cheese
1 cup low-fat cottage cheese
½ cup plain nonfat yogurt
1 tablespoon poppyseeds
1 tablespoon grated Parmesan cheese

Preheat oven to 375°. In a large nonstick skillet sauté turkey, onion, and green pepper until meat is no longer pink and vegetables are tender. Stir vigorously so turkey is in very small pieces. Add tomato sauce, Lite Salt, and pepper (sauce can be frozen at this point and thawed when ready to assemble dish).

Cook noodles in boiling water until tender; drain well. Combine ricotta, cottage cheese, yogurt, and poppyseeds. Toss with the warm noodles.

Assemble dish by putting ¾ of noodle mixture in 9-by-9-inch baking pan that has been sprayed with nonstick spray. Spoon meat mixture over noodles and add remaining noodles as final layer.

Bake covered for 30 minutes; uncover, sprinkle Parmesan cheese over top and continue baking for 10–15 minutes more. Let stand 5–10 minutes. Cut into squares and serve.

Makes 4 servings.

PER serving:

CALORIES 344	FIBER 2 gm
CSI 8	SODIUM 499 mg
FAT 9 gm	

SESAME LINGUINI WITH CHICKEN

SESAME SAUCE

2 tablespoons sesame seeds
2 cloves garlic, minced
2 teaspoons minced fresh ginger root
3 tablespoons lower-sodium soy sauce
3 tablespoons wine vinegar
1 tablespoon sherry
1½ teaspoons sugar
¼ teaspoon crushed red pepper flakes
½ cup lower-salt chicken broth

LINGUINI-CHICKEN MIXTURE

¾ cup bean sprouts
9 ounces linguini
1 teaspoon sesame oil
1½ cups sliced cucumber, halved lengthwise, seeded and sliced (⅛-inch slices)
1 cup cooked chicken, cut into one-half inch cubes, *or* 1 can (6 ounces) chicken

Toast sesame seeds in 400° oven, if desired. Prepare *Sesame Sauce* by mixing all ingredients thoroughly. Set aside.

Bring large pot of water to boil. Plunge bean sprouts into boiling water for 30 seconds. Do this using metal strainer while in boiling water so you can drain them easily. Reserve water for cooking pasta. Boil linguini until just tender, about 8 minutes. Drain and toss with 1 teaspoon sesame oil. Set aside.

Combine cucumber, chicken, bean sprouts, and *Sesame Sauce;* toss to coat completely. Add cooked linguini and toss again. Serve at room temperature.

Makes 5 servings (1½ cups each).

PER serving:

CALORIES 311	FIBER 3 gm
CSI 2	SODIUM 455 mg
FAT 5 gm	

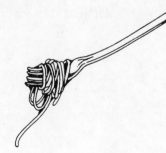

TEXAS HASH—*EASY*

Travels well to potlucks or feeds a gang of hungry teenagers. Cornbread and salad are nice additions for a casual meal.

1 tablespoon oil
3 large onions, chopped
1 large green bell pepper, chopped
½ pound ground turkey
2 cans (16 ounces each) unsalted tomatoes
2 cups uncooked macaroni
1 teaspoon chili powder
½–1 teaspoon pepper
½ teaspoon Lite Salt or less
½ cup water

Preheat oven to 350°. Heat oil in nonstick skillet. Sauté onions and green peppers, stirring often. Add ground turkey and continue to cook, stirring, until turkey browns slightly. Break up tomatoes with a spoon and add along with uncooked macaroni, seasonings, and ½ cup water. Turn into a casserole dish and bake, covered, 30 minutes; remove cover and continue baking 15–20 minutes.

Makes 4 servings (2½ cups each).

PER serving:
CALORIES 424   FIBER 5 gm
CSI 3   SODIUM 149 mg
FAT 7 gm

TURKEY-MUSHROOM SPAGHETTI SAUCE—*EASY*

Spaghetti and meat sauce! Only the cook will know that it's low-fat ground turkey.

½ cup minced onion
½ pound ground turkey
½ cup sliced fresh mushrooms *or* 1 can (4 ounces) mushrooms, drained
½ cup water
2 cloves garlic, minced
1 can (16 ounces) unsalted tomatoes
1 can (6 ounces) unsalted tomato paste
1 teaspoon parsley flakes
1 bay leaf
¾ teaspoon basil leaves
1 teaspoon oregano leaves
⅛ teaspoon pepper
¼ cup chopped green bell pepper (optional)

Sauté onions in nonstick pan. Add ground turkey and crumble with a fork. Stir until browned. Mix in mushrooms, water, garlic, tomatoes, tomato paste, parsley, bay leaf, basil, oregano, and black pepper. Simmer 1–2 hours, adding green peppers if desired for last 10 minutes of cooking. Serve over cooked spaghetti.

Makes 4 cups sauce (enough for 8 cups of pasta).

PER cup:
CALORIES 148   FIBER 3 gm
CSI 2   SODIUM 55 mg
FAT 3 gm

TURKEY TETRAZZINI

"What do I do with leftover turkey?"

12 ounces spaghetti, broken into 2-inch pieces
1 tablespoon oil
¼ cup chopped green bell pepper
2 tablespoons chopped onion
2 tablespoons chopped celery
½ pound fresh mushrooms, sliced
¼ cup flour
¼ teaspoon white pepper
¼ teaspoon nutmeg (optional)
½ teaspoon Lite Salt or less
1 cup skim milk
1 can (14½ ounces) *or* 2 cups lower-salt chicken broth
3 tablespoons dry sherry
¼ cup ripe olives, cut into large pieces
2 cups cooked, diced turkey (white meat)
1 cup frozen peas (optional for color and flavor)
2 tablespoons grated Parmesan cheese
2 tablespoons slivered almonds

Preheat oven to 350°. Cook spaghetti according to package directions in unsalted water. Drain well.

Heat oil in skillet. Sauté green pepper, onion, celery, and mushrooms. Shake flour, pepper, and Lite Salt together with skim milk in a jar until blended. Add this milk/flour mixture and chicken broth to vegetable mixture, stirring constantly. Bring to a boil and continue to boil and stir for one minute or until thickened. Blend in sherry. Add this sauce to cooked spaghetti. Add olives, turkey, and peas, if using, and put into lightly oiled 9-by-13-inch baking pan. Sprinkle with Parmesan cheese and almonds. Bake uncovered 25–30 minutes. Let stand for 10 minutes before serving.
Makes 6 servings.

PER serving:
CALORIES 422   FIBER 3 gm
CSI 4   SODIUM 444 mg
FAT 8 gm

SALADS

CHICKEN SALAD WITH YOGURT-CHIVE DRESSING

6 chicken breasts
2 cans (8 ounces each) sliced water chestnuts, drained
1 can (8 ounces) pineapple chunks, drained
½ cup chopped celery
½ cup chopped green bell pepper
Leaf lettuce
Cucumber slices for garnish

YOGURT-CHIVE DRESSING

2 cups plain nonfat yogurt
2 tablespoons light mayonnaise
2 tablespoons dry white wine
1 tablespoon chopped chives
1 teaspoon freshly squeezed lemon juice
⅛ teaspoon garlic powder
¼ teaspoon curry powder (optional)

(continued)

Preheat oven to 350°. Skin chicken and arrange in an ovenproof casserole dish. Cover loosely with foil and bake for 25–30 minutes until just tender. Cool. Remove from bones and cube chicken.

Toss in a large bowl water chestnuts, pineapple chunks, celery, green peppers, and cooked chicken cubes. Combine dressing ingredients and pour over chicken mixture. Toss. Cover and chill until serving time.

When ready to serve, arrange chicken salad on a bed of leaf lettuce and garnish with cucumber slices.

Makes 6 servings.

PER serving:
CALORIES 252   FIBER 1 gm
CSI 5   SODIUM 136 mg
FAT 5 gm

CURRIED CHICKEN AND PEANUT SALAD

This delicious main dish salad is fairly low in calories. For those with hearty appetites, serve with rolls, a vegetable (corn on the cob is great), and a favorite dessert.

DRESSING

- ¼ cup plain nonfat yogurt
- 2 tablespoons peanut butter
- 3 tablespoons skim milk
- 1½ tablespoons white wine vinegar
- 1½ teaspoons sugar
- 1 teaspoon curry powder

SALAD

- 6 cups torn mixed greens
- 2 cups diced cooked chicken (white meat)
- 2 cups shredded cabbage
- 1 can (11 ounce) mandarin orange sections, chilled and drained
- ¼ cup unsalted peanuts
- 1 tablespoon sliced green onion

Prepare dressing by combining yogurt, peanut butter, milk, vinegar, sugar, and curry. Mix well and chill (works well to put in jar and shake).

At serving time: In large salad bowl arrange the greens, chicken, cabbage, orange sections, peanuts, and green onion. Drizzle dressing over salad, toss carefully.

Makes 6 servings (1⅔ cups each).

PER serving:
CALORIES 198   FIBER 2 gm
CSI 3   SODIUM 106 mg
FAT 8 gm

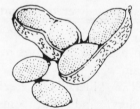

SIMPLY WONDERFUL TURKEY SALAD

A main dish salad. Fresh spinach and wild rice are a great combination. The dressing is especially delicious.

SALAD

SALAD

1 package (6 ounces) long-grain and
  wild rice mix
1 cup cubed cooked turkey (white
  meat)
¼ pound fresh mushrooms, sliced
2 cups fresh spinach leaves, cut into
  thin strips
2 green onions with tops, sliced
1 can (8 ounces) sliced water chestnuts, drained
1 cup cooked white rice, cold
10 cherry tomatoes, halved

DRESSING

⅓ cup dry white wine
2 tablespoons oil
2 tablespoons sugar
¼ teaspoon pepper

The day before: Cook wild rice mix with
seasoning packet according to package directions, omitting margarine. Cover and
chill in refrigerator. Be sure to have 1 cup
cooked white rice on hand, also.

Several hours before serving: Add cooked turkey, mushrooms, raw spinach, green onions, water chestnuts, and plain cooked
white rice to wild rice. Prepare dressing.
Add to salad; mix well. Chill in covered
container. Add tomatoes just before
serving.
  Makes 6 servings (1½ cups each).

———————————

PER serving:
CALORIES 233   FIBER 3 gm
CSI 2   SODIUM 460 mg
FAT 6 gm

STEWS AND CHOWDERS

MULLIGATAWNY STEW

A lightly seasoned stew with curry and apple. Serve in a large bowl over hot steamed
rice, if desired.

1 tablespoon margarine
1 cup chopped onion (1 medium)
1 cup diced carrot (1 medium)
1 cup diced green bell pepper (1 medium)
1 stalk celery, diced
1 cup peeled and chopped tart apple (1
  large)
2 cups cubed cooked chicken (white
  meat)
¼ cup flour
4 whole cloves
1–3 teaspoons curry powder
¼ cup minced fresh parsley
¼ teaspoon nutmeg
1 can (14½ ounces) *or* 2 cups lower-
  salt chicken broth
2 cups chopped tomatoes
Freshly ground black pepper

Melt margarine in a large saucepan over
medium-high heat. Add onion and sauté
for 5 minutes. Add carrot, pepper, celery,
and apple. Sauté, stirring often until vegetables are tender, about 10–12 minutes.
Stir in cooked chicken, sprinkle flour,
cloves, curry, parsley, and nutmeg over

(continued)

mixture in pan. Sauté 1 minute, stirring constantly. Stir in broth and tomatoes with their liquid. Season with pepper to taste. Cover, reduce heat to low, and simmer gently for about 30 minutes. If a thinner stew is desired, add water. Remove whole cloves and serve.

Makes 6 cups.

PER cup:
CALORIES 174   FIBER 3 gm
CSI 3   SODIUM 312 mg
FAT 5 gm

ROSE BOWL CHILI

After the game ends, the fun can continue with this easy, delicious dish. *Mexican Cornbread Muffins* (page 272) makes a nice accompaniment.

> 3 chicken breasts, skinned and boned
> 1 tablespoon oil
> 1 cup chopped onion
> 1 medium green bell pepper, chopped
> 2 cloves garlic, minced
> 2 cans (14½ ounces each) unsalted to-matoes
> 1 can (16 ounces) pinto beans,* drained
> ⅔ cup picante sauce
> 1 teaspoon chili powder
> 1 teaspoon ground cumin

Condiment ideas: Chopped green on-ions, diced avocado, plain nonfat yo-gurt, *or* salsa

*Use low-sodium beans if available.

Cut chicken into 1-inch cubes. Heat oil in large kettle and sauté chicken, onion, green pepper, and garlic until chicken loses its pink color. Add tomatoes, drained beans, picante sauce, chili powder, and cumin. Simmer 20 minutes or so. Ladle into bowls and serve.

Place condiments in small dishes to be spooned over top of chili.

Makes 7 cups.

PER cup including condiments:
CALORIES 213   FIBER 7 gm
CSI 2   SODIUM 479 mg
FAT 5 gm

TURKEY-VEGETABLE CHOWDER

The meatballs in this hearty soup are deli-cious and easily prepared by browning in the oven. *Poppyseed Muffins* (page 274) are a great addition.

SOUP BASE

> 1 medium onion, chopped
> 1 clove garlic, crushed
> 1 tablespoon oil
> 4 cans (16 ounces each) unsalted to-matoes, mashed
> 2 cans (8 ounces each) unsalted tomato sauce
> 2 cans (16 ounces each) pinto *or* kid-ney beans, drained*

*Use low-sodium beans if available.

1 teaspoon Worcestershire sauce
½ teaspoon Lite Salt or less
⅛ teaspoon pepper
2 teaspoons basil leaves

MEATBALLS

¼ cup grated Parmesan cheese
½ teaspoon thyme leaves
½ cup cracker crumbs
1 pound ground turkey *or* chicken

6 cups finely chopped cabbage

Sauté onions and garlic in oil in large soup kettle. Add tomatoes, tomato sauce, beans, Worcestershire sauce, Lite Salt, pepper, and basil. Simmer 30 minutes to 2 hours.

Meanwhile prepare meatballs. Combine Parmesan cheese, thyme, cracker crumbs, and ground turkey *or* chicken. Shape this mixture into thirty-six ¾-inch balls and place on nonstick baking sheet. Bake at 375° for 15 minutes to brown. Drain on paper towels. Twenty minutes before serving time add meatballs and chopped cabbage to soup. Simmer approximately 20 minutes.

Makes 10 servings (2 cups each).

PER serving:
CALORIES 280   FIBER 8 gm
CSI 3   SODIUM 433 mg
FAT 7 gm

OTHER IDEAS

ACAPULCO ENCHILADAS

A favorite recipe—this is great served with *Spanish Rice* (page 328) and tossed green salad.

12 corn tortillas
2 cups canned enchilada sauce (mild)
1 can (8 ounces) unsalted tomato sauce
3 cups diced cooked chicken or turkey (white meat)
¼ cup sliced black olives
2 tablespoons slivered almonds
½ cup grated imitation mozzarella cheese
2 cups plain nonfat yogurt *or* 2 cups *Mock Sour Cream* (page 451)
¼ cup chopped green onions

Preheat oven to 350°. Soften tortillas by wrapping in wax paper and microwaving for ½–2 minutes or by wrapping in foil and warming in conventional oven for 10 minutes. Mix enchilada sauce and tomato sauce. Mix chicken, olives, and almonds with about ½ cup sauce to moisten.

Spoon ¼ cup of chicken mixture down center of each warm tortilla. Roll and place seam side down in a 9-by-13-inch baking dish. When all are in place, cover with remaining sauce and grated cheese. Bake uncovered for 15–20 minutes. Before serv-

(continued)

ing, spoon yogurt or *Mock Sour Cream* down center of dish and sprinkle with green onions.

Makes 6 servings.

PER enchilada:
CALORIES 193   FIBER 2 gm
CSI 3   SODIUM 573 mg
FAT 5 gm

CARMEN'S CURRY

A colorful, spicy main dish. Serve with *Onion Chutney* (page 452), yogurt, and raisins in small condiment dishes for a wonderful treat. Curry flavor improves if prepared a day ahead.

  2 cups chopped onion
  1 tablespoon oil
  1 can (16 ounces) unsalted tomatoes
  1–2 tablespoons curry powder
  1 tablespoon pickling spice*
  1 bay leaf
  8 whole cloves
  ¼ teaspoon pepper
  1¼ teaspoons Lite Salt or less
  6 chicken breasts, skinned
  2 cups unsalted tomato juice
  1 cup sliced mushrooms
  1 cup cauliflower pieces
  1 cup frozen corn
  1 cup thinly sliced carrot coins
  1 cup chopped unpeeled apple
  1 tablespoon brown sugar

*To avoid serving large pieces, put pickling spice in a cheesecloth bag. Remove bag before serving.

  2 tablespoons freshly squeezed lemon juice
  1 cup frozen peas

Sauté onions in oil until golden. Add tomatoes, curry powder, pickling spice, bay leaf, cloves, pepper, and Lite Salt. Stir well and simmer 5 minutes. Add chicken breasts and tomato juice. Cook for 20 minutes. Add mushrooms, cauliflower, corn, carrots, and apple. Simmer 10 minutes. Add brown sugar and lemon juice. Remove from heat. Let cool then refrigerate overnight.

Just before serving add frozen peas and heat through (works well to put in microwave on high for 10 minutes). Serve over rice with *Onion Chutney*, golden raisins, slivered almonds, nonfat yogurt, and toasted pita bread.

Makes 6 servings.

PER serving:
CALORIES 293   FIBER 7 gm
CSI 5   SODIUM 320 mg
FAT 6 gm

CHICKEN FAJITAS SPICY-STYLE

  1½ tablespoons diced green chiles, canned or fresh
  1 medium tomato, chopped
  1 teaspoon oregano leaves
  ½ teaspoon cumin
  ½ teaspoon chili powder
  ¼ teaspoon Lite Salt or less
  1 tablespoon flour
  2 chicken breasts, skinned and boned
  2 teaspoons oil, divided

1¼ cups thinly sliced onion
1 clove garlic, minced
2 cups sliced green or red bell pepper
2 teaspoons chopped cilantro (optional)
4 flour tortillas (8-inch diameter)

Combine chiles, tomato, oregano, cumin, chili powder, and Lite Salt. Cut chicken into ½-inch strips, roll in flour, and mix into chiles/tomato mixture. Set aside to marinate briefly.

Heat 1 teaspoon oil in skillet and sauté onion and garlic for 3–4 minutes. Add green pepper and continue cooking about 5 minutes. Remove from skillet and keep warm. Cover and warm tortillas in oven or microwave.

Heat 1 teaspoon oil in skillet and sauté chicken. When no longer pink add the vegetables. Sprinkle in cilantro, if using. Fill warm tortilla with ¼ of chicken/vegetable mixture. Roll up and serve.

Makes 4 fajitas.

PER fajita:
CALORIES 290   FIBER 3 gm
CSI 4   SODIUM 336 mg
FAT 8 gm

CHICKEN FAJITAS WITH LIME

Delicious in combination with black beans.

2 chicken breasts, boned and skinned
½ cup lower-salt chicken broth
2 tablespoons freshly squeezed lime juice

¼ cup minced green onions
½ teaspoon ground coriander
½ teaspoon chili powder
2 teaspoons olive oil
2 cups thinly sliced green or red bell pepper
1½ cups thinly sliced onion
4 flour tortillas (8-inch diameter)
½ cup salsa

Half an hour before serving time: Cut chicken into 1-inch strips. Mix chicken broth, lime juice, green onions, spices, and olive oil until smooth (a blender works well for this). Pour over chicken strips; add green pepper and onion slices, and marinate for half an hour.

At cooking time: Heat broiler and drain chicken and vegetables. Place on a non-stick baking sheet. Broil chicken and vegetables until done (approximately 3–4 minutes), stir, and watch carefully to avoid burning.

While mixture is cooking, cover and warm tortillas (microwaving on low heat makes this easy).

To serve, fill warm tortillas with ¼ of chicken/vegetable mixture. Top with 2 tablespoons salsa. Roll up tortillas and serve.

Makes 4 fajitas.

PER fajita:
CALORIES 297   FIBER 3 gm
CSI 4   SODIUM 633 mg
FAT 9 gm

CHICKEN IN PASTRY

Individual chicken packets, which are very inviting. Phyllo dough* can be remarkably easy to use and these "packets" can be made ahead and frozen. Serve with broccoli and *Salad Athene* (page 292) for a lovely meal.

½ cup plain nonfat yogurt
1 tablespoon flour
2 tablespoons light mayonnaise
1 tablespoon Dijon mustard
⅛ teaspoon Worcestershire sauce
¼ teaspoon thyme leaves
⅛ teaspoon Tabasco sauce
2 tablespoons minced green onions
4 teaspoons melted margarine
8 sheets phyllo
4 chicken breasts, skinned and boned
1 tablespoon grated Parmesan cheese

Preheat oven to 375°. In a small bowl mix together yogurt and flour and then add mayonnaise, mustard, Worcestershire sauce, thyme, Tabasco sauce, and onions.

To prepare packets: Place 1 sheet of phyllo on a board and brush it with ½ teaspoon melted margarine; arrange a second sheet of phyllo on top. Spread 1 tablespoon yogurt mixture on 1 chicken breast, turn over onto corner of prepared phyllo sheet. Top with another tablespoon of yogurt mixture. Fold phyllo corner over breast. Fold each side of phyllo over breast and roll up to look like an envelope. Repeat with remaining 3 chicken breasts and yogurt sauce.

*Phyllo can be found in freezer sections of most supermarkets. Thaw unwrapped frozen dough in refrigerator 3–4 hours and work with it while it is cold. The remainder keeps well in refrigerator if tightly wrapped.

Place the 4 packets slightly apart on an ungreased baking sheet. Brush tops with remaining margarine; sprinkle with Parmesan cheese. (To freeze, pack in a single layer in a container with a tight lid. Thaw completely, covered, before baking.) Bake uncovered for 20–25 minutes or until golden brown.

Makes 4 servings.

PER serving:
CALORIES 314   FIBER 1 gm
CSI 5   SODIUM 399 mg
FAT 10 gm

SPICY CHICKEN WITH PEPPERS

½ cup ketchup
1–2 tablespoons Thai (sweet) chili sauce* (watch it, this can be hot!)
1 tablespoon oil
1 clove garlic, minced
1 large onion, cut in half and thinly sliced
1 cup thinly sliced red bell pepper
1 cup thinly sliced green bell pepper
1 stalk celery, sliced diagonally
1 whole chicken (2½–3 pounds), cut up and skinned

Preheat oven to 350°. Combine ketchup and Thai chili sauce and set aside. Heat oil in large skillet over medium heat. Add garlic and sauté until lightly golden. Add onion, red and green pepper, and celery and

*Available in Oriental grocery stores.

stir-fry until crisp tender. Add ketchup/chili sauce mixture to vegetables and remove from heat. Put chicken in baking dish. Spread vegetable mixture over chicken. Cover and bake 45 minutes. Remove cover last 5–10 minutes. Serve with steamed rice.

Makes 6 servings.

PER serving:

CALORIES 221   FIBER 1 gm
CSI 5   SODIUM 354 mg
FAT 8 gm

THAI BARBECUED CHICKEN—*EASY*

½ cup ketchup
1–3 teaspoons Thai (sweet) chili sauce*
1 whole chicken, cut up and skinned
½ cup low-calorie Italian salad dressing

*Available in Oriental grocery stores.

Heat charcoal and prepare grill. Combine ketchup and Thai chili sauce. Set aside. Place skinned chicken on rack over charcoal and brush chicken with Italian dressing while it is being barbecued. Brush ketchup–Thai chili sauce mixture on the last 10 minutes of cooking. (The grill will be easier to clean if the ketchup–Thai chili sauce mixture is brushed only on one side.)

Makes 6 servings.

PER serving:

CALORIES 191   FIBER <1 gm
CSI 5   SODIUM 513 mg
FAT 5 gm

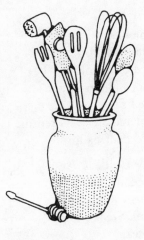

BEEF AND PORK

Would you believe there is a good recipe for a low-CSI meat loaf? There is and it tastes like Mother's. We have also included a pork and tofu recipe that is a favorite of people from Northern China—and stands a good chance of becoming one of your favorites, too.

Baked or Stewed
Old-Fashioned Meat Loaf
Pizza Rice Casserole
Pork Chops Dijon—*Easy*
Stay-Abed Stew
Stuffed Flank Steak Florentine
Vegetable Beef Soup

Stir-Fried or Grilled
Beef Broccoli Oriental
Beef-Tomato Chow Yuk
Juicy Flank Steak—*Easy*
Pepper Steak

With Beans or Pasta
Bean Hot Dish—*Easy*
Beef and Bean Ragout
Beef-Mushroom Spaghetti Sauce (with TVP)
Beef Stroganoff
"Fire" on Rice (Mao Po's Tofu)
Taco Salad
Tamale Pie

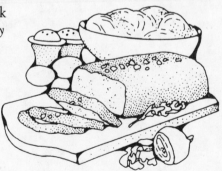

BAKED OR STEWED

OLD-FASHIONED MEAT LOAF

This tastes just like Mother's!

- ¾ cup finely chopped onion
- ¼ cup finely chopped celery
- 1 clove garlic, minced
- ¾ teaspoon thyme leaves
- 1 teaspoon oil
- ½ teaspoon Lite Salt or less
- ¼–½ teaspoon pepper
- 1 cup finely chopped mushrooms (preferably chopped in a food processor)
- ½ pound ground beef (10 percent fat)
- ½ pound ground turkey
- ½ cup fresh bread crumbs
- 2 egg whites
- 5 tablespoons chili sauce *or* ketchup (divided)
- 1 can (8 ounces) unsalted tomatoes, drained and chopped
- ⅓ cup minced parsley

In a skillet cook the onion, celery, garlic, and thyme in the oil over moderately low heat, stirring, until the onion is soft. Add Lite Salt, pepper, and mushrooms and cook the mixture over moderate heat, stirring, for 5–10 minutes, or until the mushrooms are tender and the mushroom liquid is evaporated. Transfer the mixture to a large bowl and let it cool.

Preheat oven to 350°. To the bowl add ground beef, ground turkey, bread crumbs, egg whites, 2 tablespoons of the chili sauce, drained tomatoes, and parsley and stir until it is combined well. Shape the mixture into an oval loaf in a shallow baking pan and spread the remaining 3 tablespoons chili sauce over it. Bake for 45 minutes or until done.

Makes 6 servings.

PER ⅙ recipe:
CALORIES 195
CSI 4
FAT 6 gm
FIBER 1 gm
SODIUM 375 mg

PIZZA RICE CASSEROLE

This is an all-family favorite. Great with hot French bread.

- ⅔ cup uncooked brown rice
- 1⅓ cups water (*or* use 2 cups leftover cooked rice)
- ½ pound ground beef (10 percent fat)
- 1 onion, chopped
- 2 cans (8 ounces each) unsalted tomato sauce
- ¼ teaspoon garlic powder
- 1 teaspoon sugar
- Dash pepper
- ¼ teaspoon oregano leaves
- 1 teaspoon parsley flakes
- 1½ cups low-fat cottage cheese
- ½ cup grated low-fat cheese

Preheat oven to 325°. Cook rice in water or have leftover rice ready. Brown ground beef and onion in a nonstick skillet. Drain

(continued)

fat. Add tomato sauce and spices to beef-onion mixture. Cover and simmer for 15 minutes. Combine cottage cheese and rice. Put a third of rice mixture in lightly oiled casserole dish. Top with a third of meat-tomato sauce. Continue to alternate layers, ending with tomato sauce. Sprinkle grated low-fat cheese on top. Bake for 30 minutes or until hot and bubbly.

Makes 6 servings (about 10 cups).

PER cup:
CALORIES 137   FIBER 2 gm
CSI 3   SODIUM 194 mg
FAT 3 gm

PORK CHOPS DIJON—*EASY*

Baked chops are much lower-fat than fried ones. One small delicious chop needs to be served with generous amounts of potatoes, vegetables, and salad for those with hearty appetites.

MUSTARD SAUCE

½ cup wine vinegar
¼ cup Dijon mustard
2 tablespoons minced chives *or* green onions
2 teaspoons tarragon leaves
¼ teaspoon coarsely ground black pepper

6 loin pork chops, well trimmed

Preheat oven to 425°. Combine *Mustard Sauce* ingredients and stir well. Place chops in nonstick baking pan. Spread 1 tablespoon sauce on each chop and bake for about 10 minutes. Turn chops over and spread with remaining sauce; continue baking until done, about 8–10 minutes.

Makes 6 servings.

PER serving:
CALORIES 199   FIBER trace
CSI 7   SODIUM 181 mg
FAT 10 gm

STAY-ABED STEW

This goes in a very low oven early in the morning so it can cook all day. Great with biscuits, or add dumplings on top of it.

1 pound trimmed round steak
1 onion, chopped
1 can (16 ounces) unsalted green beans, undrained
1 can (4 ounces) mushrooms, undrained
1 green bell pepper, chopped
2 medium potatoes, chunked
3 carrots, chunked
½ teaspoon Lite Salt or less
1 tablespoon parsley flakes
½ cup instant tapioca
1 can (13 ounces) unsalted tomato juice
1 cup water

Preheat oven to 250°. Trim and cube round steak and place in bottom of casserole pan. Mix vegetables, seasonings, and dry tapioca and spread over meat. Pour tomato juice and water over all. (Add more water if you want thin stew.) Bake for 6–8 hours, stirring occasionally.

Makes 4–6 servings (about 12 cups).

PER cup:
CALORIES 121
CSI 2
FAT 2 gm
FIBER 3 gm
SODIUM 215 mg

STUFFED FLANK STEAK FLORENTINE

This is nice to serve for a special occasion with *Mushroom Barley Pilaf* (page 326) and a salad.

- 2 pounds flank steak
- 3 egg whites, slightly beaten *or* ½ cup egg substitute (commercial *or Home-made Egg Substitute,* page 283)
- 2 packages (10 ounces each) frozen chopped spinach, cooked and drained
- 1 cup grated low-fat cheese
- 1 teaspoon sage
- Dash pepper
- 1½ cups bread crumbs
- 3 tablespoons flour
- 1 tablespoon oil
- 2 cans (8 ounces each) unsalted tomato sauce
- 1 cup dry red wine
- 1 cup chopped onion
- 2 cloves garlic, minced

Preheat oven to 350°. Pound steak with meat mallet to ¼-inch thickness; set aside. Combine egg whites *or* egg substitute, spin-

ach, cheese, sage, and pepper; stir in bread crumbs. Spread mixture over steak. Starting from narrow side, roll up jelly-roll fashion; tie with string. Coat lightly with flour. In large skillet, heat oil and carefully brown steak rolls on all sides. Place in 9-by-13-inch baking dish.

Combine tomato sauce, wine, onion, and garlic. Pour over meat. Cover with foil and bake for 1–1½ hours or until meat is tender. To serve meat, remove string and slice. Spoon sauce over steak rolls.

Makes 8 to 10 servings.

PER ⅛ recipe:
CALORIES 281
CSI 8
FAT 10 gm
FIBER 2 gm
SODIUM 221 mg

VEGETABLE BEEF SOUP

An old standby made with lots of vegetables and enough meat for a good flavor. Serve with *Old-Style Wheat Biscuits* (page 276) and *Berry Cobbler* (page 436).

- 1 teaspoon oil
- ½ pound beef stew meat, well trimmed
- 1 clove garlic, minced
- 1 large onion, chopped
- 2 carrots, julienned
- 3 medium potatoes, peeled and chopped
- 2 cans (16 ounces each) unsalted tomatoes
- 5 cups water
- 1½ teaspoons Lite Salt or less
- ⅛ teaspoon pepper
- ½ teaspoon basil leaves

(continued)

Heat oil in skillet. Add meat, garlic, and onions. Stir rapidly until brown. Add carrots, potatoes, tomatoes, water, Lite Salt, pepper, and basil. Bring to boil. Reduce heat. Cover and simmer at least 2 hours. Add water as needed to keep volume unchanged.

Makes 12 cups.

PER cup:

CALORIES 80   FIBER 2 gm
CSI 1   SODIUM 130 mg
FAT 2 gm

STIR-FRIED OR GRILLED

BEEF BROCCOLI ORIENTAL

1 pound trimmed round steak, partially frozen for easier slicing
2 tablespoons lower-sodium soy sauce
2 tablespoons water
1 tablespoon oyster sauce
1 teaspoon sesame oil
1 teaspoon sugar
1 teaspoon cornstarch
1 teaspoon oil
1 tablespoon minced fresh ginger root
1 tablespoon minced garlic
6 cups broccoli, cut into flowerets
3 green onions, cut into 2-inch lengths

Slice steak thinly across the grain. Combine soy sauce, water, oyster sauce, sesame oil, sugar, and cornstarch; mix well and set aside. Heat a heavy pan or wok. Add oil, ginger, and garlic and stir-fry the meat until no longer pink colored; remove from wok. Add broccoli and green onions to the wok; toss for a few minutes, then return the meat to the wok. Add sauce to the meat and stir until the sauce thickens. Serve with hot steamed rice or with *Baked Spaghetti Pie* (page 349).

Makes 4 servings.

PER serving:

CALORIES 251   FIBER 3 gm
CSI 7   SODIUM 558 mg
FAT 11 gm

BEEF-TOMATO CHOW YUK

A very attractive stir-fry dish. The fresh ginger makes it special. It's good served over steamed rice.

½ pound flank steak *or* trimmed round steak
1 slice fresh ginger root, peeled and minced*
1 clove garlic, crushed
1 teaspoon cornstarch
1 teaspoon lower-sodium soy sauce
1 egg white
1 tablespoon oil

*Chop remaining ginger root and freeze in tightly covered container, ready for the next time you need it.

1 medium green bell pepper, cut into strips
2 stalks celery, sliced
1 medium onion, cut into strips
½ cup water
¼ cup ketchup
3 tablespoons sugar (or less if tomatoes are very ripe)
1 tablespoon cornstarch
2 tablespoons water
4 medium tomatoes, peeled,† seeded, and cut into quarters

Cut the beef into very thin slices (it cuts better if partially frozen). Mix ginger root, garlic, cornstarch, soy sauce, and egg white. Add the sliced beef; stir and allow to marinate for 5 minutes.

Put the oil in a preheated skillet or wok; stir-fry the meat until the redness is gone. Remove the meat and set aside. Add the green peppers, celery, and onions to the pan along with the water. Cover and cook at medium heat for 3 minutes.

Add the ketchup and sugar; cover and cook for 2 minutes. Meanwhile, mix cornstarch with 2 tablespoons water; stir into the beef mixture and add to pan. Cook until liquid is clear and slightly thickened. Add tomatoes; cover and cook just until heated through. Serve with steamed rice.

Makes 4 servings.

†Tomatoes peel easily after plunging in boiling water for 30 seconds.

PER serving:
CALORIES 211
CSI 3
FAT 7 gm
FIBER 2 gm
SODIUM 242 mg

JUICY FLANK STEAK—*EASY*

Supper Stuffed Potatoes (page 335) and a green vegetable make nice companions for this tasty barbecued steak.

1½ pounds flank steak

MARINADE

¼ cup lower-sodium soy sauce
1–2 tablespoons white wine *or* sherry
1 teaspoon sesame oil
½–1 teaspoon black bean sauce with chili*
½ teaspoon sugar
1 green onion, finely minced
2 cloves garlic, minced
2 teaspoons minced fresh ginger root
¼ cup water

Combine marinade ingredients. Pour over flank steak and marinate for several hours, turning occasionally.

Grill over charcoal or broil on each side to desired doneness, turning once. Brush steak with marinade while cooking. Be careful not to overcook. To serve: Slice steak in thin slices, cutting on the diagonal. Serve warm.

Makes 6 servings.

*Available in Oriental grocery stores.

PER serving:
CALORIES 188
CSI 6
FAT 8 gm
FIBER trace
SODIUM 455 mg

PEPPER STEAK

An excellent stir-fry dish to prepare for people who are beginning a low-fat eating style.

> 1 pound flank steak
> 1 tablespoon Chinese rice wine *or* pale dry sherry
> 3 tablespoons lower-sodium soy sauce
> 1 teaspoon sugar
> 2 teaspoons cornstarch
> 1 tablespoon oil
> 2 medium green bell peppers, cut into ½-inch squares
> 4 slices fresh ginger root, peeled and cut ⅛ inch thick*

Cut the flank steak lengthwise into strips 1½ inches wide, then crosswise into ¼-inch slices.

In a large bowl, mix the wine, soy sauce, sugar, and cornstarch. Add the steak slices and toss with a large spoon to coat them thoroughly. The steak may be cooked at once, or marinated for as long as 6 hours.

Heat oil in a wok or large skillet over high heat for about 30 seconds. Reduce the heat to moderate if the oil begins to smoke. Immediately add the pepper squares and stir-fry for 3 minutes, or until they are tender but still crisp. Scoop them out with a slotted spoon and reserve. Add the ginger to the wok, stir for a few seconds, then add the steak mixture. Stir-fry for about 2 minutes, or until the meat shows no sign of pink. Discard the ginger. Add the pepper and cook for a minute, stirring, then trans-

fer the contents of the pan to a heated platter and serve with steamed rice.

Makes 4 servings.

PER serving:
CALORIES 217   FIBER 1 gm
CSI 5   SODIUM 538 mg
FAT 7 gm

WITH BEANS OR PASTA

BEAN HOT DISH—*EASY*

This recipe freezes well. Any combination of beans can be used. It also works well in a crockpot.

> ½ cup diced onion
> ½ pound ground beef (10 percent fat)
> ¼ cup brown sugar
> ½ cup ketchup
> 2 tablespoons vinegar
> 1 tablespoon prepared mustard
> 1 can (16 ounces) lima beans*
> 1 can (16 ounces) small red beans*
> 1 can (16 ounces) kidney beans*
> 1 can (16 ounces) butter beans*

Preheat oven to 300°. In a nonstick skillet brown diced onions and lean ground beef. Drain off fat. Drain beans and mix remain-

*Chop remaining ginger root and freeze in tightly covered container, ready for the next time you need it.

*Use low-sodium beans if available.

ing ingredients together. Add to meat and onions and bake 1½ hours in a covered baking dish.

Makes 6 servings (1½ cups each).

PER cup:
CALORIES 231 FIBER 7 gm
CSI 2 SODIUM 441 mg
FAT 3 gm

BEEF AND BEAN RAGOUT

A hearty stew with beans and beef—well liked even by people who thought they didn't like beans.

1 cup uncooked or 3 cups canned kidney beans *or* red beans*
3 cups water (omit if using canned beans)
1 pound trimmed round steak, cut in 1-inch cubes
1 tablespoon oil
3 cans (16 ounces each) unsalted tomatoes, undrained, cut up
¾ cup dry red wine
1 teaspoon sugar
2 cloves garlic, minced
½ teaspoon Lite Salt or less
½ teaspoon thyme leaves
⅛ teaspoon pepper
3 bay leaves
3 potatoes, cubed (about 3 cups)
2 medium onions, cut in wedges
1 green bell pepper, chopped

*Use low-sodium beans if available.

Rinse dried beans. Place in 3-quart saucepan with the water; soak overnight. (Or bring to boiling; reduce heat and simmer 2 minutes. Remove from heat; cover and let stand 1 hour.) Do not drain. Bring beans to boiling; reduce heat. Cover and simmer 45 minutes. Drain.

In 4-quart Dutch oven, brown meat in 1 tablespoon oil; drain. Add drained beans, the undrained tomatoes, wine, sugar, garlic, Lite Salt, thyme, pepper, and bay leaves to the meat. Bring to boiling; reduce heat. Cover and simmer 1 hour or until meat is nearly tender. Add potatoes, onions, and green peppers. Cook 30 minutes more or until meat and vegetables are tender. (The longer the mixture is simmered, the better it tastes!) Remove bay leaves before serving.

Makes 6 servings (about 13 cups).

PER cup:
CALORIES 168 FIBER 5 gm
CSI 2 SODIUM 72 mg
FAT 3 gm

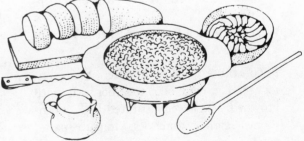

BEEF-MUSHROOM SPAGHETTI SAUCE (WITH TVP)

Textured Vegetable Protein (TVP) is very low in fat and inexpensive! We recommend combining it with lean ground beef, such as in this spaghetti sauce, when using it for the first time.

½ cup TVP reconstituted with 1 cup water
½ cup minced onion
2 ounces ground beef (10 percent fat)
½ cup sliced fresh mushrooms or 1 can (4 ounces) mushrooms, drained
2 cloves garlic, minced
1 can (16 ounces) unsalted tomatoes
1 can (6 ounces) unsalted tomato paste
1 teaspoon parsley flakes
1 bay leaf
¾ teaspoon basil leaves
½–1 teaspoon oregano leaves
⅛ teaspoon pepper
¼ cup chopped green bell pepper (optional)
¼ cup grated Parmesan cheese for topping

Reconstitute TVP with water. Sauté onions and ground beef together; stir until browned. Mix in reconstituted TVP, mushrooms, garlic, tomatoes, tomato paste, parsley, bay leaf, basil, oregano, and pepper. Simmer gently for 30 minutes. Add green peppers, if desired, the last 10 minutes of cooking. Serve over cooked spaghetti. Sprinkle with Parmesan cheese.

Makes about 4 cups of sauce.

PER cup:
CALORIES 150   FIBER 3 gm
CSI 2   SODIUM 173 mg
FAT 3 gm

BEEF STROGANOFF

A delicious low-fat version without the traditional sour cream.

1 pound trimmed round steak
2 tablespoons flour
1 teaspoon paprika
½ onion, chopped
1 clove garlic, crushed
1 tablespoon oil
1 can (4 ounces) mushrooms, undrained
1 cube beef bouillon
1 cup plain nonfat yogurt

Slice beef in thin, diagonal strips (may be easier to do if partially frozen). Mix flour and paprika, and shake beef strips in it to coat. Brown beef, onion and garlic in oil over high heat until brown. Stir in mushrooms and bouillon cube. Heat to boiling, stirring constantly. Reduce heat, cover, and simmer for 12–15 minutes. Slowly stir part of the stroganoff into the yogurt (this will prevent curdling). Return to pan and heat. Do not cover. Serve over eggless noodles or macaroni ribbons.

Makes 4 servings (about 4 cups).

PER cup:
CALORIES 242   FIBER 1 gm
CSI 6   SODIUM 442 mg
FAT 10 gm

"FIRE" ON RICE (MAO PO'S TOFU)

Szechuan-style tofu and pork.

12 ounces tofu, cut into 1-inch-square pieces (½ inch thick)
2 teaspoons oil
1 ounce finely chopped pork (use one small center-cut pork chop)
1 teaspoon chopped fresh ginger root
1 tablespoon finely minced garlic
1–2 teaspoons black bean sauce with chili* (1–2 tablespoons for fire eaters)
1 teaspoon sugar
1 teaspoon sesame oil
½ cup lower-salt chicken broth
1 tablespoon cornstarch, dissolved in ⅓ cup water
1 tablespoon chopped green onion

Heat oil in skillet. Stir-fry the chopped pork. Then add the bean paste, garlic, and ginger. Finally, add the chicken broth and tofu.

Cover skillet and cook over low heat for a few minutes (don't let tofu stick). Add sugar. Thicken the sauce with the cornstarch mixture. Place on a warm platter and sprinkle the green onions on top. Serve with steamed rice.

Makes 3 cups (3 to 4 servings).

*Available in Chinese specialty stores.

PER cup:
CALORIES 176   FIBER 1 gm
CSI 2   SODIUM 131 mg
FAT 11 gm

TACO SALAD

Summer is here!

2 cups *Baked Corn Chips* (page 262)
1 cup *Thousand Island Salad Dressing* (page 305) *or* commercial low-fat dressing
½ pound ground beef (10 percent fat)
1 can (16 ounces) kidney beans, drained*
1 teaspoon chili powder
1 large head lettuce, chopped
4 tomatoes, chopped
½ avocado, sliced
⅓ cup grated low-fat cheese
2 tablespoons hot taco sauce

Prepare *Baked Corn Chips* and *Thousand Island Salad Dressing* according to directions.

Brown ground beef in a nonstick skillet. Drain off fat. Add beans and chili powder and simmer 5 minutes. Chop vegetables and put in salad bowl.

Before serving, toss vegetables and grated cheese with bean/beef mixture and put in large salad bowl. Arrange *Corn Chips* around edge. Combine salad dressing and taco sauce. Serve in a pitcher along with salad.

Makes 6 to 8 servings (about 16 cups).

*Use low-sodium beans if available.

PER cup:
CALORIES 126   FIBER 3 gm
CSI 2   SODIUM 197 mg
FAT 4 gm

TAMALE PIE

A grain and bean staple with just a bit of beef for flavor. All that's needed to round out a meal is a salad and some fruit.

½ pound ground beef (10 percent fat)
¾ cup chopped onion
1 clove garlic, minced
½ cup chopped green bell pepper
1 can (16 ounces) unsalted whole kernel corn, drained
1 can (16 ounces) pinto, red, or kidney beans, drained*
2 cans (8 ounces each) unsalted tomato sauce
¼ cup sliced black olives, drained
2–3 tablespoons taco sauce or salsa
2 teaspoons chili powder

TOPPING

1 cup yellow cornmeal
2½ cups water

*Use low-sodium beans if available.

¼ teaspoon Lite Salt or less
½ cup grated part-skim mozzarella cheese

Preheat oven to 375°. In nonstick skillet brown ground beef with onions and garlic. Drain off fat. Add green peppers, corn, beans, tomato sauce, olives, taco sauce or salsa, and chili powder. Pour into 10-by-10-inch baking pan.

In saucepan combine cornmeal, water, and Lite Salt. Stirring constantly, bring mixture to a boil and continue cooking until it thickens slightly. Spoon over top of meat/vegetable mixture. Bake for about 45 minutes. Remove from oven and sprinkle grated mozzarella cheese on top. Return pan to oven and bake another 15 minutes.

Makes 6 servings (about 9 cups).

PER cup:
CALORIES 205   FIBER 6 gm
CSI 3   SODIUM 367 mg
FAT 4 gm

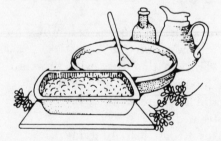

DESSERTS

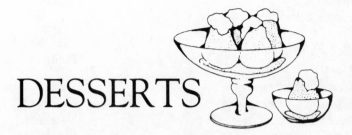

We love desserts, as you can tell by the size of this section. We've worked hard to ensure they fit into low-CSI eating. We think you'll be as happy with them as we are. And the fruit desserts are loaded with fiber as well as flavor. Note the size of the servings—when we say "serves 24," that means small pieces.

Fruit Desserts
Apple Crisp
Baked Apples
Bananas en Papillote
Berry Pavlova
Fruit-Filled Dessert Cups
Fruit Salad Alaska
Peach and Berry Meringues
Peach Cardinal
Pears in Wine
Toasted Bananas

Cookies
Carob Cookies
Crispy Spice Cookies
Forgotten Kisses
Gingies
Lace Cookies
Lebkuchen
Oatmeal Cookies

Bars
Apricot Meringue Bars
Brownies
Butterscotch Brownies

Chocolate Banana Bars
Jamocha Squares
Molasses Orange Bars
Northwest Harvest Bars
PB&J Bars
Walnut Squares

Cakes
All-Season Shortcake
Angel Quickie
Apple Loaf Cake
Baba au Rhum
Baked Doughnut Holes
Carrot Raisin Cake with Penuche Frosting
Chocolate Zucchini Cake
Cocoa Cake
Crème de Menthe Cheesecake
Depression Cake
Hot Fudge Pudding Cake
Party Carrot Cake
Pinto Fiesta Cake
Poppyseed Cake
Redheaded Shortcake
Ricotta Cheesecake

Pies and Cobblers
  Apple Strudel
  Berry Cobbler
  Berry Yogurt Pie
  Cherry Strudel
  Cranberry Squares
  Graham Cracker Crust
  Peach Almond Crisp
  Pumpkin Pie
  Swedish Pie

Upside-Down Peach Cobbler

Puddings
  Chocolate Pudding
  Pumpkin Bread Pudding

Frozen Desserts
  Cranberry Sherbet
  New and Improved Baked Alaska
  Pumpkin Frozen Yogurt
  Strawberry Ice

FRUIT DESSERTS

✕ APPLE CRISP

Crispy! Crunchy! For a larger crowd you can double the recipe and use a 9-by-13-inch baking dish.

  4 cups sliced peeled tart apples (about 4 medium)
  ⅓ cup brown sugar
  ¼ cup flour
  ¼ cup oatmeal
  ½ teaspoon cinnamon
  ¼ teaspoon nutmeg
  2 tablespoons margarine, softened
  Vanilla yogurt *or Yogurt Dessert Sauce* (page 456), optional for topping

Preheat oven to 375°. Lightly oil an 8-inch square baking pan. Place apple slices in pan. Mix remaining ingredients thoroughly. Sprinkle over apples.

Bake 30 minutes or until apples are tender and topping is golden brown. Serve warm and, if desired, with low-fat vanilla yogurt or *Yogurt Dessert Sauce.*

Makes 4–6 servings.

PER ⅙ recipe:

CALORIES 153	FIBER 2 gm
CSI <1	SODIUM 54 mg
FAT 4 gm.	

BAKED APPLES

Use tart baking apples for this classic dessert. The aroma from the cinnamon and apples is terrific!

  4 apples
  Water
  3 tablespoons brown sugar
  4 teaspoons raisins
  Dash cinnamon *or* nutmeg
  ***Yogurt Dessert Sauce* (page 456) (optional)**

Preheat oven to 350°. Wash and core apples. Peel upper ¼ of the apple to prevent the skin from splitting. Place apple upright in baking dish filled about ¼-inch deep with water. Combine brown sugar, raisins, and cinnamon. Fill the center core of the apple with the mixture. Bake 30–45 minutes or until tender. Serve hot or cold with *Yogurt Dessert Sauce* if desired.

Makes 4 servings.

PER serving:
CALORIES 125   FIBER 4 gm
CSI trace   SODIUM 5 mg
FAT <1 gm

BANANAS EN PAPILLOTE (BAKED BANANAS)

½ cup water
2 tablespoons sugar
½ cup mashed fresh fruit (apricots, berries, peaches, etc.)
½ teaspoon vanilla
4 small bananas, peeled
Fresh mint leaves, for garnish

Preheat oven to 425°. Heat water in a saucepan, add sugar, and stir to dissolve. Remove from the heat, add the mashed fruit and the vanilla. Mix well.

Fold 4 sheets of foil (12 by 8 inches) in half lengthwise. At the end of the fold, turn up and pinch the corners to make a "boat" to hold the bananas and the sauce. Put a whole banana in each "boat." Pour about 3 tablespoons of fruit sauce over the

banana. Close the foil by folding over the edges and pinching them together tightly.

Place on a baking sheet. Bake for 15–20 minutes. Serve on heated plates after having opened the foil and decorated the bananas with mint leaves.

Serve with plain nonfat yogurt and more fruit sauce, if needed.

Makes 4 servings.

PER serving:
CALORIES 127   FIBER 2 gm
CSI trace   SODIUM 1 mg
FAT <1 gm

BERRY PAVLOVA

A beautiful and tasty dessert.

3 egg whites
⅛ teaspoon Lite Salt or less
⅛ teaspoon cream of tartar
½ cup sugar
½ teaspoon vanilla
1 cup low-fat vanilla yogurt
4 cups fresh berries, washed, stemmed, and sliced

On day before: Preheat oven to 450°. Beat egg whites until foamy and add Lite Salt and cream of tartar. Beat again until very stiff; add sugar very slowly and continue beating until whites stand in stiff peaks. Carefully fold in vanilla. Put into 8-by-8-inch baking pan. Place meringue into oven and turn *off* heat immediately; leave in oven overnight. Do not open oven door for at least 8 hours.

(continued)

Early in the day: Stir yogurt until smooth. Spread yogurt on top of meringue and cover with clear plastic wrap. Refrigerate 4–6 hours, until soft. *To serve:* Cut into squares and cover with fresh berries.

Makes 9 servings (3 inches by 3 inches).

PER serving:

CALORIES 97	FIBER 2 gm
CSI trace	SODIUM 50 mg
FAT <1 gm	

FRUIT-FILLED DESSERT CUPS

An elegant dessert. Prepare shells ahead and fill at serving time. *Fresh Rhubarb Sauce* (page 455) with fresh strawberries added is especially delicious as a filling, but any fresh fruit works well.

> 1½ tablespoons sugar
> ½ teaspoon cinnamon
> 3 sheets phyllo pastry*
> 2 cups fresh fruit (nectarines, peaches, apricots, berries, kiwi)
> ½ cup nonfat plain yogurt

Preheat oven to 350°. Mix together sugar and cinnamon. Place one sheet phyllo on dry surface. Lightly spray phyllo sheet with

*A trick in handling phyllo pastry is to be sure to thaw it in the refrigerator and work with it while it is cold. If allowed to come to room temperature before unfolding, it is hard to handle. The remainder of the pastry keeps well in refrigerator if wrapped tightly.

nonstick cooking spray. Sprinkle phyllo with sugar mixture. Place second sheet of phyllo on top of the other. Repeat spraying, sprinkling, and stacking. Cut in half lengthwise and stack phyllo to form six layers.

Cut into four equal portions. Press each into muffin tin or custard cups. Edges should stand straight up while baking. Bake for 10 minutes. Cool.

When ready to serve fill each shell with fresh fruit or with *Fresh Rhubarb Sauce* and sliced fresh strawberries. Top fruit with 2 tablespoons of yogurt.

Makes 4 servings.

PER serving:

CALORIES 130	FIBER 2 gm
CSI trace	SODIUM 80 mg
FAT trace	

FRUIT SALAD ALASKA

Fruit salad with a baked meringue on top.

> 3 tablespoons orange marmalade
> 1 tablespoon Cointreau or Grand Marnier liqueur
> 1 orange, peeled and diced
> 1 can (16 ounces) pineapple chunks packed in own juice (drained) *or* 1 cup fresh pineapple cubes
> 12–16 fresh strawberries
> 1 large fresh peach, peeled and diced
> 3 egg whites
> ⅛ teaspoon cream of tartar
> 1–2 tablespoons sugar
> ½ teaspoon vanilla

Preheat oven to 450°. In a saucepan, mix the marmalade and liqueur. Bring to a boil. Let cool. Prepare the fruit. Drain well. Pour the mixed fruit into 4 individual soufflé-type baking dishes. Pour marmalade sauce over fruit. Beat the egg whites until stiff. Add the cream of tartar, beat, add the sugar, and beat until stiff. Fold in the vanilla. Spread the egg white mixture on top of the fruit salad, heaping it thick and spreading it to the edge of the dishes. Bake for 5 minutes or until the meringue is lightly browned.

Makes 4 servings.

PER serving:
CALORIES 164   FIBER 4 gm
CSI trace   SODIUM 41 mg
FAT <1 gm

PEACH AND BERRY MERINGUES

MERINGUE SHELLS

2 egg whites
⅛ teaspoon cream of tartar
¼ cup sugar

FRUIT FILLING

2 tablespoons currant jelly
1 cup fresh or frozen berries, thawed and drained
2 cups sliced fresh or canned peaches, drained
1 tablespoon amaretto (almond-flavored liqueur) *or* 1 teaspoon almond extract

Prepare meringue shells early in the day or the day before serving: Preheat oven to 250°. Line a baking sheet with parchment paper or plain brown paper. Beat egg whites and cream of tartar until frothy. Gradually add sugar, 1 tablespoon at a time, beating constantly. Beat until stiff peaks form when beater is lifted from egg whites. Divide mixture into 4 mounds on prepared baking sheet. Form each into a cup with the back of a spoon. Bake 1–1½ hours until cups just begin to brown and are not sticky. Turn off oven without removing meringues. Allow to cool 3–4 hours. If prepared ahead cover tightly.

Before serving, melt jelly in a small saucepan. Add berries. Stir gently just until berries begin to soften. Remove from heat. Cool slightly.

Place fresh or canned peaches in a bowl. Sprinkle with amaretto. Place peach slices in each meringue cup. Spoon berry sauce over top.

Makes 4 servings.

PER serving:
CALORIES 143   FIBER 3 gm
CSI trace   SODIUM 33 mg
FAT trace

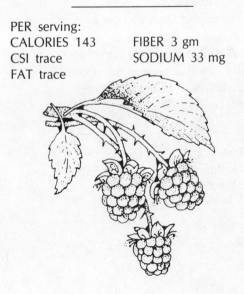

PEACH CARDINAL

Fresh peaches, poached and served with a raspberry sauce.

4 cups water
1 cup sugar
1 tablespoon vanilla
1 tablespoon freshly squeezed lemon juice
6 ripe fresh peaches, 2½-inch diameter
3 cups fresh *or* frozen raspberries
3 tablespoons sugar
Mint leaves, for decoration (optional)

Simmer water, sugar, vanilla, and lemon juice in a large saucepan. Stir until sugar has dissolved. Add unpeeled peaches to simmering syrup. Keep just below simmering point for 8 minutes, or until peaches are soft when carefully tested with a sharp knife. Remove pan from heat. Let peaches cool in syrup 20 minutes. Drain peaches. Peel while warm and arrange in serving dish or individual cups.

Put raspberries and sugar in blender and whirl until raspberries are well mashed. Pour raspberry puree over peaches. Keep chilled until serving time. Decorate with mint leaves, if desired.

Makes 6 servings.

PER serving:
CALORIES 160   FIBER 4 gm
CSI trace   SODIUM 1 mg
FAT trace

PEARS IN WINE

6 medium-size firm ripe pears
2 cups cold water
3 tablespoons freshly squeezed lemon juice, divided
2 cups red wine
½ teaspoon cinnamon
½ cup sugar
¼ cup red currant jelly
¼ cup slivered almonds, to decorate

Peel pears. They may be left whole, or cut in halves. If served whole, cut a small slice off the bottoms so that the pears will stand up easily. Carefully remove the core from the bottoms. If served in halves, cut the cores out. Drop quickly in water and 1 tablespoon of lemon juice to prevent discoloration. Bring wine, cinnamon, and rest of the lemon juice and sugar to boil in a saucepan. Drain pears and drop in boiling syrup. Reduce to simmer for 10 minutes or until pears are soft when pierced with a knife. Do not overcook. Remove pan from heat. Let cool in syrup for 20 minutes. Drain, reserving the syrup. Set pears in a serving dish or in individual cups. Continue boiling syrup until it measures ½ cup. Add red currant jelly and simmer briefly. Pour sauce over pears. Chill well and decorate with almonds.

Makes 6 servings.

PER serving:
CALORIES 244   FIBER 6 gm
CSI trace   SODIUM 8 mg
FAT 3 gm

TOASTED BANANAS

Bananas are wrapped in flour tortillas, seasoned with spices, and served warm with *Orange Sauce* or chocolate syrup. An unusual fruit dessert that is very easy to prepare. Children can easily help make these and love the results!

ORANGE SAUCE

¼ cup sugar
1 tablespoon cornstarch
1 cup orange juice
1 tablespoon margarine
1 tablespoon freshly squeezed lemon juice

Mix together sugar and cornstarch; add orange juice and cook, stirring until thickened. Stir in margarine and lemon juice. Serve warm over toasted bananas.

6 large firm, ripe bananas*
3 tablespoons freshly squeezed lemon juice
12 flour tortillas (8-inch diameter)
⅔ cup sugar
1 teaspoon cinnamon
⅛ teaspoon nutmeg
¼ cup skim milk

Preheat oven to 400°. Peel bananas and cut in half lengthwise; dip in lemon juice. Place each slice at one end of a tortilla. Stir together sugar, cinnamon, and nutmeg; sprinkle over bananas (reserve a small amount for top). Roll each tortilla around

*Applesauce or apple pie filling can also be used. Spread ½ cup fruit on tortilla, sprinkle with cinnamon/sugar, and roll up.

banana and secure with a wooden pick. Brush tortilla lightly with milk and sprinkle with remaining cinnamon/sugar mixture. Place on a lightly oiled, nonstick baking sheet and bake for 15 minutes. Remove from baking sheet immediately and serve while warm with warm *Orange Sauce*.

Makes 12 servings.

PER serving:
CALORIES 226   FIBER 2 gm
CSI 1   SODIUM 126 mg
FAT 4 gm

COOKIES

CAROB COOKIES

Substituting carob powder for cocoa decreases the CSI considerably.

1½ cups white flour
1½ cups whole wheat flour
½ cup carob powder
1 tablespoon powdered instant coffee (decaffeinated works well)
½ teaspoon baking soda
1½ teaspoons baking powder
1 cup sugar
5 egg whites
¾ cup oil
1 teaspoon vanilla
¼ cup chopped nuts

Preheat oven to 375°.
Mix dry ingredients together. Beat egg

(continued)

whites slightly and add oil and vanilla; add to dry ingredients. Add chopped nuts and form into small balls. Bake for 15 minutes.

Makes 48 cookies.

PER cookie:
CALORIES 83   FIBER <1 gm
CSI <1   SODIUM 23 mg
FAT 4 gm

CRISPY SPICE COOKIES

3 cups flour
2 teaspoons ground ginger
1½ teaspoons cinnamon
1 teaspoon ground cloves
¾ cup margarine
½ cup sugar
½ cup dark corn syrup

Preheat oven to 350°. Sift first 4 ingredients. Cream margarine and sugar; stir in corn syrup. Mix in flour. Roll out ⅛-inch thick on floured surface. Cut into shapes. Place on baking sheet. Bake about 10 minutes. Decorate, if desired.

Makes 54 cookies (2 inches each).

PER cookie:
CALORIES 62   FIBER trace
CSI trace   SODIUM 36 mg
FAT 3 gm

FORGOTTEN KISSES

These are pretty cookies suitable for parties. This recipe makes two kinds of cookies: one with coffee flavoring and the other with lemon and nuts.

2 egg whites
⅛ teaspoon Lite Salt or less
½ teaspoon cream of tartar
¾ cup sugar
½ teaspoon vanilla
½ teaspoon powdered instant coffee
Dash nutmeg
¼ cup finely chopped walnuts
¼ teaspoon grated lemon peel

Preheat oven to 350°. Beat egg whites until fluffy. Add Lite Salt and cream of tartar and beat. Add sugar slowly, beating all the time. Continue beating until mixture is glossy and stands in stiff peaks. Add vanilla. Place half the mixture in small bowl and fold in coffee powder and nutmeg. Fold nuts and lemon peel into remaining mixture. Drop by tablespoons onto unoiled baking sheet. Put in 350° oven. Turn *off* oven heat immediately. Leave cookies until cool (at least 2 hours). Do not open oven door. Remove onto racks.

Makes 36 small kisses.

PER cookie:
CALORIES 23   FIBER trace
CSI trace   SODIUM 12 mg
FAT <1 gm

GINGIES

⅓ cup margarine
1 cup brown sugar
1½ cups dark molasses
½ cup cold water
3 cups whole wheat flour
3 cups white flour
1 teaspoon allspice
1 teaspoon ground ginger
1 teaspoon ground cloves
1 teaspoon cinnamon
2 teaspoons baking soda
1 tablespoon cold water

Mix the margarine, brown sugar and molasses together thoroughly. Stir in ½ cup cold water. Sift the flours and spices together and add to above mixture. Dissolve the baking soda in 1 tablespoon cold water and add to dough. Mix well, cover bowl, and chill dough.

When ready to bake, preheat oven to 350°. Roll out cookie dough thick (½ inch). Cut with 2½-inch round cutter. Place far apart on lightly oiled baking sheet. Bake until no imprint remains when touched lightly with finger, about 15–18 minutes.

Makes 45 large, puffy cookies.

PER cookie:
CALORIES 110   FIBER 1 gm
CSI trace   SODIUM 59 mg
FAT 2 gm

LACE COOKIES

A *great* low-fat cookie!

1 cup sugar
⅓ cup margarine, softened
¼ cup commercial egg substitute *or* *Homemade Egg Substitute* (page 283)
½ teaspoon vanilla
¼ teaspoon baking soda
1 cup uncooked oatmeal
3 tablespoons flour

Preheat oven to 350°. Combine sugar, margarine, egg substitute, vanilla, baking soda, oatmeal, and flour and mix well. Spray cookie sheets with nonstick spray.

Drop dough by one-teaspoonful amounts, 2 inches apart, on the prepared cookie sheets. Bake for 6–10 minutes or until light brown.

To have flat cookies: Allow to cool on the cookie sheet before peeling cookies off.

To have cylinder-shaped cookies: While still warm, roll cookies carefully around handle of a wooden spoon as they are removed from the cookie sheet.

Store cookies in an airtight container.

Makes 84 cookies (about 2¼ inches each).

PER cookie:
CALORIES 20   FIBER trace
CSI trace   SODIUM 14 mg
FAT <1 gm

LEBKUCHEN

Let these cookies "rest" for one week prior to eating them; it improves the flavor and texture.

- 2¾ cups flour
- 1 teaspoon cinnamon
- 1 teaspoon ground cloves
- 1 teaspoon allspice
- 1 teaspoon nutmeg
- ½ teaspoon baking soda
- ½ cup honey
- ½ cup molasses
- ¾ cup brown sugar
- 2 egg whites
- 1 tablespoon freshly squeezed lemon juice
- 1 teaspoon freshly grated lemon rind
- ⅓ cup finely chopped nuts
- ⅓ cup candied fruit peel

GLAZE

- ½ cup powdered sugar
- 2 tablespoons cornstarch
- 1–3 tablespoons hot water
- ½ teaspoon vanilla *or* brandy

Sift flour with spices and baking soda; set aside. Heat the honey, molasses, and brown sugar to a boil; cool to lukewarm. Stir in egg whites and juice, and grate the lemon rind into the mixture. Stir in flour in several additions, then work in nuts and peel. Cover and chill *overnight*.

Preheat oven to 400° and lightly oil baking sheets. On a floured board roll dough ¼-inch thick in small batches (keep rest chilled), and cut into rectangles 1½ by 2½ inches. Place 1 inch apart and bake 10–12 minutes.

Mix ingredients for glaze together (make a thick, smooth paste), and brush cookies while still hot (using a pastry brush). Decorate with more candied fruit if desired. Store cookies in airtight tins to age at least a week before eating.

Makes about 60 cookies.

PER cookie:
CALORIES 58   FIBER trace
CSI trace   SODIUM 11 mg
FAT <1 gm

OATMEAL COOKIES

These are cholesterol-free but not low in fat, so they should be eaten only occasionally.

- 1 cup shortening
- 1 cup brown sugar
- 1 cup granulated sugar
- 3 egg whites
- 1 teaspoon vanilla
- 1½ cups flour
- 1 teaspoon baking soda
- 3 cups oatmeal
- 1 cup raisins

Thoroughly cream shortening and sugars. Add egg whites and vanilla. Beat well. Sift together flour and soda; add to creamed mixture. Stir in oatmeal and raisins. Mix well. Form dough in rolls 1–1½ inches in diameter. Wrap in foil or plastic. Freeze thoroughly.

Preheat oven to 350°. With sharp knife, slice cookies about ¼ inch thick. Bake on ungreased baking sheet for 10 minutes or until lightly browned.

Makes about 90 cookies.

PER cookie:
CALORIES 62   FIBER trace
CSI <1   SODIUM 12 mg
FAT 3 gm

BARS

APRICOT MERINGUE BARS

A very dainty and sweet cookie.

2½ cups flour
½ teaspoon baking soda
½ cup margarine
2 egg whites
¼ cup sugar
½ teaspoon vanilla
1 cup apricot jam

Preheat oven to 375°. Sift flour and baking soda. Cream margarine, egg whites, sugar, and vanilla. Combine flour mixture and creamed mixture. Press out onto an un-oiled baking sheet, about ¼ inch thick. Spread the apricot jam evenly on the dough. Bake for 15 minutes or until very lightly browned. Remove bars from oven and turn oven down to 300°.

MERINGUE TOPPING

2 egg whites
2 tablespoons flour
½ cup sugar
½ cup finely chopped walnuts

Beat egg whites until stiff. Stir in the flour and sugar. Spread meringue topping over the slightly cooked jam and the bars and sprinkle with the walnuts. Return to the 300° oven and bake for 15 minutes.

Makes 42 bars (about 2 by 2 inches).

PER bar:
CALORIES 91   FIBER trace
CSI <1   SODIUM 42 mg
FAT 3 gm

BROWNIES

A true winner! See *Redheaded Shortcake* (page 435) for a fancier version!

⅔ cup sugar
⅓ cup water
3 tablespoons oil
½ teaspoon vanilla
3 egg whites, lightly beaten
½ cup flour
¼ cup cocoa powder
¾ teaspoon baking powder
1 teaspoon sifted powdered sugar (optional)

Preheat oven to 350°. Combine sugar, water, oil, and vanilla; stir well. Add egg whites and beat. Combine flour, cocoa, and baking powder. Add to sugar mixture, stirring well.

(continued)

Pour batter into a lightly oiled 8-inch-square baking pan. Bake for 20 minutes or until wooden pick inserted in center comes out clean. Sprinkle with powdered sugar, if desired. Cool and cut into squares.

Makes 9 servings (2½ by 2½ inches).

PER serving:
CALORIES 133   FIBER 1 gm
CSI 1   SODIUM 41 mg
FAT 5 gm

BUTTERSCOTCH BROWNIES

2 tablespoons oil
1 tablespoon molasses
⅔ cup sugar
½ cup egg substitute (commercial or Homemade Egg Substitute, page 283)
2 teaspoons vanilla
1 cup wheat germ
½ cup powdered nonfat milk
½ teaspoon baking powder
¼ cup chopped walnuts

Preheat oven to 350°. Combine first 5 ingredients and stir well. Mix dry ingredients together in a separate bowl. Add walnuts to dry ingredients.

Combine the wet and dry ingredients, stirring only enough to blend. Spread in an 8-by-8-inch pan that has been completely lined with wax paper. Bake for 30 minutes. Turn out of pan and remove wax paper immediately. Cut into bars while hot.

Makes 12 bars.

PER bar:
CALORIES 133   FIBER 2 gm
CSI <1   SODIUM 47 mg
FAT 5 gm

CHOCOLATE BANANA BARS

Children (of any age) love these.

¼ cup cocoa
1 tablespoon water
2 very ripe small bananas
1½ cups sugar
6 egg whites or 1 cup egg substitute (commercial or Homemade Egg Substitute, page 283)
1 teaspoon vanilla
1 cup oatmeal or oat bran
¼ cup flour
¼ teaspoon Lite Salt or less
¼ cup chopped walnuts

Preheat oven to 350°. Place the cocoa, water, and bananas in a blender or a large bowl and mix until liquified. Add the sugar, egg whites or egg substitute, and vanilla. Stir in the oatmeal or oat bran, flour, Lite Salt, and nuts. Pour into a 9-by-13-inch pan sprayed lightly with nonstick spray. Bake for 45 minutes. Cool and cut into squares.

Makes 24 servings (2¼ by 2 inches).

PER bar:
CALORIES 86   FIBER 1 gm
CSI trace   SODIUM 23 mg
FAT 1 gm

JAMOCHA SQUARES

⅓ cup margarine
3 tablespoons cocoa powder
½ cup brown sugar
½ teaspoon vanilla
1 cup flour
1 teaspoon baking powder
3 egg whites
1½ teaspoons instant coffee granules
¼ cup Kahlua *or* other coffee-flavored liqueur*

Preheat oven to 350°. Melt margarine in small saucepan. Remove from heat, add cocoa, and mix well. Stir in sugar and vanilla. Set aside.

Combine flour and baking powder and set aside. Add egg whites, one at a time to cocoa mixture, beating well after each addition. Dissolve coffee granules in liqueur; add to chocolate mixture. Mix well. Add flour and baking powder gradually.

Pour batter into a lightly oiled 8-inch-square baking pan. Bake for 15–20 minutes. Cool completely. Dust top of cake with powdered sugar if desired. Cut into squares.

Makes 16 squares.

*Small 1.5 ounce bottles can be purchased at liquor stores.

PER square:
CALORIES 103   FIBER 1 gm
CSI <1   SODIUM 81 mg
FAT 4 gm

MOLASSES ORANGE BARS

1 can (6 ounces) frozen orange juice concentrate, thawed
½ cup oatmeal
1 cup raisins
½ cup margarine
½ cup sugar
½ cup molasses
2 egg whites
2 cups flour
1½ teaspoons baking soda
1 teaspoon ground ginger
1 teaspoon cinnamon

Preheat oven to 325°. Combine orange juice, oatmeal and raisins and set aside. Cream margarine, sugar, and molasses until fluffy. Blend in egg whites. Mix together flour, baking soda, and spices and add to molasses mixture. Add raisin mixture and mix well. Pour into lightly oiled 9-by-13-inch baking pan. Bake 45 minutes. Cool, then cut into bars.

Makes 28 bars (about 2 by 2 inches).

PER bar:
CALORIES 123   FIBER <1 gm
CSI <1   SODIUM 90 mg
FAT 4 gm

NORTHWEST HARVEST BARS

A delicious low-fat bar.

¼ cup margarine
⅔ cup brown sugar
2 tablespoons hot water mixed with 1
  packet Butter Buds (optional)
4 egg whites
¾ cup flour
½ teaspoon baking powder
½ teaspoon Lite Salt or less
½ teaspoon cinnamon
½ teaspoon nutmeg
½ teaspoon ground ginger
¼ teaspoon baking soda
⅔ cup canned pumpkin
½ cup raisins
½ teaspoon vanilla

Preheat oven to 350°. Spray a 9-inch square baking pan with nonstick coating. In large saucepan, melt margarine over low heat. Remove from heat and stir in brown sugar, water, and Butter Buds, if used; beat in egg whites. Add dry ingredients and mix until well blended. Stir in pumpkin, raisins, and vanilla. Pour into prepared pan and bake 25–30 minutes. Cool and cut into bars.

Makes 16 bars (about 2¼ by 2¼ inches).

———————————————

PER bar:
CALORIES 102   FIBER <1 gm
CSI <1   SODIUM 109 mg
FAT 3 gm

PB&J BARS

Peanut butter and jam make for a fun dessert.

¾ cup brown sugar
¼ cup margarine
½ cup creamy peanut butter
¼ cup egg substitute (commercial or
  Homemade Egg Substitute, page 283)
  or 2 egg whites
1½ cups flour
1 cup uncooked oatmeal
½ teaspoon baking powder
½ teaspoon baking soda
¾ cup jam or preserves (berry works
  well)

Heat oven to 375°. Beat together brown sugar and margarine until light and fluffy. Blend in peanut butter and egg substitute or whites. Stir in flour, oatmeal, baking powder, and baking soda. Mix well. Set aside 1 cup of cookie dough and press remaining mixture evenly into bottom of ungreased 13-by-9-inch baking pan. Bake 8 to 10 minutes; cool.

Spread jam or preserves over partially baked crust. Crumble and sprinkle remaining cup of dough over jam. Return to oven and continue baking 20 minutes or until golden brown. Cool and cut into bars with sharp knife.

Makes 32 bars (1½ by 2¼ inches).

———————————————

PER bar:
CALORIES 106   FIBER 1 gm
CSI <1   SODIUM 62 mg
FAT 4 gm

WALNUT SQUARES

Sweet and nutty, these bars make good tea cookies.

- 1 cup finely ground whole wheat bread crumbs
- ¾ cup brown sugar
- 4 egg whites
- ½ teaspoon cream of tartar
- 1 teaspoon vanilla
- ½ cup chopped walnuts

Preheat oven to 350°. Mix together bread crumbs and sugar. In a separate bowl, beat egg whites with cream of tartar until stiff.

Gently fold the vanilla, crumb mixture, and walnuts (in order listed) into the egg whites. Bake in an unoiled 8-by-8-inch square pan for 20 minutes, then reduce heat to 300° and bake an additional 10 minutes. Cut into small squares.

Makes about 30 squares (1½ inches each).

PER square:
CALORIES 40   FIBER trace
CSI trace   SODIUM 21 mg
FAT 1 gm

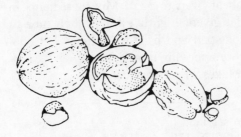

CAKES

Good

ALL-SEASON SHORTCAKE

Serve this easy shortcake all year long with berries, nectarines, or peaches and vanilla yogurt.

- 3 egg whites
- ¾ cup sugar
- 1 teaspoon grated orange peel
- ½ teaspoon vanilla
- ½ cup skim milk
- 1 tablespoon margarine
- 1 cup flour
- 1 teaspoon baking powder
- ¼ teaspoon Lite Salt or less
- ¼ teaspoon ground nutmeg

- 6 cups fresh fruit, sliced as for short-cake
- ½ cup sugar
- 3 cups low-fat vanilla yogurt *or* Dream Whip prepared with skim milk

Cut a piece of waxed paper to fit the bottom of a 9-inch square baking pan. Lightly oil pan sides and paper.

Preheat oven to 350°. With a mixer, beat together the egg whites, sugar, orange peel, and vanilla until very light and fluffy. In a small saucepan, heat the milk and margarine until hot, then stir into the egg mix-

(continued)

ture. In a bowl, stir together the flour, baking powder, Lite Salt, and nutmeg. Add to the batter and stir to blend well. Pour batter into prepared pan.

Bake cake for 15 minutes, until center springs back when touched. Cook in pan for 5 minutes, then run a knife around sides to loosen. Turn out onto rack, peel off paper, and cool completely.

When ready to serve, slice shortcake in half horizontally and place ½ on serving platter. Layer with 1½ cups yogurt or Dream Whip and 3 cups prepared fruit. Top with remaining cake half, 1½ cups yogurt or Dream Whip, and 3 cups fresh fruit. Cut in squares to serve.

Makes 9 servings.

PER serving:
CALORIES 292   FIBER 2 gm
CSI 1   SODIUM 141 mg
FAT 3 gm

ANGEL QUICKIE

Tastes and looks wonderful! No need for a frosting. Leftover slices are very good toasted under the broiler and topped with fruit.

1 package angel food cake mix
⅓ cup cocoa
2 teaspoons powdered instant coffee (instant espresso is delicious)

Preheat oven to 350°. Follow directions on angel food mix package, stirring cocoa and coffee powder into dry mix. Beat 1½ minutes, scraping bowl often. Bake 40–50 minutes in *unoiled* tube pan. Invert and cool thoroughly.

Makes 10 servings.

PER serving:
CALORIES 186   FIBER 2 gm
CSI <1   SODIUM 205 mg
FAT 1 gm

APPLE LOAF CAKE

½ cup apple juice *or* water
½ cup oil
2 cups sugar
3 egg whites *or* ½ cup egg substitute (commercial *or* *Homemade Egg Substitute,* page 283)
1 teaspoon vanilla
3 cups chopped unpeeled apples
¼ cup chopped nuts
2 cups white flour
1 cup whole wheat flour
¾ teaspoon nutmeg
¾ teaspoon cinnamon
1½ teaspoons baking soda

Preheat oven to 325°. Mix ingredients in order given. Lightly oil a 10-inch tube or Bundt pan and bake for 1 hour. Let cool before removing from pan.

Makes 24 servings.

PER serving:
CALORIES 179   FIBER 1 gm
CSI <1   SODIUM 53 mg
FAT 6 gm

BABA AU RHUM (SAVARIN)

A rum-flavored yeast cake with red berry sauce served over it.

- 2 packages yeast
- 1 cup skim milk, lukewarm
- 4 cups white flour
- 6 egg whites
- 2 teaspoons sugar
- ½ teaspoon Lite Salt or less
- 5 tablespoons melted margarine

Dissolve yeast in lukewarm milk. In a large bowl, mix flour, egg whites, and dissolved yeast. The dough should be smooth. Cover and let rise in a warm place for at least 1 hour and until the dough has doubled in volume.

Add sugar, Lite Salt, and melted margarine to the dough. Mix well. It will be a soft, sticky dough this time. Oil a 12-cup mold (a ring mold works well) or a Bundt cake pan. Put the dough in the pan to fill about halfway to the top. Let rise again, in the mold, from 1–2 hours.

Bake in a 375° oven. If the top becomes too brown, cover for a while with foil. Bake 30 minutes or until "baba" pulls away from sides of pan.

Unmold while still warm. After cooling, put back in the mold to soak up the *Rum Syrup.*

RUM SYRUP

- 2 cups sugar
- 2 cups water
- 1 cup rum

Dissolve sugar in water. Bring to a boil and simmer for about 5 minutes, then add rum. Pour over the cooked and cooled baba, a tablespoon at a time, until all syrup is absorbed.

Unmold and serve with *Strawberry or Raspberry Sauce* (page 455) or any sauce of your choice to spoon over the top of each serving.

Makes 24 servings.

PER serving:
CALORIES 190   FIBER <1 gm
CSI <1   SODIUM 67 mg
FAT 3 gm

BAKED DOUGHNUT HOLES

Everyone loves these lower-fat little cakes. The fresher they are the better!

- 2 tablespoons oil
- ½ cup sugar
- 2 egg whites *or* ¼ cup egg substitute (commercial *or Homemade Egg Substitute,* page 283)
- 1 teaspoon vanilla
- ⅔ cup skim milk
- 2 cups white flour
- 1 tablespoon baking powder
- ½ teaspoon nutmeg

TOPPING

- 1½ tablespoons margarine
- ½ cup sugar
- 2 teaspoons cinnamon

(continued)

Preheat oven to 400°. Cream oil, ½ cup sugar, and egg whites *or* egg substitute. Add vanilla and skim milk; stir well. Sift dry ingredients and add gradually to the creamed mixture. Lightly oil *small* muffin tins and fill ⅔ full with batter. Bake 15–18 minutes.

While doughnuts are baking, prepare topping. Melt margarine and place in a small bowl. Mix sugar and cinnamon together in another small bowl. Brush warm doughnuts lightly with the melted margarine and then roll in the cinnamon-sugar mixture.

Makes 36 doughnuts.

PER doughnut hole:

CALORIES 59	FIBER trace
CSI trace	SODIUM 39 mg
FAT 1 gm	

CARROT RAISIN CAKE WITH PENUCHE FROSTING

A rich spice cake with a wonderful frosting! Surprisingly easy to make.

1½ cups sugar
2⅔ cups water
1 cup raisins
4 cups grated carrots (about 4 medium)
2 tablespoons margarine
1 teaspoon cinnamon
½ teaspoon cloves
½ teaspoon nutmeg
4 cups flour
2 teaspoons baking powder
2 teaspoons baking soda
½ cup chopped walnuts

Combine sugar, water, raisins, grated carrots, margarine, cinnamon, cloves, and nutmeg in a saucepan and cook for 10 minutes. Cool to room temperature.

Preheat oven to 325°. Combine flour, baking powder, and baking soda in separate bowl. Add dry ingredients to carrot/raisin mixture. Fold in chopped walnuts. Bake in lightly oiled 9-by-13-inch pan for 45 minutes or until wooden pick inserted in center comes out clean. Cool in pan and frost.

PENUCHE FROSTING

½ cup brown sugar
¼ cup skim milk
2 tablespoons margarine
1½ cups sifted powdered sugar (sifted before measuring)
1 teaspoon vanilla

Combine brown sugar, milk, and margarine in saucepan and cook for 3 minutes. Cool for about 10 minutes and add sifted powdered sugar and vanilla. Beat until smooth and spread over cooled cake.

Makes 20 servings (about 2¼ by 2½ inches).

PER serving:

CALORIES 271	FIBER 2 gm
CSI <1	SODIUM 156 mg
FAT 4 gm	

Eye.

CHOCOLATE ZUCCHINI CAKE

A very nice cake that does not need to be frosted.

    1 teaspoon vanilla
    ½ cup oil
    1½ cups sugar
    4 egg whites
    ½ cup skim milk
    1 teaspoon baking soda
    1¼ cups white flour
    1¼ cups whole wheat flour
    ¼ cup cocoa powder
    ½ teaspoon cinnamon
    ½ teaspoon nutmeg
    ¼ teaspoon Lite Salt or less
    2 cups grated zucchini

Preheat oven to 350°. Combine vanilla, oil, sugar, egg whites, and skim milk. Sift together baking soda, flours, cocoa, cinnamon, nutmeg, and Lite Salt. Add dry ingredients alternately with zucchini to the first mixture.

Bake for 60–65 minutes in a lightly oiled Bundt pan, or about 45 minutes in a 9-by-13-inch pan.

Makes 24 servings (about 2 by 2 inches).

PER serving:
CALORIES 142   FIBER 2 gm
CSI <1   SODIUM 54 mg
FAT 5 gm

COCOA CAKE

This is very versatile—can be made into cupcakes or into a cake. Serve unfrosted or top it with berries.

    1½ cups flour
    1 cup sugar
    1 teaspoon baking soda
    3 tablespoons cocoa powder
    3 tablespoons oil
    1 teaspoon vanilla
    1 tablespoon vinegar
    1 cup cold water

Preheat oven to 350°. Sift dry ingredients together. Pour the liquid ingredients over the dry ingredients and stir until smooth. If making cupcakes, turn into 12 paper-lined muffin tins, and bake for 25–30 minutes. For a cake, bake in ungreased 9-inch square pan for 35 minutes. Cool.

Makes 9 servings of cake or 12 cupcakes.

PER ⅑ recipe:
CALORIES 205   FIBER 1 gm
CSI 1   SODIUM 92 mg
FAT 5 gm

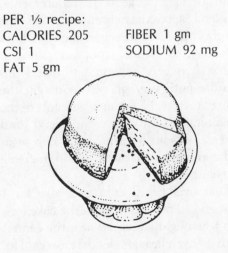

CRÈME DE MENTHE CHEESECAKE

A beautiful treat!

1 cup chocolate cookie crumbs (use Nabisco's "Famous Wafers"); reserve 2 tablespoons for topping
1 teaspoon sugar
2 tablespoons melted margarine
2½ cups part-skim ricotta cheese
⅔ cup plain nonfat yogurt
4 egg whites
¾ cup sugar
1 tablespoon cornstarch
⅓ cup crème de menthe

Preheat oven to 350°. To prepare crumbs, grind cookies in a blender (save 2 tablespoons for topping). Combine remaining chocolate crumbs, 1 teaspoon sugar, and melted margarine in a small mixing bowl. Press firmly into the bottom of a 10-inch springform pan. Bake for 10 minutes; cool.

Blend approximately a third of the ricotta cheese, all the yogurt and egg whites in a covered blender until very smooth. (Note: It is very important to blend this mixture until very smooth to obtain the desired texture.) Add small amounts of the remaining ricotta cheese and blend until smooth. Gradually blend in ¾ cup sugar and cornstarch. Beat well. Blend in crème de menthe.

Pour over baked crust and bake for 1 hour and 10 minutes or until the cake feels firm when lightly touched near the center. Turn off oven heat and let the cake cool for 2 hours in the oven with the door ajar. (Note: The cake will fall to approximately half its height.) Chill. Release sides of pan. Sprinkle 2 tablespoons remaining chocolate crumbs over top.
Makes 12 servings.

PER serving:
CALORIES 210   FIBER 0 gm
CSI 5   SODIUM 156 mg
FAT 8 gm

DEPRESSION CAKE

From the days when sugar and eggs were scarce—now, it means healthful food.

1 cup raisins
2 cups water
2 tablespoons oil
1 cup brown sugar
1 cup white flour
1 cup whole wheat flour
1½ teaspoons baking soda
1 teaspoon cinnamon
1 teaspoon nutmeg

Preheat oven to 325°. Cook raisins in water. Simmer until 1 cup liquid remains. Set aside to cool. Cream sugar and oil. Add raisins and liquid. Beat with a spoon. Add flours, baking soda, spices and beat well. Bake in a lightly oiled 9-inch-square pan for 30–40 minutes.
Makes 9 servings (3 by 3 inches).

PER serving:
CALORIES 263   FIBER 3 gm
CSI <1   SODIUM 135 mg
FAT 4 gm

HOT FUDGE PUDDING CAKE

A delicious treat!

- 1 cup flour
- 2 teaspoons baking powder
- ¾ cup sugar
- 2 tablespoons cocoa powder
- ½ cup skim milk
- 1 tablespoon oil
- ¼ cup chopped walnuts

TOPPING

- ¼ cup cocoa powder
- 1 cup brown sugar
- 1¾ cups *hot* water

Preheat oven to 350°. Sift together first 4 ingredients. Stir in skim milk and oil and then walnuts. Spread in a 9-inch-square unoiled pan. Prepare topping. Combine cocoa and brown sugar and sprinkle over batter. Pour the hot water over entire batter and topping. Bake for 45 minutes. During baking the cake mixture rises to the top and the chocolate sauce settles to the bottom. Invert square of pudding on dessert plates. Dip sauce from pan over each. Or, the entire pudding can be inverted in a deep serving platter.

Makes 9 servings (about 3 by 3 inches).

PER serving:
CALORIES 259　　FIBER 2 gm
CSI 1　　　　　　SODIUM 93 mg
FAT 5 gm

PARTY CARROT CAKE

Exc.

- 2 cups sugar
- ½ cup oil
- 1½ cups whole wheat flour
- 1½ cups white flour
- 2½ teaspoons baking soda
- 2½ teaspoons cinnamon
- ½ teaspoon Lite Salt or less
- 2 cups shredded carrots
- 2 teaspoons vanilla
- 1 can (11 ounces) mandarin oranges, undrained
- 5 egg whites

Preheat oven to 350°. In large bowl, combine all cake ingredients. Beat 2 minutes at high speed. Pour into lightly oiled 9-by-13-inch pan. Bake 50–60 minutes or until wooden pick inserted in center comes out clean and cake pulls away from sides of pan. Cool. Cake can be removed from pan after 30 minutes.

"CREAM" CHEESE FROSTING

Make half the frosting recipe if sides of cake are not to be frosted.

- ½ package (4 ounces) light cream cheese or Neufchâtel, softened
- 1 teaspoon vanilla
- 2 cups powdered sugar

Blend ingredients in medium bowl; beat until smooth. Adjust powdered sugar as desired for proper firmness. Spread over cake. Store frosted cake in refrigerator.

Makes 24 servings (about 2 by 2 inches).

(continued)

PER serving:
CALORIES 224   FIBER 1 gm
CSI 2   SODIUM 130 mg
FAT 6 gm

PINTO FIESTA CAKE

An unusual use of legumes, to say the least!

1 cup sugar
¼ cup margarine
2 egg whites, lightly beaten
2 cups cooked pinto beans, mashed, *or*
  refried beans*
1 cup flour
1 teaspoon baking soda
1 teaspoon cinnamon
½ teaspoon ground cloves
½ teaspoon allspice
2 cups diced raw apples
1 cup raisins
¼ cup chopped walnuts
2 teaspoons vanilla

Preheat oven to 375°. Cream sugar and margarine, add beaten egg whites. Add mashed beans. Mix well. Sift all dry ingredients (including spices) together and add to sugar mixture. Add apples, raisins, chopped walnuts, and vanilla. Pour into lightly oiled 10-inch tube or Bundt cake pan and bake for 45 minutes.

Makes 16 servings.

*Use low-sodium beans if available.

PER serving:
CALORIES 182   FIBER 4 gm
CSI <1   SODIUM 101 mg
FAT 5 gm

POPPYSEED CAKE

2 ounces poppyseeds (½ cup)
1 cup skim milk
½ cup egg substitute (commercial *or*
  Homemade Egg Substitute, page 283)
  or 3 egg whites
⅓ cup oil
1 cup sugar
1 teaspoon almond extract
Grated rind of 1 lemon
2 cups whole wheat flour
¼ cup powdered nonfat milk
½ teaspoon cinnamon
¼ teaspoon nutmeg
2½ teaspoons baking powder

Soak poppyseeds in skim milk for 1 hour. Preheat oven to 350°. Add egg whites, oil, sugar, almond extract, and lemon rind to poppyseeds. Mix well, and combine with remaining ingredients, stirring only to just moisten the batter. Pour in lightly oiled 9-by-5-inch loaf pan. Bake 45–60 minutes. Prepare glaze and spread over warm cake.

GLAZE

2 tablespoons powdered sugar (approximate)
½ teaspoon vanilla, rum *or* brandy extract, *or* freshly squeezed lemon juice
1 tablespoon cornstarch
1–2 tablespoons hot water (depends on desired thickness)

Blend ingredients and cook until glaze is clear.

Makes 16 servings (½ inch each).

PER serving:
CALORIES 180   FIBER 2 gm
CSI 1   SODIUM 88 mg
FAT 7 gm

REDHEADED SHORTCAKE

A colorful and fun dessert.

1 recipe *Brownies* (page 423)
4½ cups fresh berries (sliced strawberries *or* raspberries work very well)
3 cups low-fat vanilla yogurt

Prepare *Brownies*, cool, and cut into 9 squares. Arrange on serving plates. Cover each with ½ cup berries and ⅓ cup vanilla yogurt. Serve immediately.

Makes 9 servings.

PER serving:
CALORIES 241   FIBER 3 gm
CSI 2   SODIUM 89 mg
FAT 7 gm

RICOTTA CHEESECAKE

Made with ricotta cheese and egg whites, this cheesecake tastes light and delicious.

1 cup graham cracker crumbs
2 tablespoons sugar
¼ teaspoon cinnamon
2 tablespoons melted margarine
2½ cups part-skim ricotta cheese

1 cup plain nonfat yogurt
4 egg whites
1 cup sugar
1 tablespoon cornstarch
1 teaspoon vanilla
3 tablespoons freshly squeezed lemon juice
Yogurt Dessert Sauce (page 456), optional for topping

Preheat oven to 350°. In a small bowl combine the cracker crumbs, sugar, cinnamon, and margarine. Press firmly into the bottom of a 10-inch springform pan. Bake for 10 minutes. Cool.

Blend approximately a third of the ricotta cheese and all the yogurt and egg whites in a covered blender until very smooth. (*Note:* It is very important to blend this mixture until very smooth to obtain the desired texture.) Add small amounts of the remaining ricotta cheese and blend until smooth. Gradually blend in sugar and cornstarch. Beat well. Blend in vanilla and lemon juice.

Pour over crust in prepared pan and bake for 1 hour and 10 minutes or until the cake feels firm when lightly touched near the center. Turn off oven heat and let the cake cool for 2 hours in the oven with the door ajar. (*Note:* The cake will fall to approximately half its height.) Chill. Release sides of pan and place on serving dish.

If a topping is desired, *Yogurt Dessert Sauce* or a fruit sauce works well.

Makes 12 servings.

PER serving:
CALORIES 211   FIBER trace
CSI 4   SODIUM 179 mg
FAT 7 gm

PIES AND COBBLERS

APPLE STRUDEL

2 tart apples, peeled and cut into small
  pieces (2 cups)
⅓ cup raisins
2 tablespoons chopped walnuts
¼ cup sugar
½ teaspoon cinnamon
3 sheets phyllo*
1 teaspoon melted margarine
1 tablespoon dry bread crumbs

Heat oven to 375°. Lightly spray cookie
sheet with nonstick spray. In bowl combine apples, raisins, walnuts, sugar and cinnamon.

Place 1 phyllo sheet on large piece of
plastic wrap. Brush lightly with melted
margarine and crumbs. Repeat layering 2
more times. Spread ⅓ apple mixture evenly
along shorter side of phyllo. Using plastic
wrap, lift phyllo and carefully roll it around
mixture, jelly-roll fashion. Do not seal
ends. Place roll seam side down on pre-

*Phyllo (or filo) can be found in the freezer section of most
supermarkets. Thaw the unwrapped frozen dough in the
refrigerator for 3–4 hours and work with it while it is cold.
The remainder of the pastry keeps well in refrigerator if
wrapped tightly.

pared cookie sheet; discard plastic wrap.
Brush top lightly with remaining melted
margarine. Bake for 35 minutes or until
golden brown.

Makes 6 to 8 servings.

PER ⅙ recipe:
CALORIES 133   FIBER 2 gm
CSI trace   SODIUM 57 mg
FAT 2 gm

BERRY COBBLER

FILLING

4 cups blueberries, or another favorite
  variety
¼ cup firmly packed brown sugar
1 tablespoon cornstarch (for juicier
  berries, use 3 tablespoons)
1 teaspoon freshly squeezed lemon juice
½ teaspoon cinnamon

TOPPING

¼ cup uncooked oatmeal
1 cup flour
1 tablespoon sugar
2 teaspoons baking powder
2 tablespoons margarine
½ cup skim milk
2 egg whites

Heat oven to 350°. Combine berries,
brown sugar, cornstarch, lemon juice, and
cinnamon. Place in bottom of 9-by-9-inch
square baking dish. Place in oven and bake
15 minutes until hot and bubbling.

While berries are baking, combine topping ingredients. Mix oatmeal, flour, sugar, and baking powder. Add margarine and cut into mixture with a fork until it looks like coarse bread crumbs. Add milk and egg whites, stirring only until moistened.

Drop 6 spoonfuls of dough onto hot berries and return to oven. Continue baking 25 minutes or until topping is golden brown.

Makes 6 servings.

PER serving:
CALORIES 233   FIBER 4 gm
CSI <1   SODIUM 184 mg
FAT 5 gm

While blender is running, dissolve gelatin by first sprinkling over 1 tablespoon cold water, then stirring in 3 tablespoons boiling water. Add dissolved gelatin to blender and blend well. Add 1 cup sliced strawberries or raspberries and blend. Pour into bowl containing remaining 2 cups berries and stir carefully. Chill until slightly set (1 hour); spoon into cooled pie shell. Cover and chill for several hours or until set.

Makes 8 servings.

PER serving:
CALORIES 196   FIBER 2 gm
CSI 1   SODIUM 237 mg
FAT 4 gm

BERRY YOGURT PIE

When strawberries or raspberries are at their peak, think of making this pie!

One 9-inch _Graham Cracker Crust_ (page 439)

¾ cup plain nonfat yogurt
¾ cup low-fat cottage cheese
6 tablespoons sugar
1 teaspoon vanilla
¼ cup water
1 envelope unflavored gelatin
3 cups sliced fresh strawberries _or_ whole raspberries

Earlier in the day, prepare _Graham Cracker Crust_. Bake 10 minutes and cool.

To prepare filling, combine yogurt, cottage cheese, sugar, and vanilla in blender.

CHERRY STRUDEL

Much lower in fat than cherry pie and equally delicious!

1 can (16 ounces) pie cherries, well-drained
⅓ cup sugar
½ cup dry bread crumbs
1 teaspoon almond extract _or_ 1 tablespoon sherry or kirsch
3 sheets phyllo*
2 teaspoons melted margarine
1 tablespoon dry bread crumbs

*Phyllo (or filo) can be found in the freezer section of most supermarkets. Thaw the unwrapped frozen dough in the refrigerator for 3–4 hours and work with it while it is cold. The remainder of the pastry keeps well in refrigerator if wrapped tightly.

(continued)

Heat oven to 375°. In medium bowl combine cherries, sugar, ½ cup bread crumbs, and almond extract or liqueur.

Place 1 sheet of phyllo on large piece of plastic wrap (this helps with moving it later). Brush phyllo lightly with melted margarine and sprinkle with crumbs. (Use 1 tablespoon crumbs for all 3 sheets phyllo.) Place another sheet of phyllo on top and continue layering with margarine and crumbs 2 more times.

Spread cherry mixture evenly along shorter side of phyllo (cover about ⅙ of the dough). Using plastic wrap, lift phyllo and carefully roll it around cherry mixture, jelly-roll fashion. Do not seal ends. Place finished roll seam side down on cookie sheet; discard plastic wrap. Brush top lightly with remaining melted margarine. Bake 20 minutes or until golden brown. Serve while warm.

Makes 6 servings.

PER serving:
CALORIES 148   FIBER 1 gm
CSI trace   SODIUM 124 mg
FAT 2 gm

CRANBERRY SQUARES

1½ cups cranberries (6 ounces)
½ cup raisins
½ cup peeled, chopped apple
½ cup unsweetened apple juice
2 teaspoons sugar
¾ cup whole wheat flour
½ cup uncooked oatmeal

2 tablespoons brown sugar
½ teaspoon cinnamon
¼ cup light molasses
2 tablespoons oil
2 tablespoons sliced almonds

Nonfat vanilla yogurt or frozen yogurt

Combine cranberries, raisins, chopped apple, apple juice, and sugar in saucepan. Bring to a boil and cook 5 minutes or until cranberries begin to pop, stirring occasionally. Reduce heat and simmer, uncovered 10 minutes; stir occasionally. Cool completely.

Preheat oven to 350°. Combine flour, oatmeal, brown sugar, cinnamon, molasses, and oil in a bowl. Toss with a fork until mixture resembles coarse meal.

Lightly spray 8-by-8-inch baking pan with nonstick spray. Press 1 cup of the flour mixture into bottom of pan. Top with cooled cranberry mixture and spread evenly. Sprinkle remaining flour mixture over cranberry layer and press lightly. Add nuts as last layer. Bake for 35 minutes or until golden.

Cut into squares and serve warm topped with vanilla yogurt or frozen yogurt. If you wish to serve as a bar-type cookie, cool completely before cutting into squares. Cover loosely to store.

Makes 12 servings.

PER serving:
CALORIES 125   FIBER 2 gm
CSI trace   SODIUM 6 mg
FAT 3 gm

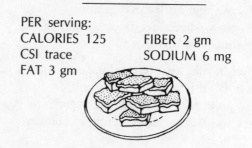

GRAHAM CRACKER CRUST

1½ cups graham cracker crumbs
2 tablespoons honey
1 tablespoon oil

Preheat oven to 350°. Blend graham cracker crumbs, honey, and oil and mix well. Pat into 9-inch pie pan. Bake for 10 minutes. Allow shell to cool before filling.

Makes one 9-inch crust.

PER ⅙ of 9-inch crust:
CALORIES 142   FIBER <1 gm
CSI 1   SODIUM 176 mg
FAT 5 gm

PEACH ALMOND CRISP

Streusel topping with almonds makes a tasty dessert that is a much lower-fat choice than pie.

3 cans (16 ounces each) sliced peaches, drained (use juice packed)
½ cup oatmeal
¼ cup brown sugar
¼ cup flour
½ teaspoon cinnamon
¼ teaspoon ginger
2 tablespoons melted margarine
1 tablespoon sliced almonds
Frozen nonfat yogurt (optional)

Heat oven to 375°. Spoon drained peaches evenly into 8-inch baking dish. Combine oatmeal, sugar, flour, and spices. Add margarine and mix with a fork until crumbly. Sprinkle topping evenly over peaches. Bake 15–20 minutes or until golden brown. Serve warm and topped with frozen yogurt, if desired.

Makes 6 servings.

PER serving:
CALORIES 158   FIBER 2 gm
CSI <1   SODIUM 54 mg
FAT 5 gm

PUMPKIN PIE

A harvest special!

1 9-inch *Graham Cracker Crust* (see above)

2 cups canned or cooked pumpkin
1½ cups evaporated skim milk
¼ cup brown sugar
½ cup white sugar
1 teaspoon cinnamon
½ teaspoon ground ginger
¼ teaspoon nutmeg *or* allspice
⅛ teaspoon ground cloves
3 egg whites

Yogurt Dessert Sauce (page 456)

Earlier in the day, prepare *Graham Cracker Crust.* Bake 10 minutes and cool.

To prepare filling, preheat oven to 350° and mix all the ingredients until well blended. Pour mixture into cooled pie

(continued)

shell. Bake 1 hour or until an inserted knife comes out clean.

Serve with *Yogurt Dessert Sauce.*

Makes 6 servings.

___

PER serving:
CALORIES 327   FIBER 3 gm
CSI 1   SODIUM 275 mg
FAT 5 gm

SWEDISH PIE

This simple apple dessert can be easily assembled, baked during dinner, and enjoyed warm.

- ¾ cup sugar
- ½ cup flour
- ¼ cup egg substitute (commercial *or* *Homemade Egg Substitute,* page 283)
- 1 teaspoon baking powder
- 1 teaspoon vanilla
- ¾ cup peeled, chopped apples (1 large)
- ¼ cup chopped walnuts

Preheat oven to 350°. Beat together the first five ingredients. Fold in chopped ap-

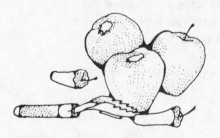

ples and nuts. Pour into 9-inch pie plate that has been sprayed with nonstick spray. Bake 20–30 minutes or until it resembles a light brown crust. Cut into 2-inch wedges. Serve while warm, topped with frozen non-fat vanilla yogurt.

Makes 8 servings.

___

PER serving:
CALORIES 130   FIBER <1 gm
CSI trace   SODIUM 52 mg
FAT 2 gm

UPSIDE-DOWN PEACH COBBLER

This dessert is delicious when made with any kind of fruit.

- 2 tablespoons melted margarine
- ½ cup sugar
- 1 cup flour
- 2 teaspoons baking powder
- ¾ cup skim milk
- 4 cups sliced peaches (fresh *or* canned and drained)
- ¼ teaspoon cinnamon
- ¼ teaspoon nutmeg

Preheat oven to 375°. Place margarine in 8-by-8-inch pan and put in oven to melt (2 minutes or so). Mix together sugar, flour, baking powder, and skim milk and spoon over melted margarine. Do not mix. Place sliced peaches on top of batter and sprinkle cinnamon and nutmeg over the top. Bake for 30 minutes. Serve warm with low-fat vanilla yogurt, if desired.

Makes 6 servings.

PER serving:
CALORIES 226   FIBER 2 gm
CSI <1   SODIUM 164 mg
FAT 4 gm

PUDDINGS

CHOCOLATE PUDDING

3 tablespoons cornstarch
1½ tablespoons cocoa powder
2 cups skim milk
½ cup sugar
1 teaspoon vanilla

Combine cornstarch and cocoa. Add milk slowly and stir until blended. Cook over medium heat, stirring continuously, until smooth and thick.

Remove from heat and stir in sugar and vanilla. Be sure the sugar is completely dissolved in the hot pudding. Pour into dessert dishes and chill.

Makes 6 servings (about 3 cups).

PER ½ cup:
CALORIES 115   FIBER <1 gm
CSI trace   SODIUM 43 mg
FAT <1 gm

PUMPKIN BREAD PUDDING

For bread pudding lovers! Serve warm or cold with *Yogurt Dessert Sauce* (page 456).

8 slices whole wheat bread
1 cup egg substitute (commercial *or Homemade Egg Substitute*, page 283)
2¼ cups skim milk
1 can (16 ounces) pumpkin
1 cup brown sugar
1½ teaspoons cinnamon
1½ teaspoons pumpkin pie spice
½ teaspoon nutmeg
1 teaspoon vanilla
¾ cup raisins

Preheat oven to 375°. Crumble bread by hand or in a blender or food processor to make bread crumbs. Combine egg substitute, skim milk, pumpkin, brown sugar, cinnamon, spices, and vanilla; add raisins and combine with bread crumbs in a lightly oiled 2-quart casserole dish.

Set 2-quart casserole dish in larger baking dish filled partially with hot water. Bake 1 hour or until knife inserted in center comes out clean.

Makes 12 servings (about 6 cups).

PER ½ cup:
CALORIES 184   FIBER 3 gm
CSI trace   SODIUM 164 mg
FAT <1 gm

FROZEN DESSERTS

CRANBERRY SHERBET

Surprise everyone with a delicious home-made sherbet. This one does not require an ice cream freezer.

4 cups fresh cranberries
1¾ cups water
1 cup sugar
1 cup water
2 teaspoons unflavored gelatin
¼ cup cold water
2 egg whites, stiffly beaten

Simmer cranberries in 1¾ cups water until soft. Cool slightly and put in electric blender and mix. Return to saucepan.

Add sugar and 1 cup water and boil, covered 5 minutes, without stirring. Soak gelatin in ¼ cup water. Dissolve gelatin in the hot juice. Chill. Fold beaten egg whites into cooled fruit mixture.

Put mixture in a covered shallow container and freeze. After about 4 hours, or when fairly frozen, blend mixture until smooth. Return to freezer. If you prefer a smoother texture (smaller ice crystals), blend mixture 2 or 3 times while sherbet is freezing.

Makes 6 cups.

OTHER SERVING SUGGESTIONS
Sherbets are particularly delectable when served in fruit shells. Fancy cut and hollow out lemons, oranges, or tangerines. Fill with sherbet. Refreeze. Garnish with leaves.

For an even fancier touch, put a dollop of meringue (egg whites stiffly beaten) on top. Pop in a 500° oven for a few seconds just before serving.

PER cup:
CALORIES 162   FIBER 3 gm
CSI 0   SODIUM 19 mg
FAT trace

NEW AND IMPROVED BAKED ALASKA

This really is a quickie and will delight your guests! Combine cake and frozen desserts ahead and freeze. At dessert time, spread with meringue and pop in a hot oven for a couple of minutes.

1 small (6½-inch diameter) angel food cake
1 cup chocolate nonfat frozen yogurt
1 cup strawberry sorbet

MERINGUE

5 egg whites, room temperature
½ teaspoon cream of tartar
1 teaspoon vanilla
2 tablespoons sugar

Slice angel food cake into three layers. Place 1 layer on a plate or tray. Spread slightly softened chocolate frozen yogurt on cake, cover with second layer of cake. Put in freezer. Spread slightly softened sorbet on top layer of cake. Remove cake from freezer and invert top layer on it. Cover with plastic and put in freezer for several hours or overnight.

Just before serving preheat oven to 475°. Beat egg whites until foamy. Add cream of tartar and vanilla. Beat until soft peaks form. Gradually add sugar, beating until stiff. Remove cake from freezer, place on ovenproof serving dish, and quickly spread meringue over entire surface, making sure edges are sealed with meringue to serving dish. Bake for 2–3 minutes or until meringue peaks are lightly browned. Slice and serve immediately.

Makes 8 to 10 servings.

PER ¹⁄₁₀ recipe:

CALORIES 156	FIBER trace
CSI trace	SODIUM 162 mg
FAT trace	

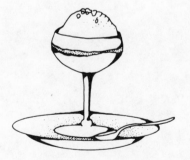

PUMPKIN FROZEN YOGURT

"You won't believe it's low-fat!" A very creamy, rich flavor. For a fancier dessert, spoon one-half of the yogurt mixture into *Graham Cracker Crust* (page 439), cover, and store in freezer. Remove from freezer 20 minutes before serving.

½ cup egg substitute (commercial or use *Homemade Egg Substitute,* page 283)
¾ cup sugar
¾ cup brown sugar
½ teaspoon cinnamon
¼ teaspoon allspice
⅛ teaspoon ginger
Dash ground cloves
1 quart plain nonfat yogurt
1 cup pumpkin
1 teaspoon vanilla

Beat egg substitute and all sugars together until sugars are dissolved. Add remaining ingredients and mix well. Pour into shallow container or ice cream freezer to freeze.

Makes 9 cups frozen.

VARIATION

For a less "yogurty-tasting" dessert, use 1 quart softened nonfat vanilla frozen yogurt and omit the white sugar.

PER cup:

CALORIES 208	FIBER <1 gm
CSI trace	SODIUM 116 mg
FAT trace	

STRAWBERRY ICE (SORBET)

¾ cup sugar
1 cup hot water
2 tablespoons freshly squeezed lemon juice
1 tablespoon orange juice
1 pint strawberries, hulled

Dissolve sugar in hot water and cool. Add juices. Put strawberries and sugar syrup into the blender and whirl until it is smooth. Place in a freezer-proof dish, and freeze until firm-ish, then whirl in blender again. Freeze until hard.

Makes 3 cups.

PER 1 cup:
CALORIES 240   FIBER 2 gm
CSI 0   SODIUM 4 mg
FAT <1 gm

BEVERAGES

Our favorite beverage is water, of course.
We did want to include a few ideas for
special occasions.

_____

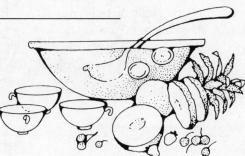

Eggnog
Orange Frosty
Orange Iced Tea
Quick Hot Spiced Cider
Strawberry Banana Smoothie

EGGNOG

½ cup egg substitute (commercial *or Homemade Egg Substitute,* page 283)
2–4 tablespoons sugar
1 can (13 ounces) evaporated skim milk
¾ cup skim milk
1 teaspoon vanilla
1 teaspoon rum flavoring, *or* 3 ounces of rum *or* dry sherry
Nutmeg

Whip egg substitute and sugar together and combine with the two kinds of milk, vanilla, and rum flavoring (*or* rum *or* dry sherry). Mix well. Chill. Top with nutmeg. The flavor is enhanced by chilling overnight.
Makes 3 cups.

PER ½ cup:
CALORIES 100   FIBER 0 gm
CSI trace   SODIUM 134 mg
FAT trace

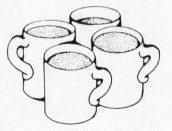

ORANGE FROSTY

1 can (6 ounces) orange juice concentrate
1 cup skim milk
½ cup water
½ cup sugar
1 tablespoon vanilla

Blend; add 1 tray crushed ice and blend again.
Makes 5 cups.

PER cup:
CALORIES 168   FIBER <1 gm
CSI trace   SODIUM 27 mg
FAT trace

ORANGE ICED TEA

A tasty thirst-quencher fancy enough, for parties. The sugar brings out the fruit and mint flavors.

7 tea bags
12 large fresh mint leaves
½–1 cup sugar
3 cups boiling water
2 cups orange juice
¼ cup freshly squeezed lemon juice
7 cups cold water

Place tea bags, mint leaves, and sugar in large bowl or glass jar. Pour boiling water over them and steep until cool (about 1 hour). Remove tea bags and mint. Add fruit juices and cold water to cooled tea. Chill and serve over ice.

　　Makes 12 cups.

PER cup:
CALORIES 67　　FIBER trace
CSI trace　　　SODIUM 5 mg
FAT trace

QUICK HOT SPICED CIDER

Put the amount of cider you want to serve into a kettle. Sprinkle top with ground cinnamon and cloves. Stir and taste. Heat to just below boiling. Serve warm.

PER ½ cup:
CALORIES 61　　FIBER trace
CSI 0　　　　　SODIUM 4 mg
FAT trace

STRAWBERRY BANANA SMOOTHIE

1 cup buttermilk
½ ripe banana
2 tablespoons frozen or fresh strawberries (sweetened)
1 tablespoon orange juice concentrate

Combine all ingredients in an electric blender; mix for a few seconds or until mixture is uniform in color and consistency.

　　Makes 2 cups.

PER cup:
CALORIES 102　　FIBER 1 gm
CSI 1　　　　　SODIUM 130 mg
FAT 1 gm

Mulled Cider
1-3 qt. cider in kettle
Whole cloves into orange & add
1 long or 2 shorter pieces cinnamon
Heat to just below boiling.
Reduce heat to simmer for 30 min.
or until cider tastes spicy. Serve
4-12 cups　　　　　　warm.

SAUCES AND GRAVIES

A good sauce can make a dish. The sauces in this section will do a lot to add the special touch to other recipes. For example, we think the *Onion Chutney* is a treasure we were lucky to find and pass on. Serve it with curry dishes.

For Pasta and Vegetables
Basic White Sauce
Beef-Mushroom Spaghetti Sauce (see page 410 in "Beef and Pork" section)
Clam Sauce for Pasta (see page 367 in "Fish and Shellfish" section)
Homemade Enchilada Sauce
Light Mushroom Sauce for Pasta
Marinara Sauce
Mock Hollandaise Sauce
Mock Sour Cream
Onion Chutney
Savory Eggplant Pasta Sauce
Turkey-Mushroom Spaghetti Sauce (see page 392 in "Chicken and Turkey" section)

For Fish and Poultry
Baked Cranberry-Nut Relish
Cucumber-Dilly Sauce
Tartar Sauce
Turkey Gravy

For Falafel
Tahini Dressing (see page 320 in "Sandwiches" section)
Yogurt Dressing (see page 320 in "Sandwiches" section)

For Rolls, Pancakes, Waffles, or Desserts
Fresh Rhubarb Sauce
Strawberry or Raspberry Sauce
Whipped Honey-Orange Spread
Yogurt Dessert Sauce

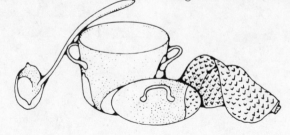

FOR PASTA AND VEGETABLES

BASIC WHITE SAUCE

A white sauce can be prepared in a "low-fat" style. Serve over vegetables for "creamed" or "scalloped" dishes or as a base for "creamed" soups.

> 2 tablespoons margarine
> 2 tablespoons flour
> ¼ teaspoon Lite Salt or less
> ¼ teaspoon pepper
> 2 cups skim milk

Melt margarine in small saucepan over low heat. Add flour, Lite Salt, and pepper, stirring until mixture is smooth and bubbly. Remove from heat. Add skim milk. Heat to boiling, stirring constantly. The consistency should be like heavy cream.

Makes 2¼ cups.

OTHER USES

This typical white sauce can be used in many ways. A number of spices or ingredients can be added to it to create interesting and varied dishes. Add:

—½ teaspoon curry powder as an accompaniment for chicken, rice or shrimp.

—½ teaspoon dill weed as an accompaniment for fish.

PER cup:
CALORIES 189   FIBER trace
CSI 2   SODIUM 334 mg
FAT 11 gm

HOMEMADE ENCHILADA SAUCE

A "no oil" version that is very quickly prepared and much lower in salt than canned.

> 1 tablespoon chili powder
> 1½ tablespoons flour
> 1½ cups water
> 1 teaspoon vinegar
> ½ teaspoon garlic powder
> ½ teaspoon onion powder
> ½ teaspoon Lite Salt or less
> ¼ teaspoon oregano leaves

Combine in a small saucepan chili powder, flour, and 2 tablespoons water. Mix until smooth. Add remaining water gradually to make a smooth sauce (a wire whisk makes this easy). Add vinegar, garlic powder, onion powder, Lite Salt, and oregano. Bring to a boil. Lower heat; simmer uncovered for about 3 minutes.

Makes 1⅓ cups.

PER cup:
CALORIES 55   FIBER 2 gm
CSI trace   SODIUM 428 mg
FAT 1 gm

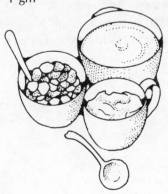

LIGHT MUSHROOM SAUCE FOR PASTA

For mushroom lovers who enjoy a thin, light sauce over fresh cooked pasta! Very attractive when served over fresh spinach pasta.

1 pound small mushrooms
1 tablespoon margarine
1 clove garlic, minced
2 tablespoons flour
2 cups skim milk
¼ cup chopped parsley
½ teaspoon Lite Salt or less
¼ teaspoon pepper
1 tablespoon freshly squeezed lemon juice
¼ cup freshly grated Parmesan cheese
Fresh pasta for 4

Wash and dry mushrooms thoroughly and slice thin. Melt margarine in a large skillet. Sauté garlic. Add sliced mushrooms and sauté over high heat until mushrooms are brown and liquid is mostly evaporated. Stir in flour and cook for a few minutes, then add milk, parsley, Lite Salt, and pepper. Stir and cook for 5 minutes or until it begins to thicken. Add lemon juice.

Fill a large saucepan ⅔ full with water. Bring to a boil. Add pasta. Bring water back to a boil and cook uncovered until pasta is tender, but firm to bite. Drain pasta and mix with sauce. Sprinkle with ¼ cup Parmesan cheese. Serve immediately.

Makes 4 cups sauce (enough for 8 cups pasta).

PER cup:
CALORIES 140   FIBER 1 gm
CSI 2   SODIUM 312 mg
FAT 5 gm

MARINARA SAUCE (TOMATO SAUCE)

This is wonderful over fresh pasta or whenever you need a nicely flavored tomato sauce. Double the recipe and keep some in the freezer.

1 clove garlic, minced
1 tablespoon olive oil *Hc.*
2 cans (16 ounces each) unsalted tomatoes
1 2 cans (8 ounces each) unsalted tomato sauce
1 teaspoon oregano leaves
1 tablespoon chopped or dried parsley

Sauté garlic in olive oil. Add tomatoes and tomato sauce slowly. Stir in oregano and parsley. Bring to a boil and simmer covered for 20 minutes to 2 hours. (The longer the better!) Break up the tomatoes with a potato masher and stir sauce occasionally.

This sauce has great versatility. Use it as a pizza sauce and in any other dishes calling for tomato sauce. For Mexican flavors, add ground cumin (½–1 teaspoon) and hot sauce.

Makes about 4 cups.

PER cup:
CALORIES 117   FIBER 4 gm
CSI <1   SODIUM 41 mg
FAT 4 gm

MOCK HOLLANDAISE SAUCE

Serve this sauce over *"Eggs" Benedict* (page 281) for a special meal.

1 tablespoon cornstarch
1 cup lower-salt chicken broth
4 teaspoons freshly squeezed lemon juice
2 tablespoons margarine
¼ cup grated low-fat cheese

Mix cornstarch with a little broth to a smooth paste. Add the remaining broth, lemon juice, and margarine. Heat slowly to boiling, stirring constantly. Cook 3 minutes longer, stirring occasionally; add cheese and stir until melted.

Makes about 1 cup.

PER ¼ cup:
CALORIES 90   FIBER trace
CSI 2   SODIUM 310 mg
FAT 7 gm

MOCK SOUR CREAM

May be used for sour cream in any recipe that doesn't require heating.

1 cup low-fat cottage cheese
2 tablespoons buttermilk
½–1 teaspoon freshly squeezed lemon juice

Blend cottage cheese, buttermilk, and lemon juice in blender or with mixer until smooth. Scrape sides of container often with rubber spatula while blending.

Makes 1 cup.

USES

As a dip for crackers, pretzels, breadsticks, fresh vegetables, or berries; as a dressing for fruit or vegetable salads; as a topping for potatoes, cooked vegetables, tortillas, etc; as a spread for bagels.

NOTE: If a recipe requires the sour cream to be heated, use *plain nonfat yogurt* directly from the carton.

PER ¼ cup:
CALORIES 55   FIBER 0 gm
CSI 1   SODIUM 238 mg
FAT 1 gm

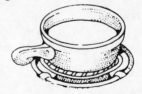

ONION CHUTNEY

Chutney is to curry dishes what salsa is to Mexican food. This recipe is large enough to be a condiment for 3 or 4 meals with curry dishes—so freeze the excess.

> 4 green tomatoes
> 3 tart apples, unpeeled
> 1 onion, peeled
> 1 cup vinegar
> 1 cup sugar
> ¼ teaspoon cayenne pepper
> 2 teaspoons finely minced fresh ginger root
> ¼ teaspoon turmeric
> ¼ teaspoon Lite Salt or less

Chop tomatoes, apples, and onion until very fine (a food processor works best). Combine vinegar, sugar, cayenne, ginger, turmeric, and Lite Salt and bring to boil. Add the chopped tomato/onion/apple mixture and simmer for 30 minutes. Remove from heat and let cool. Refrigerate what you plan to use and freeze the rest.

Serve cold as a side dish with curry dishes, turkey, or other favorites of your choice.

Makes 3 cups.

PER 2 tablespoons:
CALORIES 56   FIBER 1 gm
CSI trace   SODIUM 13 mg
FAT trace

SAVORY EGGPLANT PASTA SAUCE

> ½ eggplant, cut in 1-inch cubes (3½ cups cubed)
> 2 tablespoons flour
> 2 cans (16 ounces each) unsalted tomatoes, finely chopped or mashed
> 1 can (6 ounces) unsalted tomato paste
> 2 cloves garlic, finely minced
> ¼ cup chopped onions
> 2 teaspoons oregano leaves
> 2 teaspoons basil leaves
> 1 teaspoon dried parsley
> ⅛ teaspoon black pepper
> 2 cups sliced mushrooms
> ¼ cup grated Parmesan cheese

Preheat oven to broil. Put eggplant cubes in colander and rinse. Put flour in a small bag; add damp eggplant and shake to coat with flour. Pour onto cookie sheet. Broil until slightly browned on all sides. Remove from oven.

Mix together in a large pan tomatoes, tomato paste, garlic, onion, and spices and bring to a boil. Add eggplant and mushrooms. Reduce heat, cover, and simmer for 1½ hours. Serve over spaghetti or other pasta. Sprinkle 1 tablespoon Parmesan cheese over each serving.

Makes 5 cups (about 4 servings).

PER cup:
CALORIES 131   FIBER 5 gm
CSI 1   SODIUM 439 mg
FAT 3 gm

FOR FISH AND POULTRY

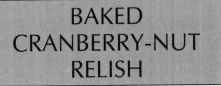

BAKED CRANBERRY-NUT RELISH

This relish freezes well so can be made early for a special dinner.

1 package (12 ounces) cranberries
¾ cup sugar
¼ cup walnuts, chopped into large pieces
½ cup orange marmalade
2 tablespoons freshly squeezed lemon juice

Preheat oven to 350°. In shallow baking pan combine cranberries and sugar. Cover well and bake 1 hour. Meanwhile toast nuts on cookie sheet in oven for 12 minutes or until golden.

When cranberries are baked, combine with toasted nuts, marmalade, and lemon juice. Serve warm or cold.

Makes 2¼ cups.

PER ¼ cup:
CALORIES 152   FIBER 2 gm
CSI trace   SODIUM 4 mg
FAT 2 gm

CUCUMBER-DILLY SAUCE

A delicious sauce to serve with any fish, especially salmon.

3 cups grated cucumber (3 large cucumbers)
2 tablespoons light mayonnaise
1 cup plain nonfat yogurt
1½ teaspoons dill weed
½ teaspoon Lite Salt or less

Peel, seed, and coarsely grate cucumbers. Drain well and squeeze until dry. Set aside. Combine mayonnaise and yogurt and mix thoroughly with wire whisk. Add herbs, Lite Salt, and grated cucumber. Mix well. Cover and refrigerate for several hours before serving.

Makes 3 cups.

PER ¼ cup:
CALORIES 30   FIBER 1 gm
CSI trace   SODIUM 75 mg
FAT <1 gm

TARTAR SAUCE

Especially nice served with *Skinny Sole* (page 378).

1 cup low-fat cottage cheese
2 tablespoons buttermilk
3 tablespoons chopped onion
3 tablespoons chopped parsley
3 tablespoons chopped sweet pickle *or* drained sweet pickle relish

(continued)

Combine cottage cheese and buttermilk in blender until smooth. Add this mixture to chopped vegetables in bowl and mix.

Makes 1¾ cups.

PER tablespoon:
CALORIES 10   FIBER 0 gm
CSI trace   SODIUM 41 mg
FAT trace

TURKEY GRAVY

You can get your turkey gravy base all made ahead of time, which will save you that much fussing at the last minute. This is a white wine turkey stock thickened at the end with cornstarch. When the turkey is done and the roaster degreased, blend the gravy base into the roasting juices.

Turkey neck and gizzard
2 tablespoons oil
1 cup chopped onion
1 cup chopped carrots
1 cup dry white wine *or* ⅔ cup dry white vermouth
2 cups lower-salt chicken broth
Water as needed
½ teaspoon Lite Salt or less
1 bay leaf
½ teaspoon thyme leaves *or* sage
3 tablespoons cornstarch blended with ¼ cup port or cold low-sodium chicken broth

Early in the day: Chop neck into 2-inch pieces and quarter the gizzard. Dry on paper towels. Heat oil in a heavy 3-quart saucepan, stir in the neck and gizzard, and brown rapidly on all sides. Remove them and stir the vegetables into the pan. Cover and cook slowly 5–8 minutes, or until tender. Uncover, raise heat and brown lightly for several minutes. Return neck and gizzard to pan, add the wine, broth, and enough water to cover ingredients by an inch. Add Lite Salt and herbs and simmer partially covered for 2½–3 hours. Strain and return stock to pan. There should be about 3 cups. Beat in cornstarch mixture and simmer 2–3 minutes. Liquid will be lightly thickened. When cool, cover and refrigerate until turkey is done.

Finishing the sauce or gravy: When the turkey is roasted, skim all fat out of roasting pan and discard. Pour remaining drippings into saucepan with thickened turkey stock and stir over moderately high heat for several minutes. Pour into a warm gravy bowl.

Makes about 4 cups.

PER ¼ cup:
CALORIES 32   FIBER <1 gm
CSI trace   SODIUM 136 mg
FAT 2 gm

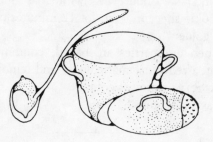

FOR ROLLS, PANCAKES, WAFFLES, OR DESSERTS

FRESH RHUBARB SAUCE

A wonderful dessert sauce or topping for waffles or pancakes. The addition of fresh berries makes it special.

4 cups rhubarb, cut into 1-inch pieces
½ cup water
½ cup sugar
1 teaspoon cinnamon
½ cup fresh strawberries, sliced (optional)

Place prepared rhubarb and water in saucepan. Simmer about 10 minutes or until rhubarb is tender and slightly transparent. Remove from heat and add sugar and cinnamon. Stir until sugar is dissolved. Store in refrigerator. If adding fresh strawberries, fold into cooked sauce when cool. Store in refrigerator.
Makes 2 cups.

PER ½ cup:
CALORIES 100   FIBER 3 gm
CSI trace   SODIUM 3 mg
FAT trace

STRAWBERRY OR RASPBERRY SAUCE

This can be used as a topping for *Baba au Rhum* (page 429), frozen desserts, fruit desserts, pancakes, waffles, etc.

1 quart of strawberries or raspberries
⅓ cup (or less) sugar according to taste
Juice of 1 lemon *or* 2 tablespoons sherry

Stem, wash, and drain berries. Put berries in an electric blender and puree until smooth (or push berries through a food mill). Add sugar, lemon juice *or* sherry and mix all together.
Makes 4 cups.

PER ¼ cup:
CALORIES 31   FIBER <1 gm
CSI 0   SODIUM 1 mg
FAT trace

WHIPPED HONEY-ORANGE SPREAD

A small amount on *Fruit Scones* (page 275) is great! This spread has more texture than when made with cream cheese, but is still delicious.

1 cup low-fat ricotta cheese, room temperature
2–3 tablespoons honey
1 tablespoon grated orange peel

(continued)

In a small bowl beat ricotta cheese, honey, and orange peel until light, fluffy and very smooth. Serve immediately or cover and chill for several days.

Makes 1⅓ cups.

PER 1 tablespoon:
CALORIES 23   FIBER trace
CSI <1   SODIUM 14 mg
FAT 1 gm

YOGURT DESSERT SAUCE

This light sauce can be used with *Pumpkin Bread Pudding* (page 441), *Baked Apples* (page 414), *Apple Crisp* (page 414), or any other fruit dessert. Wonderful over fresh strawberries!

2 cups plain nonfat yogurt
1 teaspoon vanilla extract
¼ cup sugar

Combine all ingredients and stir well.

Makes enough topping for 8 servings (about 2 cups).

PER ¼ cup:
CALORIES 61   FIBER 0 gm
CSI <1   SODIUM 40 mg
FAT <1 gm

APPENDIX
THE CSI TABLE OF FOODS

APPETIZERS/SNACKS
(SELECT CSIs OF 2 OR LOWER PER SERVING)

	SERVING SIZE		CSI	FAT (GM)	CALORIES
DIPS AND SPREADS					
Baba Ganouj	¼ cup	(61 gm)	tr.	1	18
Hummous	¼ cup	(65 gm)	tr.	3	106
Salmon Mousse	¼ cup	(47 gm)	1	4	70
Liver Pâté	¼ cup	(68 gm)	14	12	144
Bean Dip	¼ cup	(64 gm)	tr.	1	59
Bean dip	¼ cup	(69 gm)	2	3	82
Chowchow	¼ cup	(53 gm)	tr.	3	49
Chunky Avocado Dip	¼ cup	(61 gm)	<1	5	72
Guacamole	¼ cup	(60 gm)	1	5	62
Salsa	¼ cup	(63 gm)	tr.	tr.	24
Dill Dip	¼ cup	(52 gm)	1	3	66
Sour cream dip	¼ cup	(52 gm)	8	11	111
Popeye's Spinach Dip	¼ cup	(53 gm)	<1	1	37
Spinach dip	¼ cup	(54 gm)	4	13	138
Clam dip	¼ cup	(52 gm)	6	7	87
Cheese dip	¼ cup	(41 gm)	8	10	118
Shrimp dip	¼ cup	(47 gm)	8	8	99
"Egg" Salad Sandwich Spread	¼ cup	(53 gm)	tr.	3	55
POCKET BREAD FILLERS					

Spicy Black Bean Salad	¼ cup	(43 gm)	tr.	1	57
Chili Bean Salad	¼ cup	(55 gm)	tr.	1	64
Southern Caviar	¼ cup	(52 gm)	tr.	1	68
Steamed Buns	1 bun	(41 gm)	<1	3	73
Eggroll (with shrimp and pork)	1 roll	(101 gm)	6	11	158
Marinated Mushrooms	¹⁄₁₀ recipe	(43 gm)	tr.	3	39
Snappy Clams	⅛ recipe	(50 gm)	<1	2	39
Zucchini Toast	2 toasts	(55 gm)	<1	2	51
Spinach Triangles	3 triangles	(22 gm)	1	2	54
Rumaki	3 pieces	(40 gm)	6	4	68
Oysters Rockefeller	3 oysters	(79 gm)	10	12	162
Swedish meatballs	3 meatballs	(131 gm)	12	21	287

BAKERY GOODS
(SELECT CSIs OF 2 OR LOWER PER SERVING)

BISCUITS

Old-style Wheat Biscuit	One	(34 gm)	<1	4	86
Canned	One 2"	(21 gm)	<1	3	68
Baking powder	One 2"	(28 gm)	2	5	118
Scone	One 4"	(56 gm)	6	12	294

The abbreviation *tr.* stands for trace (less than 0.5); the symbol <1 stands for less than one (0.5 to 0.9). Recipes in **bold italics** can be found in Part III.

459

BAKERY GOODS (continued)

	SERVING SIZE		CSI	FAT (GM)	CALORIES
BISCUIT OR BAKING MIX					
Baking Mix, modified	1 cup	(121 gm)	4	17	491
Typical (Bisquick)	1 cup	(113 gm)	10	17	475
SWEET ROLLS					
Poptart	One	(50 gm)	2	6	196
Brioche	One	(30 gm)	4	6	119
Sweet roll, cinnamon	One 4"	(69 gm)	5	11	276
Maple bar	One	(42 gm)	6	12	192
Danish	One 4"	(58 gm)	8	18	235
Croissant	One	(55 gm)	9	12	167
Sunday Morning Sticky Buns	⅑ recipe	(60 gm)	<1	3	214
Sticky nut roll	One 4"	(102 gm)	13	20	444
DOUGHNUTS					
Baked Doughnut Holes	Two	(40 gm)	tr.	3	118
Doughnut, cake (unfrosted)	One 3"	(36 gm)	4	6	153
Doughnut, cake (frosted)	One 3"	(67 gm)	5	10	279
Doughnut, cake (frosted, with coconut)	One 3"	(73 gm)	7	12	309
COFFEE CAKES					
Sunrise Cake	¹⁄₁₆ of cake	(68 gm)	<1	4	161
Coffee cake, streusel topping	3" x 3" x 2"	(94 gm)	6	12	316
SPECIALTY ITEMS					

Twinkie, Hostess	One	(48 gm)	3	4	163
Ho Ho, Hostess	One	(25 gm)	4	6	118
Cupcake, Hostess	One	(57 gm)	4	7	219
Ding Dong, Hostess	One	(38 gm)	6	10	186
Eclair, chocolate	One 4" x 2"	(113 gm)	10	10	201
Cream puff	One 2½"	(87 gm)	12	8	173

BEANS (LEGUMES) COOKED
(SELECT CSIs OF 1 OR LOWER)

Beans, no fat added (navy, pinto, kidney, black, etc.)	½ cup	(90 gm)	tr.	1	106
Lentils, split peas, no fat added	½ cup	(100 gm)	tr.	1	115
Garbanzo (chick peas), black-eyed peas	½ cup	(124 gm)	tr.	3	212
Soybeans	½ cup	(90 gm)	<1	5	117
Tofu (bean curd)	½ cup	(110 gm)	<1	5	79
Pork and beans (canned)	½ cup	(128 gm)	1	4	155
BAKED					
Rancher's Beans	½ cup	(119 gm)	tr.	tr.	171
Classic Baked Beans	½ cup	(95 gm)	tr.	1	115
Baked beans with ham	½ cup	(128 gm)	3	6	192

The abbreviation *tr.* stands for trace (less than (0.5); the symbol <1 stands for less than one (0.5 to 0.9). Recipes in **bold italics** can be found in Part III.

461

BEANS (LEGUMES) COOKED (continued)

	SERVING SIZE		CSI	FAT (GM)	CALORIES
REFRIED					
Black Beans with 1000 Uses	½ cup	(106 gm)	tr.	tr.	63
Refried Beans	½ cup	(87 gm)	<1	3	113
Refried beans (canned)	½ cup	(121 gm)	<1	2	124
Refried beans (typical restaurant)	½ cup	(122 gm)	6	14	243
DIPS					
Bean Dip	¼ cup	(64 gm)	tr.	1	59
Jalapeño dip	¼ cup	(69 gm)	2	4	83
SOUPS					
Greek Lentil	1 cup	(255 gm)	tr.	1	149
Greek-Style Garbanzo	1 cup	(217 gm)	tr.	4	156
Navy Bean	1 cup	(163 gm)	tr.	<1	79
Split Pea	1 cup	(240 gm)	tr.	1	106
Black Bean Chili	1 cup	(244 gm)	<1	4	277
Minestrone	1 cup	(244 gm)	1	3	83
Rose Bowl Chili	1 cup	(267 gm)	2	5	213
Split pea, lentil, etc.	1 cup	(250 gm)	2	6	170

BEVERAGES: ALCOHOLIC
(SELECT CSIs OF 0 PER SERVING)

Beer, light	12 ounces	(353 gm)	0	0	96
Beer or ale	12 ounces	(353 gm)	0	0	145
Wine, table (Chablis, Burgundy, Champagne)	4 ounces	(116 gm)	0	0	91
Wine, dessert or aperitif (port, sherry, sweet vermouth)	4 ounces	(116 gm)	0	0	158
Liquor (gin, whiskey, vodka, rum, cognac)	1½ ounces	(42 gm)	0	0	105
MIXED COCKTAILS					
Bloody Mary	6 ounces	(179 gm)	0	tr.	129
Gimlet	6 ounces	(184 gm)	0	0	335
Mai Tai	6 ounces	(171 gm)	0	0	374
Manhattan	6 ounces	(170 gm)	0	0	342
Martini	6 ounces	(170 gm)	0	0	363
Margarita, Daiquiri	6 ounces	(176 gm)	0	tr.	402
Old-Fashioned	6 ounces	(192 gm)	0	0	516
Brandy Alexander	6 ounces	(173 gm)	9	12	417
Crème de Menthe or Grasshopper	6 ounces	(197 gm)	9	12	537
Piña Colada	6 ounces	(191 gm)	13	14	323
LIQUEURS					
Cordials, fruit type	1 ounce	(28 gm)	0	0	80

The abbreviation *tr.* stands for trace (less than 0.5); the symbol <1 stands for less than one (0.5 to 0.9). Recipes in ***bold italics*** can be found in Part III.

BEVERAGES: ALCOHOLIC (continued)

	SERVING SIZE		CSI	FAT (GM)	CALORIES
Coffee-flavored (Kahlua)	1 ounce	(38 gm)	0	0	88
Irish Cream	1 ounce	(34 gm)	3	2	92

BEVERAGES: COLD
(SELECT CSIs OF 2 OR LOWER PER SERVING)

	SERVING SIZE		CSI	FAT (GM)	CALORIES
FRUIT-TYPE DRINKS					
Apple cider	1 cup	(248 gm)	0	0	116
Lemonade	1 cup	(240 gm)	0	0	110
Fruit juice, average	1 cup	(240 gm)	tr.	tr.	120
Orange Iced Tea	1 cup	(240 gm)	tr.	tr.	67
Orange Frosty	1 cup	(239 gm)	tr.	tr.	168
Strawberry Banana Smoothie	1 cup	(390 gm)	1	1	102
MILK SHAKES					
All flavors (McDonald's)	16 ounces	(231 gm)	5	7	304
All flavors (most restaurants including other fast-food restaurants)	16 ounces	(360 gm)	8	11	442
All flavors (specialty ice cream stores)	16 ounces	(384 gm)	32	39	671
POP DRINKS					
Non-cola, sweetened	12 ounces	(360 gm)	0	0	111
Cola, sweetened	12 ounces	(360 gm)	0	0	155

Diet pop	12 ounces		0	0	4
Root beer float	1½ cups	(307 gm)	6	7	241
MILK DRINKS					
Milk, skim	1 cup	(245 gm)	<1	tr.	85
Milk, 1%	1 cup	(244 gm)	2	3	102
Milk, 2%	1 cup	(244 gm)	4	5	122
Milk, whole	1 cup	(244 gm)	7	8	149
Buttermilk	1 cup	(245 gm)	2	2	98
Chocolate milk (2%)	1 cup	(250 gm)	5	7	194
Instant Breakfast, all flavors					
made with skim milk	1 cup	(285 gm)	1	1	215
made with whole milk	1 cup	(279 gm)	7	9	279
Egg Nog	1 cup	(246 gm)	tr.	tr.	200
Egg Nog, commercial (no alcohol)	1 cup	(254 gm)	16	19	340
OTHERS					
Club soda, carbonated water, seltzer	1 cup	(240 gm)	0	0	0
Gatorade	1 cup	(240 gm)	0	0	58
Tea, unsweetened	1 cup	(240 gm)	0	0	0

The abbreviation *tr.* stands for trace (less than 0.5); the symbol <1 stands for less than one (0.5 to 0.9). Recipes in **bold italics** can be found in Part III.

BEVERAGES: HOT
(SELECT CSIs OF 2 OR LOWER PER SERVING)

	SERVING SIZE		CSI	FAT (GM)	CALORIES
Quick Hot Spiced Cider	1 cup	(250 gm)	0	tr.	122
Postum	1 cup	(240 gm)	0	0	15
Tea, unsweetened	1 cup	(240 gm)	0	0	0
Coffee, black	1 cup	(240 gm)	0	tr.	5
Coffee with ½ ounce skim milk	1 cup	(255 gm)	<1	<1	10
Coffee with ½ ounce Mocha Mix	1 cup	(255 gm)	<1	2	24
Coffee with ½ ounce half-and-half	1 cup	(255 gm)	1	2	25
Coffee, specialty (cappuccino, mocha, Vienna, au lait)	1 cup	(249 gm)	3	3	85
Cocoa with skim milk, sugar-free	1 cup	(260 gm)	2	2	68
Cocoa with skim milk, (Swiss Miss, from vending machine)	1 cup	(264 gm)	2	2	154
Cocoa with whole milk	1 cup	(263 gm)	8	10	217

BREADS AND TORTILLAS
(SELECT CSIs OF 1 OR LOWER PER SERVING)

YEAST BREADS					
White	1 slice	(25 gm)	tr.	<1	68

Whole wheat	1 slice	(29 gm)	tr.	<1	70
Raisin	1 slice	(23 gm)	tr.	<1	61
Rye	1 slice	(29 gm)	tr.	tr.	70
Pumpernickel	1 slice	(25 gm)	tr.	tr.	62
English muffin	One	(57 gm)	tr.	1	135
Whole Wheat French Bread	⅕ loaf	(38 gm)	tr.	<1	125
Grape-nut Bread	1 slice or roll	(42 gm)	tr.	1	99
French, Italian, sourdough	4¼" x 2¾" x 1"	(30 gm)	tr.	tr.	83
Pita or pocket	One	(64 gm)	tr.	<1	180
Boston brown	1 slice	(48 gm)	tr.	<1	101
Cinnamon swirl	1 slice	(22 gm)	tr.	<1	59
Egg	1 slice	(33 gm)	2	2	89
Cheese	1 slice	(29 gm)	2	3	87
Challah	1 slice	(33 gm)	2	2	89
Focaccia	⅙ loaf	(60 gm)	1	5	190
Boboli	⅛ loaf	(60 gm)	2	8	183
YEAST ROLLS					
Hard	1 small	(25 gm)	tr.	<1	77
Kaiser	One	(50 gm)	tr.	2	153
Caraway Dinner Roll	One	(48 gm)	tr.	<1	108
Pan or dinner-type	One	(28 gm)	<1	2	83
Poor boy or submarine	3" x 11½"	(135 gm)	1	4	385
Crescent	One	(28 gm)	3	6	101

The abbreviation *tr.* stands for trace (less than 0.5); the symbol <1 stands for less than one (0.5 to 0.9). Recipes in **bold italics** can be found in Part III.

BREADS AND TORTILLAS (continued)

	SERVING SIZE		CSI	FAT (GM)	CALORIES
Croissant	One	(55 gm)	9	12	167
TORTILLAS					
Corn, plain	5¾" diameter	(23 gm)	tr.	<1	52
Taco or tostada shell, fried	5½" diameter	(14 gm)	1	3	63
Flour, plain	7½" diameter	(38 gm)	1	3	118
Flour, fried	7½" diameter	(43 gm)	3	8	162
BAGELS					
Plain or flavored	One	(75 gm)	tr.	2	225
Egg	One	(75 gm)	2	4	225
MUFFINS AND SCONES					
Blueberry Bran Muffin	One	(89 gm)	tr.	<1	146
Cereal Bran Muffin	One	(59 gm)	<1	4	116
A Barrel of Muffins	One	(43 gm)	<1	4	105
Poppyseed Muffin	One	(62 gm)	<1	5	163
Nutty Orange Muffin	One	(63 gm)	<1	5	167
Mexican Cornbread Muffin	One	(74 gm)	<1	4	165
Pumpkin Oat Muffin	One	(82 gm)	<1	4	177
Applesauce Oatmeal Muffin	One	(59 gm)	<1	5	157
Dutchy Crust Muffins or Coffee Cake	One	(64 gm)	<1	5	181
Cinnamon Rhubarb Muffin	One	(50 gm)	<1	4	140
Typical plain muffin	One	(55 gm)	2	6	149
Oatmeal Raisin Muffin	One	(47 gm)	<1	4	137

Oatmeal raisin muffin, typical	One	(61 gm)	2	6	164
Yogurt Scone	One	(60 gm)	<1	3	136
Fruit Scone	One	(39 gm)	<1	4	107
QUICK BREADS					
Grandma Kirschner's Date Nut Bread	½" slice	(61 gm)	tr.	4	209
Pumpkin Harvest Loaf	½" slice	(38 gm)	<1	4	163
Lemon Nut Bread	½" slice	(58 gm)	<1	5	153
Cornbread	2" x 4" x 2"	(78 gm)	<1	6	180
Fruit Bread	½" slice	(55 gm)	<1	4	151
Orange Walnut Bread	½" slice	(55 gm)	<1	4	166
Banana Nut Bread	½" slice	(66 gm)	<1	4	142
Whole Wheat Quick Bread	½" slice	(36 gm)	<1	2	93
Nut bread	½" slice	(58 gm)	2	10	199
Zucchini bread (no nuts)	½" slice	(45 gm)	3	9	172
Pumpkin bread (no nuts)	½" slice	(45 gm)	4	5	161
Cornbread, typical	3" x 3" x 1"	(59 gm)	5	8	190
MISCELLANEOUS					
Breadstick, plain	One 7½"	(11 gm)	tr.	tr.	30
Hamburger or hot dog bun	One	(40 gm)	<1	2	114
Breadcrumbs, commercial	½ cup	(50 gm)	<1	2	195
Lefse	1 serving	(38 gm)	1	3	78
Croutons, commercial	½ cup	(18 gm)	3	4	89
Popover	One	(40 gm)	5	4	92

The abbreviation *tr.* stands for trace (less than 0.5); the symbol <1 stands for less than one (0.5 to 0.9). Recipes in **bold italics** can be found in Part III.

BREAKFAST DISHES
(SELECT CSIs OF 4 OR LOWER PER SERVING)

	SERVING SIZE		CSI	FAT (GM)	CALORIES
PANCAKES					
Cornmeal Pancakes	Two 5"	(136 gm)	<1	3	178
Cornmeal pancakes, typical	Two 5"	(139 gm)	7	9	228
Oatmeal Buttermilk Pancakes	Three 4"	(162 gm)	1	3	228
Modified pancakes (made with oil, skim milk, no yolks)	Three 4"	(143 gm)	1	6	212
Typical pancakes (made from mix)	Three 4"	(138 gm)	8	10	258
German Oven Pancake	½ pancake	(369 gm)	2	10	373*
Dutch Baby (typical)	½ pancake	(183 gm)	29	22	402
Crepe Blintz	One	(216 gm)	4	7	239
Blintz, typical	One	(115 gm)	12	14	227
Crepe	One	(35 gm)	tr.	2	62
Crepe, typical	One	(68 gm)	5	4	116
WAFFLES					
Orange Waffles	One 7"	(111 gm)	1	8	197
Cinnamon Waffles	One 7"	(111 gm)	2	8	197
Modified waffles (made with oil, no yolks, skim milk)	One 7"	(113 gm)	2	8	192
Typical waffles	One 7"	(113 gm)	8	13	249

*Contains fruit.

470

FRENCH TOAST

French Toast	¼ recipe	(56 gm)	tr.	1	95
Modified (made with skim milk, egg substitute)	One	(75 gm)	<1	4	116
Typical	One	(72 gm)	5	6	131

OMELETS

Spanish Omelet	⅙ recipe	(183 gm)	tr.	1	93
Vegetable Frittata	½ recipe	(272 gm)	2	7	232
Omelet, plain	2 eggs	(128 gm)	27	20	244
Omelet, cheese	2 eggs	(154 gm)	34	28	350
Omelet, ham & cheese	2 eggs	(190 gm)	36	32	413

EGGS

Whites	Two	(66 gm)	0	0	32
Whole	One	(50 gm)	12	6	79
Yolks	Two	(34 gm)	25	11	125

EGG SUBSTITUTES

Egg Beaters	¼ cup	(60 gm)	0	0	30
Second Nature	¼ cup	(60 gm)	0	2	49
Scramblers	¼ cup	(60 gm)	0	4	68
Homemade Egg Substitute	¼ cup	(60 gm)	<1	4	70

OTHER EGG DISHES

Scrambled Whites	½ cup	(99 gm)	0	0	48

The abbreviation *tr.* stands for trace (less than 0.5); the symbol <1 stands for less than one (0.5 to 0.9). Recipes in **bold italics** can be found in Part III.

BREAKFAST DISHES (continued)

	SERVING SIZE		CSI	FAT (GM)	CALORIES
Scrambled Egg Substitute	½ cup	(114 gm)	2	8	127
Scrambled Eggs, typical	½ cup, 2 eggs	(124 gm)	27	20	244
Egg McMuffin	One	(138 gm)	16	16	340
Sausage McMuffin with egg	One	(165 gm)	24	33	517
Egg, fried with margarine	One	(55 gm)	13	9	113
Two fried eggs and four slices bacon	One serving	(138 gm)	32	32	387
"Eggs" Benedict	One	(193 gm)	4	11	238
Eggs Benedict, typical	One	(132 gm)	30	25	721

CANDIES, CHOCOLATES, AND OTHER SWEETS
(SELECT CSIs OF 2 OR LOWER PER SERVING)

CANDY BARS

Bit O' Honey	2 ounces	(57 gm)	1	3	206
Payday	2 ounces	(57 gm)	2	10	256
M & M's (peanut)	2 ounces	(57 gm)	2	10	268
Twix	2 ounces	(57 gm)	4	9	243
Zagnut	2 ounces	(57 gm)	4	9	254
Milky Way	2 ounces	(57 gm)	5	8	237
Baby Ruth	2 ounces	(57 gm)	5	13	283
Butterfinger	2 ounces	(57 gm)	5	11	264

472

Mars Bar	2 ounces	(57 gm)	5	8	237
M & M's (plain)	2 ounces	(57 gm)	5	11	266
Oh Henry	2 ounces	(57 gm)	5	13	283
Power House	2 ounces	(57 gm)	5	13	283
Snicker	2 ounces	(57 gm)	5	13	283
Three Musketeers	2 ounces	(57 gm)	5	8	237
Reese's Peanut Butter Cup	2 ounces	(57 gm)	6	16	296
Mounds	2 ounces	(57 gm)	7	10	250
Almond Joy	2 ounces	(57 gm)	8	15	274
Granola Bar	2 ounces	(57 gm)	9	10	254
Heath	2 ounces	(57 gm)	9	18	286
Hershey with almonds	2 ounces	(57 gm)	10	20	303
Krackel	2 ounces	(57 gm)	10	17	292
Mr. Goodbar	2 ounces	(57 gm)	10	22	310
Nestle (chocolate, almonds)	2 ounces	(57 gm)	10	20	303
Summit	2 ounces	(57 gm)	10	17	292
Hershey (plain) or Kisses	2 ounces	(57 gm)	11	18	296
NUT-TYPE CANDY					
Divinity	2 ounces	(64 gm)	<1	8	235
Nut brittle	2 ounces	(57 gm)	2	15	302
Pecan praline	2 ounces	(57 gm)	3	9	243
Bridge mix	2 ounces	(57 gm)	3	9	252
Fudge with walnuts	2 ounces	(60 gm)	3	10	257

The abbreviation *tr.* stands for trace (less than (0.5); the symbol <1 stands for less than one (0.5 to 0.9). Recipes in **bold italics** can be found in Part III.

CANDIES, CHOCOLATES, AND OTHER SWEETS (*continued*)

	SERVING SIZE		CSI	FAT (GM)	CALORIES
Rocky road (chocolate, nuts, and marshmallows)	2 ounces	(57 gm)	6	14	232
Almond Roca	2 ounces	(57 gm)	9	21	305
MISCELLANEOUS CANDY					
Gumdrops	1 ounce	(28 gm)	0	tr.	98
Hard candy	1 ounce	(28 gm)	0	tr.	109
Jelly beans	1 ounce	(28 gm)	0	tr.	104
Licorice	1 ounce	(28 gm)	tr.	tr.	100
Mints, non-chocolate	1 ounce	(28 gm)	tr.	1	103
Taffy	1 ounce	(28 gm)	tr.	2	103
Cracker Jack	⅔ cup	(28 gm)	0	3	120
Ayd's (diet candy)	1 ounce	(28 gm)	2	2	107
Toffee	1 ounce	(28 gm)	2	3	113
Sugar Babies	1 ounce	(28 gm)	3	5	116
Caramels, plain & chocolate	1 ounce	(28 gm)	3	5	116
Malted milk balls	1 ounce	(28 gm)	4	7	135
Carob-coated raisins	1 ounce	(28 gm)	<1	4	112
Carob-coated peanuts	1 ounce	(28 gm)	1	8	140
Chocolate-covered cherries	1 ounce	(28 gm)	3	5	123
Chocolate-covered creams	1 ounce	(28 gm)	3	5	123
Chocolate-covered raisins	1 ounce	(28 gm)	3	5	120
Chocolate Easter eggs	1 ounce	(28 gm)	3	5	120
Yogurt-coated peanuts	1 ounce	(28 gm)	4	9	129

	1 ounce	(28 gm)	4	5	
Yogurt-coated raisins	1 ounce	(28 gm)			101
OTHER SWEETS					
Honey	½ cup	(168 gm)	0	0	511
Honey	1 tablespoon	(21 gm)	0	0	64
Jam, jelly, typical	½ cup	(160 gm)	tr.	tr.	437
Jam, jelly, typical	1 tablespoon	(20 gm)	tr.	tr.	55
Jam, jelly, low-sugar	½ cup	(160 gm)	0	0	223
Jam, jelly, low-sugar	1 tablespoon	(20 gm)	0	0	30
Marshmallows, plain	½ cup	(25 gm)	0	0	80
Marshmallows, chocolate-covered	½ cup	(28 gm)	3	6	145
Marshmallow Creme	½ cup	(69 gm)	0	0	217
Molasses	½ cup	(160 gm)	0	0	371
Sugar, brown	½ cup	(110 gm)	0	0	410
Sugar, powdered	½ cup	(64 gm)	0	0	247
Sugar, granulated	½ cup	(96 gm)	0	0	370
Syrup, maple-flavored	½ cup	(168 gm)	0	0	487
Coconut, sweetened	½ cup	(37 gm)	12	13	185

The abbreviation *tr.* stands for trace (less than (0.5); the symbol <1 stands for less than one (0.5 to 0.9). Recipes in **bold italics** can be found in Part III.

CEREALS
(SELECT CSIs OF 2 OR LOWER PER CUP)

READY-TO-EAT	SERVING SIZE		CSI	FAT (GM)	CALORIES
Wheat Bran, unprocessed	1 tablespoon	(4 gm)	tr.	<1	7
All-Bran	1 cup	(85 gm)	tr.	2	212
Bran Buds	1 cup	(84 gm)	tr.	2	217
Branflakes	1 cup	(39 gm)	tr.	<1	127
Branflakes with Raisins	1 cup	(57 gm)	tr.	1	175
Cheerios/Wheaties	1 cup	(29 gm)	tr.	tr.	101
Chex, Corn & Rice	1 cup	(28 gm)	tr.	tr.	110
Corn Flakes/Rice Krispies	1 cup	(23 gm)	tr.	tr.	89
Grape-nuts	1 cup	(112 gm)	tr.	tr.	403
Grape-nut Flakes	1 cup	(32 gm)	tr.	tr.	115
Kashi	1 cup	(22 gm)	tr.	<1	74
Presweetened, variety of brands	1 cup	(28 gm)	tr.	<1	110
Puffed Rice	1 cup	(14 gm)	0	tr.	56
Puffed Wheat	1 cup	(12 gm)	tr.	tr.	44
Shredded Wheat	1 biscuit/25 bite-size	(24 gm)	tr.	<1	86
Special K	1 cup	(21 gm)	tr.	tr.	82
Captain Crunch	1 cup	(37 gm)	2	3	156
Muesli	1 cup	(84 gm)	tr.	2	280

Granola, low-fat commercial (Golden Temple)	1 cup	(57 gm)	<1	6	250
Granola, commercial with soy oil (Vita Crunch)	1 cup	(113 gm)	3	18	495
Granola, commercial with coconut oil	1 cup	(113 gm)	17	20	503

COOKED

Farina, Cream of Wheat, Ralston, Roman Meal, Malt-O-Meal	1 cup	(233 gm)	tr.	tr.	126
Oat bran	1 cup	(240 gm)	tr.	2	103
Oatmeal, regular	1 cup	(234 gm)	tr.	2	145
Oatmeal, instant	1 cup	(207 gm)	tr.	3	217

CHEESES
(SELECT CSIs OF 4 OR LOWER PER OUNCE OR 19 OR LOWER PER CUP GRATED)

COTTAGE-TYPE CHEESES

Cottage cheese, dry curd	½ cup	(73 gm)	tr.	tr.	62
Tofu (bean curd)	½ cup	(110 gm)	<1	5	79
Cottage cheese, low-fat (1%)	½ cup	(113 gm)	<1	1	81
Cottage cheese, low-fat (2%)	½ cup	(113 gm)	2	2	102
Cottage cheese, regular (4%)	½ cup	(105 gm)	4	5	111

CHEDDAR AND JACK-TYPE CHEESES

Dorman's Light*	1 ounce	(28 gm)	<1	5	70

The abbreviation *tr.* stands for trace (less than 0.5); the symbol <1 stands for less than one (0.5 to 0.9). Recipes in **bold italics** can be found in Part III.

CHEESES (continued)

	SERVING SIZE		CSI	FAT (GM)	CALORIES
Scandic Mini Chol or Swedish low-fat*	1 ounce	(28 gm)	2	9	113
Olympia's Low-Fat	1 ounce	(28 gm)	4	5	72
Green River Part Skim	1 ounce	(28 gm)	4	5	72
Heidi Ann Low Fat Ched-Style Cheese, Kraft Light Naturals Mild Cheddar	1 ounce	(28 gm)	4	5	80
Swiss	1 ounce	(28 gm)	6	8	107
Cheddar, Monterey Jack, Colby, Havarti, Long Horn	1 ounce	(28 gm)	8	9	114
CHEESE SLICES					
Lite-line	1 ounce	(28 gm)	2	2	51
Lite 'n' Lively	1 ounce	(28 gm)	3	4	74
Kraft Light Naturals (Swiss Reduced Fat)	1 ounce	(28 gm)	4	5	90
American	1 ounce	(28 gm)	7	9	106
VELVEETA-TYPE CHEESES					
Mini Chol*	1 ounce	(28 gm)	2	9	113
Velveeta	1 ounce	(28 gm)	5	7	88
CREAM-TYPE CHEESES					
Gardenia ricotta, low-fat	2 tablespoons	(30 gm)	<1	1	32
Whipped Honey-Orange Spread	2 tablespoons	(28 gm)	1	2	46
Part-skim ricotta	2 tablespoons	(30 gm)	2	2	39
Light Philadelphia cream cheese	1 ounce	(28 gm)	4	5	60
Neufchâtel (lower-fat cream cheese)	1 ounce	(28 gm)	5	7	74

Cream cheese including whipped	1 ounce	(28 gm)	8	10	99
PIZZA-TYPE CHEESES					
Imitation mozzarella*	1 ounce	(28 gm)	1	6	80
Lite part-skim mozzarella	1 ounce	(28 gm)	2	2	60
Part-skim mozzarella	1 ounce	(28 gm)	4	5	72
SNACK AND PARTY-TYPE CHEESES					
Hickory Farms Lyte*	1 ounce	(28 gm)	1	6	90
Scandic Mini Chol or Swedish low-fat*	1 ounce	(28 gm)	2	9	113
Reduced Calories Laughing Cow	1 ounce	(28 gm)	2	3	45
String, Lappi	1 ounce	(28 gm)	4	5	72
Cheese spread (jars)	1 ounce	(28 gm)	5	7	88
Brie	1 ounce	(28 gm)	6	8	95
Gruyère	1 ounce	(28 gm)	6	8	107
Edam, Limburger, Port du Salut	1 ounce	(28 gm)	8	9	114
Roquefort or blue	1 ounce	(28 gm)	8	9	114
Feta	1 ounce	(28 gm)	8	9	114
GRATED					
Dorman's Light*	1 cup	(114 gm)	2	20	285
Imitation mozzarella*	1 cup	(110 gm)	5	23	310
Scandic Mini Chol*	1 cup	(114 gm)	6	36	454
Kraft Light Naturals Cheddar	1 cup	(114 gm)	16	20	322

* Cheese made with skim milk and vegetable oil, thus the fat is less saturated than in regular cheeses.

The abbreviation tr. stands for trace (less than 0.5); the symbol <1 stands for less than one (0.5 to 0.9). Recipes in **bold italics** can be found in Part III.

CHEESES (continued)

	SERVING SIZE	CSI	FAT (GM)	CALORIES
Part-skim mozzarella	1 cup (114 gm)	15	18	290
Green River Part Skim or Olympia's Low-Fat	1 cup (140 gm)	18	22	356
Parmesan	2 tablespoons (10 gm)	2	3	46
Parmesan	1 cup (80 gm)	19	24	365
Cheddar or Monterey Jack	1 cup (140 gm)	37	46	564

CHIPS, CRACKERS, AND POPCORN
(SELECT CSIs OF 2 OR LOWER PER SERVING)

CRACKERS

		CSI	FAT (GM)	CALORIES
Very Low–Fat Varieties:	(average nutrient values) (40 gm)	tr.	tr.	134
Armenian Crackerbread	1 large			
Breadsticks, plain	3½ sticks			
Cracklesnax	24			
Crispy Cakes (Squared Rice Cakes)	7 squares			
Crokine	8 slices			
Kavli	4 slices			
Matzo	1⅓			
Rice Cakes	4			

480

Ry Krisp, Natural	6			
Siljans Knacke (Swedish Crispbread)	½			
"Sunshine" Krispy (soda crackers)	14			
Wasa Lite Rye	5			
Low-Fat Varieties: (average nutrient values)	(40 gm)	2	5	172
Soda crackers (most brands)	13			
Stoned Wheat Thins	6			
Ak Mak	7			
Melba Rounds	13			
Ry Krisp, Seasoned	6			
Carr's Table Water Crackers	12			
Bremner	17			
Pretzel Goldfish	60			
Harvest Crisps	18			
High-Fat Varieties: (average nutrient values)	(40 gm)	3	9	192
Wheat Thins	20			
Triscuits	9			
Ritz	12			
Chicken in a Biskit	20			
Most "party" varieties	12–20			
Pretzels	20 twists/ 1 cup sticks	(40 gm)	1	2	156

The abbreviation *tr.* stands for trace (less than (0.5); the symbol <1 stands for less than one (0.5 to 0.9). Recipes in **bold italics** can be found in Part III.

CHIPS, CRACKERS, AND POPCORN (continued)

	SERVING SIZE		CSI	FAT (GM)	CALORIES
POPCORN					
Air-popped (no fat)	3 cups	(18 gm)	tr.	<1	69
Air-popped (plus 1 teaspoon margarine)	3 cups	(23 gm)	<1	5	105
Microwave (selected brands):					
Redenbacher's Gourmet, Natural Flavor	3 cups	(28 gm)	<1	5	105
Betty Crocker Pop-Secret, Butter Flavor	3 cups	(28 gm)	1	8	140
Jolly Time, Natural Flavor	3 cups	(28 gm)	2	10	130
Cracker Jack	3 cups	(120 gm)	2	13	510
Commercially popped, plain- or cheese-flavored	3 cups	(28 gm)	5	6	116
Caramel corn	3 cups	(105 gm)	5	21	468
CHIPS					
Baked Corn Chips	2 cups	(57 gm)	<1	5	228
Pita Chips	2 cups	(45 gm)	tr.	1	268
Tortilla chips:					
fried in vegetable oil	2 cups	(57 gm)	2	12	282
fried in lard	2 cups	(57 gm)	5	12	282
fried in palm or coconut oil	2 cups	(57 gm)	10	12	282
Cheese puffs	2 cups	(34 gm)	3	12	190
Corn chips	2 cups	(70 gm)	4	22	370
Potato chips	2 cups	(53 gm)	5	19	277
Pork rinds	2 cups	(28 gm)	5	9	150
Pringles	2 cups	(50 gm)	6	22	295

MISCELLANEOUS

Party mix, low-fat (cereal, pretzels, few nuts, oil)	1 cup	(59 gm)	2	14	185
Party mix, typical (cereal, nuts, butter)	1 cup	(64 gm)	8	23	334
Trail mix, commercial (peanuts, sunflower seeds, raisins, carob)	1 cup	(150 gm)	6	39	704
Cornnuts	1 cup	(92 gm)	6	14	419

CHOCOLATE (BAKING)
(SELECT CSIs OF 5 OR LOWER PER SERVING)

BAKING CHIPS

Carob chips	1 cup	(170 gm)	5	10	695
Chocolate chips	1 cup	(170 gm)	36	60	898
Butterscotch chips	1 cup	(170 gm)	43	53	903

BAKING CHOCOLATE

Carob powder	¼ cup	(28 gm)	0	tr.	106
Cocoa powder, unsweetened	¼ cup	(28 gm)	4	7	84
Cocoa powder plus oil (to equal one ounce chocolate)	3 Tbsp. cocoa & 1 Tbsp. oil	(35 gm)	5	19	187
Chocolate, baking (sweet/German)	1 ounce	(28 gm)	6	10	148
Chocolate, baking (unsweetened)	1 ounce	(28 gm)	9	15	143

CHOCOLATE SAUCE

Syrup type (canned)	¼ cup	(76 gm)	<1	2	211
Fudge type	¼ cup	(76 gm)	7	10	251

The abbreviation tr. stands for trace (less than (0.5); the symbol <1 stands for less than one (0.5 to 0.9). Recipes in **bold italics** can be found in Part III.

DESSERTS: CAKES
(SELECT CSIs OF 5 OR LOWER PER SERVING)

	SERVING SIZE	CSI	FAT (GM)	CALORIES
CARROT CAKES, FROSTED				
Carrot-Raisin Cake with Penuche Frosting	(112 gm)	<1	4	271
Party Carrot Cake (smaller piece)	(81 gm)	2	6	224
Party Carrot Cake (larger piece)	(161 gm)	3	12	449
Carrot cake, typical	(197 gm)	14	29	662
APPLE CAKES, UNFROSTED				
Pinto Fiesta Cake	1/16 of cake	<1	5	182
Apple Loaf Cake (smaller piece)	1/24 of cake	<1	6	179
Apple Loaf Cake (larger piece)	1/12 of cake	2	11	359
Apple cake, typical	1/12 of cake	6	23	457
CHIFFON-TYPE CAKES, UNFROSTED				
Angel food cake, plain	1/10 of cake	0	0	170
Angel Quickie (chocolate angel food)	1/10 of cake	<1	1	186
Chiffon	1/10 of cake	9	14	336
Sponge	1/10 of cake	12	4	279
PUDDING CAKES, UNFROSTED				
Hot Fudge Pudding Cake	3" x 3"	1	5	259
White pudding cake, typical	3" x 3"	3	9	238

Description	Serving	Weight			
Yellow, chocolate, spice, or apple-sauce pudding cake, typical	3" x 3"	(82 gm)	7	10	254
ZUCCHINI CAKES, UNFROSTED					
Chocolate Zucchini Cake (smaller piece)	1/24 of cake	(51 gm)	<1	5	142
Chocolate Zucchini Cake (larger piece)	1/2 of cake	(101 gm)	2	10	284
Zucchini cake, typical	1/2 of cake	(85 gm)	6	9	285
POUND CAKES					
***Poppyseed Cake* (glazed)**	5" x 3" x 1/2"	(62 gm)	1	7	180
Pound cake, typical (unglazed)	5" x 3" x 1/2"	(42 gm)	7	9	178
Chocolate, typical (unglazed)	5" x 3" x 1/2"	(53 gm)	9	13	250
JELLY ROLL CAKES					
All flavors except chocolate (jelly filling)	4" diameter, 1" thick	(71 gm)	4	1	198
Chocolate (cream filling)	4" diameter, 1" thick	(56 gm)	9	7	192
CHOCOLATE CAKES					
Cocoa Cake (unfrosted)	3" x 3" x 2"	(50 gm)	1	5	205
Cocoa Cake (seven minute frosting)	3" x 3" x 2"	(69 gm)	1	5	254
Cocoa Cake (Cocoa frosting)	3" x 3" x 2"	(82 gm)	2	9	331
Chocolate cake, typical (seven minute frosting)	3" x 3" x 2"	(100 gm)	5	7	271
Chocolate cake, typical (Chocolate fudge frosting)	3" x 3" x 2"	(115 gm)	8	12	346

The abbreviation *tr.* stands for trace (less than (0.5); the symbol <1 stands for less than one (0.5 to 0.9). Recipes in **bold italics** can be found in Part III.

DESSERTS: CAKES (continued)

	SERVING SIZE		CSI	FAT (GM)	CALORIES
Devil's Food, typical (Seven Minute frosting)	3" x 3" x 2"	(107 gm)	10	15	378
Devil's Food, typical (Chocolate fudge frosting)	3" x 3" x 2"	(122 gm)	13	19	453
German chocolate (frosted)	3" x 3" x 2"	(118 gm)	17	24	472
SPICE-TYPE CAKES					
Depression Cake	3" x 3" x 2"	(73 gm)	<1	4	263
Spice-cake, typical (unfrosted)	3" x 3" x 2"	(83 gm)	4	6	203
Gingerbread, typical	3" x 3" x 2"	(117 gm)	7	12	330
WHITE CAKES					
From mix with water, egg whites (Cocoa frosting)	3" x 3" x 2"	(120 gm)	3	9	319
From mix with water, egg whites (Chocolate fudge frosting)	3" x 3" x 2"	(122 gm)	5	10	317
Homemade with milk and butter (Chocolate fudge frosting)	3" x 3" x 2"	(119 gm)	8	14	380
CHEESECAKES					
"Royal" No-bake Cheesecake Mix made with skim milk	1/8	(100 gm)	3	10	270
made with whole milk	1/8	(100 gm)	4	12	280
Ricotta Cheesecake	1/12 of 10"	(116 gm)	4	7	211
Crème de Menthe Cheesecake	1/12 of 10"	(106 gm)	5	8	210
Cheesecake, typical	1/12 of 10"	(110 gm)	22	25	355
SHORTCAKES					
All-Season Shortcake	3" x 3"	(242 gm)	1	3	292

	Portion	Weight	CSI	Fat (gm)	Cal
Red-headed Shortcake	2½" x 2½"	(206 gm)	2	7	241
Strawberry Shortcake, typical	⅙ of 8"	(286 gm)	19	31	616
OTHERS					
New and Improved Baked Alaska	1/10 recipe	(71 gm)	tr.	tr.	156
Baba au Rhum	1/24 of cake	(67 gm)	<1	3	190
Trifle (pound cake, fruit, jam, custard)	½ cup	(130 gm)	14	20	290
Fruitcake, typical	3" x 3" x 2"	(221 gm)	17	30	769

DESSERTS: COOKIES AND BARS
(SELECT CSIs OF 3 OR LOWER PER SERVING)

	Portion	Weight	CSI	Fat (gm)	Cal
HOMEMADE COOKIES					
Modified:					
Forgotten Kisses	3 cookies	(21 gm)	tr.	2	70
Lace Cookies	3 cookies	(14 gm)	tr.	2	60
Lebkuchen	2 cookies	(36 gm)	tr.	1	115
Gingies	1 large	(33 gm)	tr.	2	110
Carob	2 large	(41 gm)	1	8	166
Crispy Spice	3 large	(44 gm)	1	8	187
Oatmeal	2 medium	(24 gm)	1	5	124
Typical:					
Oatmeal	2 cookies	(53 gm)	2	9	186

The abbreviation *tr.* stands for trace (less than 0.5); the symbol <1 stands for less than one (0.5 to 0.9). Recipes in **bold italics** can be found in Part III.

DESSERTS: COOKIES AND BARS (*continued*)

	SERVING SIZE		CSI	FAT (GM)	CALORIES
Peanut butter	2 cookies	(37 gm)	4	9	166
Sugar	2 cookies	(33 gm)	4	6	134
Chocolate chip	2 cookies	(40 gm)	6	11	186
COMMERCIAL COOKIES					
Fortune cookies	3 cookies	(23 gm)	1	2	103
Gingersnaps	Six 2"	(42 gm)	2	4	176
Animal	16 small	(43 gm)	2	4	181
Graham crackers	6 squares	(42 gm)	2	4	176
Vanilla wafers	Twelve 1½"	(45 gm)	3	4	189
Fig bars	Three 1½"	(47 gm)	3	4	197
Pecan shortbread	Three 2"	(43 gm)	4	10	204
Oatmeal	Three 3"	(41 gm)	4	10	204
Oreos	Four 2"	(44 gm)	5	10	219
Chocolate chip	Four 2"	(44 gm)	5	10	219
Chocolate chip, typical deli	One 3¼"	(58 gm)	6	13	289
Chocolate chip, giant size	One 5¼"	(128 gm)	14	30	637
BAR COOKIES					
Brownies:					
Jamocha Squares	2" x 2"	(28 gm)	<1	4	103
Butterscotch Brownies	2" x 2½"	(39 gm)	<1	5	133
Brownies	2½" x 2½"	(41 gm)	1	5	133
Cocoa Cake, unfrosted	3" x 3"	(50 gm)	1	5	205

	Size	Weight			
Brownies from mix, unfrosted (with oil, no nuts, egg whites)	3" x 3"	(76 gm)	1	8	294
Brownies from scratch, unfrosted (with shortening, egg whites, chocolate, nuts)	3" x 3"	(124 gm)	8	30	519
Brownies, typical, unfrosted (with shortening, chocolate, nuts, whole eggs)	3" x 3"	(124 gm)	15	33	543
Brownies, typical, frosted	3" x 3"	(169 gm)	20	42	721
Chocolate Banana Bars	2" x 2¼"	(35 gm)	tr.	1	86
Apricot Meringue Bars	2" x 2"	(26 gm)	<1	3	91
Northwest Harvest Bars	2¼" x 2¼"	(42 gm)	<1	3	102
Molasses Orange Bars	2" x 2"	(58 gm)	<1	4	123
PB & J Bars	1½" x 2¼"	(24 gm)	<1	4	106
Rice Krispie bar, no chocolate	3" x 3"	(21 gm)	<1	4	98
Rice Krispie bar, with chocolate	3" x 3"	(50 gm)	5	11	228
Date bar, typical	2" x 2"	(59 gm)	3	6	188
Pumpkin bar, typical	2" x 2"	(47 gm)	5	8	164
Lemon bar, typical	2" x 2"	(37 gm)	6	6	140
Walnut Squares	1½" x 1½"	(14 gm)	tr.	1	40
Baklava	2" x 2"	(78 gm)	8	29	428

The abbreviation *tr.* stands for trace (less than 0.5); the symbol <1 stands for less than one (0.5 to 0.9). Recipes in ***bold italics*** can be found in Part III.

DESSERTS: FRUIT
(SELECT CSIs OR 1 OR LOWER PER SERVING)

	SERVING SIZE		CSI	FAT (GM)	CALORIES
Baked Apples	1 apple	(145 gm)	tr.	<1	125
Bananas en Papillote	1 banana	(128 gm)	tr.	<1	127
Berry Pavlova	3" x 3"	(114 gm)	tr.	<1	97
Berry Pavlova, typical	3" x 3¼"	(147 gm)	10	13	294
Fruit-Filled Dessert Cups	¼ recipe	(109 gm)	tr.	tr.	130
Fruit Salad Alaska	¼ recipe	(223 gm)	tr.	<1	164
Peach Cardinal	1 peach	(174 gm)	tr.	tr.	160
Peach and Berry Meringues	¼ recipe	(166 gm)	tr.	tr.	143
Pears in Wine	1 pear	(204 gm)	tr.	3	244
Apple Strudel	⅙ recipe	(64 gm)	tr.	2	133
Cherry Strudel	⅙ recipe	(76 gm)	tr.	2	148
Toasted Bananas	1/12 recipe	(125 gm)	1	4	226

490

DESSERTS: ICE CREAM AND OTHER FROZEN DESSERTS
(SELECT CSIs OF 3 OR LOWER PER CUP)

Soft-serve sorbet (Vitari)	1 cup	(153 gm)	0	0	160
Cranberry Sherbet	1 cup	(160 gm)	0	tr.	162
Sno-cone, Slushie, fruit ice, sorbet	1 cup	(193 gm)	0	0	255
Strawberry Ice	1 cup	(190 gm)	0	<1	240
Frozen yogurt, nonfat	1 cup	(184 gm)	tr.	tr.	224
Pumpkin Frozen Yogurt	1 cup	(234 gm)	tr.	tr.	208
Lite Lite Tofutti	1 cup	(238 gm)	<1	<1	180
Low, Lite 'n' Luscious (Baskin-Robbins)	1 cup	(208 gm)	2	3	214
Frozen yogurt, low-fat	1 cup	(150 gm)	3	4	227
Sherbet	1 cup	(193 gm)	3	4	270
Tofutti*	1 cup	(170 gm)	3	24	420
Ice Milk, typical soft-serve	1 cup	(175 gm)	4	5	224
Mocha Mix Frozen Dessert*	1 cup	(158 gm)	4	14	280
Frozen yogurt, cream added	1 cup	(167 gm)	6	7	240
Light ice cream (ice milk)	1 cup	(150 gm)	6	8	236
Ice cream, store brands (10% fat)	1 cup	(163 gm)	15	18	329
Ice cream, rich (12% fat)	1 cup	(208 gm)	19	24	480
Ice cream, extra rich (18% fat)	1 cup	(208 gm)	30	38	580
Popsicle	One	(75 gm)	0	0	99
Fudgesicle	One	(73 gm)	tr.	tr.	91

* Made with vegetable oil instead of butterfat.

The abbreviation *tr.* stands for trace (less than 0.5); the symbol <1 stands for less than one (0.5 to 0.9). Recipes in **bold italics** can be found in Part III.

491

DESSERTS: ICE CREAM AND OTHER FROZEN DESSERTS (continued)

	SERVING SIZE		CSI	FAT (GM)	CALORIES
Jell-O Pudding Pops	One	(1.8 fl. oz.)	2	2	80
Dreamsicle	One	(66 gm)	2	3	104
Ice cream sandwich	One	(62 gm)	4	5	173
Drumstick, Nutti-Buddie	One	(61 gm)	6	10	189
Ice cream bar (chocolate covered)	One	(85 gm)	12	13	224
Ice cream cone (cone only)	One	(12 gm)	tr.	tr.	45

DESSERTS: PIES AND COBBLERS
(SELECT CSIs OF 2 OR LOWER PER SERVING)

FILLING & CRUSTS

Fruit/Nut:			CSI	FAT (GM)	CALORIES
Swedish Pie	⅛ of recipe	(51 gm)	tr.	2	130
Cranberry Squares	¹⁄₁₂ of recipe	(46 gm)	tr.	3	125
Upside-Down Peach Cobbler	⅙ of recipe	(147 gm)	<1	4	226
Berry Cobbler	⅙ of recipe	(170 gm)	<1	5	233
Apple Crisp (crumb topping)	⅙ of recipe	(99 gm)	<1	4	153
Peach Almond Crisp	⅙ of recipe	(174 gm)	<1	5	158
Apple or cherry cobbler (biscuit topping)	1 cup	(144 gm)	2	8	272
Glazed fruit pie (single crust)	⅙ of 9"	(165 gm)	5	12	309

	Serving	Weight			
Mincemeat pie (single crust)	1/6 of 9"	(147 gm)	6	13	330
Fruit pie (double crust)	1/6 of 9"	(181 gm)	11	27	504
Pecan pie (single crust)	1/6 of 9"	(156 gm)	15	41	682
Cream:					
Berry Yogurt Pie (graham cracker crust)	1/8 of 9"	(151 gm)	1	4	196
Pumpkin Pie (graham cracker crust)	1/6 of 9"	(220 gm)	1	5	327
Pumpkin pie (single crust)	1/6 of 9"	(220 gm)	14	19	418
Lemon meringue pie (single crust)	1/6 of 9"	(178 gm)	14	20	452
Custard pie (single crust)	1/6 of 9"	(154 gm)	15	18	345
Banana cream pie (single crust)	1/6 of 9"	(173 gm)	20	26	447
Grasshopper pie (single crumb crust)	1/6 of 9"	(182 gm)	22	35	575
Chocolate cream pie (single crust)	1/6 of 9"	(192 gm)	23	30	491
Coconut cream pie (single crust)	1/6 of 9"	(179 gm)	25	29	455
PIE CRUSTS (SINGLE)					
Meringue	3"	(24 gm)	0	0	70
Graham cracker:					
Graham Cracker Crust	1/6 of 9"	(36 gm)	1	5	142
Commercial	1/6 of 9"	(45 gm)	6	15	237
Conventional:					
Made with oil	1/6 of 9"	(34 gm)	2	12	184
Made with shortening	1/6 of 9"	(33 gm)	4	14	189
Commercial	1/6 of 9"	(34 gm)	5	12	173
Made with lard	1/6 of 9"	(31 gm)	5	12	172

The abbreviation *tr.* stands for trace (less than 0.5); the symbol <1 stands for less than one (0.5 to 0.9). Recipes in **bold italics** can be found in Part III.

DESSERTS: PIES AND COBBLERS (*continued*)

	SERVING SIZE		CSI	FAT (GM)	CALORIES
Made with whole eggs	⅙ of 9"	(40 gm)	8	14	212
Chocolate Crumb	⅙ of 9"	(33 gm)	7	16	198
TURNOVERS AND TARTS					
Apple Strudel	⅙ recipe	(64 gm)	tr.	2	133
Cherry Strudel	⅙ recipe	(76 gm)	tr.	2	148
Turnover, fruit-filled, commercial	5" folded	(64 gm)	5	19	229
Pie tart, commercial	One	(86 gm)	7	15	275

DESSERTS: PUDDINGS
(SELECT CSIs OF 2 OR LOWER PER SERVING)

			CSI	FAT (GM)	CALORIES
PUDDINGS FROM MIXES					
All flavors (with skim milk)	1 cup	(260 gm)	<1	1	251
All flavors (with whole milk)	1 cup	(260 gm)	6	8	307
PUDDINGS, HOMEMADE					
Chocolate Pudding	1 cup	(210 gm)	<1	<1	230
Lemon	1 cup	(200 gm)	4	2	114
Tapioca	1 cup	(200 gm)	15	9	255
Rice	1 cup	(265 gm)	17	11	365

BREAD PUDDINGS

Pumpkin Bread	1 cup	(300 gm)	<1	2	367
Bread pudding, typical	1 cup	(265 gm)	16	16	441

OTHER PUDDINGS

Gelatin, flavored (low-sugar)	1 cup	(240 gm)	0	0	16
Gelatin, flavored (Jell-O)	1 cup	(240 gm)	0	0	142
Pudding Pops	One	(52 gm)	2	2	80
Chocolate soufflé	1 cup	(59 gm)	8	8	127
Custard, baked	1 cup	(281 gm)	22	14	300
Chiffon, all flavors	1 cup	(165 gm)	25	12	414
Plum pudding	1 cup	(230 gm)	30	47	895
Chocolate mousse	1 cup	(191 gm)	33	31	380
Bavarian cream	1 cup	(152 gm)	37	35	388

DESSERTS: SAUCES
(SELECT CSIs OF 1 OR LOWER PER SERVING)

Yogurt Dessert Sauce	¼ cup	(64 gm)	<1	<1	61
Custard sauce	¼ cup	(68 gm)	9	5	93
Caramel or butterscotch (flavored sauce)	¼ cup	(85 gm)	0	0	264

The abbreviation *tr.* stands for trace (less than [0.5]); the symbol <1 stands for less than one (0.5 to 0.9). Recipes in *bold italics* can be found in Part III.

DESSERTS: SAUCES (*continued*)

	SERVING SIZE		CSI	FAT (GM)	CALORIES
Caramel (homemade)	¼ cup	(82 gm)	2	7	291
Chocolate sauce (syrup type)	¼ cup	(76 gm)	<1	2	211
Chocolate sauce (fudge type)	¼ cup	(76 gm)	7	10	251
Fresh Rhubarb Sauce	¼ cup	(69 gm)	tr.	tr.	50
Strawberry or Raspberry Sauce	¼ cup	(44 gm)	0	tr.	31

EGGS AND EGG DISHES
(*SELECT CSIs OF 2 OR LOWER PER SERVING*)

EGGS			CSI	FAT (GM)	CALORIES
Whites	Two	(66 gm)	0	0	32
Whole	One	(50 gm)	12	6	79
Yolks	Two	(34 gm)	25	11	125

EGG SUBSTITUTES					
Egg Beaters	¼ cup	(60 gm)	0	0	30
Second Nature	¼ cup	(60 gm)	0	2	49
Scramblers	¼ cup	(60 gm)	0	4	68
Homemade Egg Substitute	¼ cup	(60 gm)	<1	4	70

EGG DISHES

Scrambled whites	½ cup	(99 gm)	0	0	48
Scrambled egg substitute	½ cup	(114 gm)	2	8	127
Scrambled eggs, typical	½ cup, 2 eggs	(124 gm)	27	20	244
Egg McMuffin	One	(138 gm)	16	16	340
Sausage McMuffin with egg	One	(165 gm)	24	33	517
Egg, poached or fried with margarine	One	(55 gm)	13	9	113
Spanish Omelet	⅙ recipe	(183 gm)	tr.	1	93
Vegetable Frittata	½ recipe	(272 gm)	2	7	232
Egg omelet, plain	2 eggs	(128 gm)	27	20	244
Egg omelet, cheese	2 eggs	(154 gm)	34	28	349
Egg omelet, ham & cheese	2 eggs	(190 gm)	36	32	413
Deviled egg, made with *"Egg" Salad Sandwich Spread*	½ egg white, 2 teaspoons filling	(26 gm)	tr.	tr.	17
Deviled egg, typical	½ egg	(28 gm)	8	6	65

EGG SANDWICHES

"Egg" Salad Sandwich Spread	½ cup	(105 gm)	<1	5	110
Tofu "Egg" Salad	½ cup	(75 gm)	<1	5	66
Egg salad (with mayonnaise)	½ cup	(111 gm)	24	23	252

The abbreviation *tr.* stands for trace (less than (0.5); the symbol <1 stands for less than one (0.5 to 0.9). Recipes in **bold italics** can be found in Part III.

FAST-FOOD DISHES

	SERVING SIZE		CSI	FAT (GM)	CALORIES
BREAKFAST					
English muffin (with butter)	One	(63 gm)	3	5	186
Hash brown potatoes	1 serving	(55 gm)	3	9	144
Hot cakes (with butter and syrup)	1 serving	(214 gm)	6	10	500
Danish:					
Raspberry	One	(117 gm)	5	16	414
Apple	One	(115 gm)	5	18	389
Cinnamon-raisin	One	(110 gm)	6	21	445
Iced cheese	One	(110 gm)	8	22	395
Biscuit:					
with spread	One	(85 gm)	8	18	330
with sausage	1 serving	(121 gm)	14	31	467
with bacon, egg, & cheese	1 serving	(145 gm)	23	32	483
with sausage & egg	1 serving	(175 gm)	29	40	585
Sausage, pork	1 serving	(53 gm)	9	19	210
Sausage McMuffin	1 serving	(138 gm)	13	26	427
Egg McMuffin	1 serving	(138 gm)	19	16	340
Sausage McMuffin with egg	1 serving	(165 gm)	27	33	517
Eggs, scrambled	1 serving	(98 gm)	31	13	180
SANDWICHES					
Chicken McNuggets	1 serving	(109 gm)	8	20	323
Filet o' Fish	1 sandwich	(143 gm)	8	26	435

Item	Serving	Weight			Calories
Hamburger	1 serving	(100 gm)	9	11	263
Cheeseburger	1 serving	(114 gm)	9	16	318
Quarter Pounder	1 serving	(160 gm)	13	24	427
Big Mac	1 serving	(200 gm)	16	35	570
Quarter Pounder, cheese	1 serving	(186 gm)	18	32	525
Mc DLT	1 serving	(254 gm)	20	44	680

SIDE ORDERS

Item	Serving	Weight			Calories
Soft-serve/cone	1 cone	(115 gm)	3	5	189

Sundae:

Item	Serving	Weight			Calories
strawberry	1 serving	(164 gm)	5	9	320
caramel	1 serving	(165 gm)	5	10	361
hot fudge	1 serving	(164 gm)	7	11	357
French fries	1 serving	(68 gm)	5	12	220
Apple pie	1 serving	(85 gm)	5	14	253
Cookies, McDonaldland	1 serving	(67 gm)	5	11	308
Choclaty Chip	1 serving	(69 gm)	9	16	342

Milk shake:

Item	Serving	Weight			Calories
vanilla	16 fl. ounces	(231 gm)	5	7	287
strawberry	16 fl. ounces	(231 gm)	5	7	279
chocolate	16 fl. ounces	(231 gm)	5	7	304

The abbreviation *tr.* stands for trace (less than (0.5); the symbol <1 stands for less than one (0.5 to 0.9). Recipes in **bold italics** can be found in Part III.

FATS AND SPREADS

OILS (SELECT CSIs OF 18 OR LOWER PER ½ CUP)

	SERVING SIZE		CSI	FAT (GM)	CALORIES
Rapeseed (Puritan-Canola)	½ cup	(109 gm)	9	109	981
Safflower (Saffola)	½ cup	(109 gm)	10	109	981
Walnut	½ cup	(109 gm)	10	109	981
Sunflower (Sunlite)	½ cup	(109 gm)	11	109	981
Corn (Mazola)	½ cup	(109 gm)	14	109	981
Olive	½ cup	(108 gm)	15	108	972
Sesame	½ cup	(109 gm)	16	109	981
Soybean (Crisco, My-te-Fine, Western Family, Wesson)	½ cup	(109 gm)	16	109	981
Cottonseed/Soybean Mix	½ cup	(109 gm)	17	109	981
Avocado	½ cup	(109 gm)	18	109	981
Peanut (Planter's)	½ cup	(108 gm)	18	108	972
Palm	½ cup	(109 gm)	54	109	981
Coconut	½ cup	(109 gm)	95	109	981

MARGARINE AND BUTTER (SELECT CSIs OF 15 OR LOWER PER ½ CUP, OR 0.7 OR LOWER PER TEASPOON)

	SERVING SIZE		CSI	FAT (GM)	CALORIES
Margarine, diet (40% fat, not recommended for baking)	½ cup	(115 gm)	7	45	400
Margarine, table spread (60% fat, Country Crock)	½ cup	(115 gm)	11	70	621
Margarine, liquid (squeeze type)	½ cup	(113 gm)	15	91	812

Food	Amount				
Margarine, tub or soft stick (Saffola, Mazola, Fleischmann's)	½ cup	(114 gm)	15	91	809
Margarine, hard stick (inexpensive store brands)	½ cup	(114 gm)	19	91	809
Butter	½ cup	(114 gm)	71	92	817
Margarine, diet (40% fat)	1 teaspoon	(5 gm)	0.3	2	17
Margarine, table spread (60% fat)	1 teaspoon	(5 gm)	0.5	3	27
Margarine, liquid (squeeze type)	1 teaspoon	(5 gm)	0.7	4	35
Margarine, tub or soft stick	1 teaspoon	(5 gm)	0.7	4	35
Margarine, hard stick (inexpensive store brands)	1 teaspoon	(5 gm)	0.8	4	35
Butter	1 teaspoon	(5 gm)	3.1	4	36
Peanut butter	1 tablespoon	(16 gm)	1.4	8	95

MAYONNAISE AND MIRACLE WHIP (SELECT CSIs OF 0.8 OR LOWER PER TABLESPOON)

Food	Amount				
Miracle Whip, Light Salad Dressing	1 tablespoon	(14 gm)	0.6	4	45
Miracle Whip Salad Dressing, Cholesterol-free	1 tablespoon	(14 gm)	1.1	7	70
Miracle Whip Salad Dressing, Regular	1 tablespoon	(14 gm)	1.3	7	70
Mayonnaise, Light (Heart Beat)	1 tablespoon	(14 gm)	0.5	4	40
Mayonnaise, Light (Best Foods, Kraft)	1 tablespoon	(14 gm)	0.8	5	50
Mayonnaise (Best Foods, Kraft, Saffola), Cholesterol-free	1 tablespoon	(14 gm)	1.7	11	101
Mayonnaise (Best Foods, Kraft, Saffola), Regular	1 tablespoon	(14 gm)	2.1	11	101

OTHER FATS (SELECT CSIs OF 26 OR LOWER PER ½ CUP)

Food	Amount				
Peanut Butter	½ cup	(129 gm)	11	66	762

The abbreviation *tr.* stands for trace (less than (0.5); the symbol <1 stands for less than one (0.5 to 0.9). Recipes in **bold italics** can be found in Part III.

FATS AND SPREADS (continued)

	SERVING SIZE		CSI	FAT (GM)	CALORIES
Shortening (Crisco)	½ cup	(103 gm)	26	103	927
Shortening (Fluffo, Snowdrift)	½ cup	(102 gm)	34	103	927
Bacon grease	½ cup	(102 gm)	40	103	927
Lard	½ cup	(102 gm)	46	102	918
Suet (beef fat)	½ cup	(102 gm)	55	102	869

FRUITS
(SELECT CSIs OF LESS THAN 1)

	SERVING SIZE		CSI	FAT (GM)	CALORIES
Fruits, most varieties:	1 medium piece, 1 cup melon or berries, ½ cup grapes, ½ cup canned fruit, ½ cup juice, ¼ cup dried	(100 gm)	tr.	tr.	60
Avocado	¼	(50 gm)	1	8	84
Olives, green	½ cup	(70 gm)	1	9	81
Olives, black	½ cup	(70 gm)	1	10	97
Coconut, raw	½ cup	(40 gm)	12	13	142

502

GRAINS (COOKED)
(SELECT CSIs OF 1 OR LOWER PER CUP)

RICE					
White	1 cup	(205 gm)	tr.	tr.	223
Brown	1 cup	(150 gm)	tr.	<1	179
Wild	1 cup	(212 gm)	tr.	<1	189
WHEAT					
Couscous	1 cup	(146 gm)	tr.	tr.	164
Bulgur	1 cup	(135 gm)	tr.	<1	227
Macaroni or spaghetti	1 cup	(130 gm)	tr.	<1	192
Lasagna or manicotti noodles	1 cup	(87 gm)	tr.	tr.	129
Egg noodles	1 cup	(160 gm)	3	2	200
MISCELLANEOUS					
Barley	1 cup	(150 gm)	tr.	<1	203
Millet	1 cup	(135 gm)	tr.	2	262
Chow mein noodles	1 cup	(45 gm)	4	11	220
FLOUR					
Wheat, white	1 cup	(115 gm)	tr.	1	419
Whole wheat	1 cup	(120 gm)	tr.	2	400
Rye	1 cup	(88 gm)	tr.	2	308
Cornmeal	1 cup	(138 gm)	tr.	2	491

The abbreviation *tr.* stands for trace (less than (0.5); the symbol <1 stands for less than one (0.5 to 0.9). Recipes in **bold italics** can be found in Part III.

MAIN ENTRÉES: ASIAN DISHES
(SELECT CSIs OF 9 OR LOWER PER SERVING)

	SERVING SIZE		CSI	FAT (GM)	CALORIES
Beef-Tomato Chow Yuk	1½ cups	(270 gm)	3	7	211
Beef Broccoli Oriental	¼ recipe	(230 gm)	7	11	251
CHOW MEIN DISHES					
Pinto Bean Chow Mein	1 cup	(156 gm)	tr.	2	96
Bean Sprout Tuna Chow Mein	1 cup	(134 gm)	1	3	91
Chicken chow mein, typical	1 cup	(69 gm)	4	9	224
Pork chow mein, typical	1 cup	(69 gm)	7	15	270
Stir-Fried Mushrooms and Broccoli	⅛ recipe	(101 gm)	<1	3	69
"Fire" on Rice	1 cup	(200 gm)	2	11	176
Turkey Lettuce Stir-Fry	¼ recipe	(185 gm)	2	5	147
Cashew Chicken	1¾ cups	(288 gm)	4	10	242
Spicy Chicken with Peppers	⅙ recipe (2 pieces)	(245 gm)	5	8	221
Zesty Stir-Fried Chicken	¼ recipe	(315 gm)	5	9	266
Thai Barbecued Chicken	⅙ recipe	(133 gm)	5	5	191
Seafood Teriyaki and Kabobs	¼ recipe	(183 gm)	6	3	258
Wonderful Oriental Steamed Fish	¼ recipe	(326 gm)	7	4	268
Peppers and Prawns	¼ recipe	(200 gm)	9	5	174
Egg foo Yong	1 serving	(78 gm)	10	12	131
Tempura	6 prawns	(124 gm)	14	14	272

Food	Serving	(gm)			
Fried rice	1 cup	(260 gm)	18	14	338
Chinese Noodles	2¼ cups	(338 gm)	tr.	3	192
Top Raamen	1 cup	(227 gm)	2	8	161

MAIN ENTRÉES: BEEF AND PORK DISHES
(SELECT CSIs OF 9 OR LOWER PER SERVING)

Food	Serving	(gm)			
Beef Stroganoff	1 cup	(185 gm)	6	10	242
Beef stroganoff, typical	1 cup	(242 gm)	27	44	571
Beef and Bean Ragout	1 cup	(243 gm)	2	3	168
Bean Hot Dish	1 cup	(186 gm)	2	3	231
Stay-Abed Stew	1 cup	(190 gm)	2	2	121
Beef vegetable stew	1 cup	(245 gm)	8	14	246
Cabbage Roll with rice and tofu	1 roll	(130 gm)	tr.	<1	80
Cabbage roll with rice and cheese	1 roll	(87 gm)	3	8	117
Cabbage roll with ground beef and rice	1 roll	(139 gm)	5	9	176
Black Bean Chili	1 cup	(244 gm)	<1	4	277
Rick's Chili	1 cup	(215 gm)	<1	3	126
Chicken chili with beans	1 cup	(213 gm)	1	4	190
Rose Bowl Chili	1 cup	(267 gm)	2	5	213
Chili con carne with beans	1 cup	(255 gm)	8	14	282

The abbreviation *tr.* stands for trace (less than (0.5); the symbol <1 stands for less than one (0.5 to 0.9). Recipes in **bold italics** can be found in Part III.

MAIN ENTRÉES: BEEF AND PORK DISHES (continued)

	SERVING SIZE	CSI	FAT (GM)	CALORIES
Chili con carne without beans	1 cup (255 gm)	11	18	282
Pizza Rice Casserole	1 cup (144 gm)	3	3	137
Hamburger Helper with ground beef	1 cup (231 gm)	11	18	356
Hamburger rice casserole	1 cup (240 gm)	12	24	385
Meat loaf, 10% fat ground beef, egg white (smaller piece)	1 thin slice (2½" x 5" x ¾") (101 gm)	3	4	126
Old-Fashioned Meat Loaf	⅙ recipe (130 gm)	4	6	195
Meat loaf, 10% fat ground beef, egg white (larger piece)	1 slice (2½" x 5" x 1½") (202 gm)	7	7	253
Meat loaf, typical	1 slice (2½" x 5" x 1½") (199 gm)	17	25	391
Pepper Steak	¼ recipe (199 gm)	5	7	217
Juicy Flank Steak	⅙ recipe (76 gm)	6	8	188
Stuffed Flank Steak Florentine	⅛ recipe (3 oz. cooked meat) (243 gm)	8	10	281
HAMBURGERS				
Very Skinny Burgers	One (156 gm)	5	10	288
Skinny Burgers	One (212 gm)	8	15	375
''Hamburger'' (typical, at home): 5 oz. (cooked) ground beef (30% fat), 1 Tbsp. ketchup, 3 slices dill pickle, 1 Tbsp. mayonnaise, lettuce, tomato, onion, bun	One (236 gm)	25	50	763
Quarter Pounder	One (160 gm)	13	24	427
Quarter Pounder, cheese	One (186 gm)	18	32	525
Pork Chops Dijon	⅙ recipe (112 gm)	7	10	199

MAIN ENTRÉES: CHICKEN AND TURKEY DISHES
(SELECT CSIs OF 9 OR LOWER PER SERVING)

Dish	Serving	Weight	CSI	Fat (gm)	Calories
Chicken Cacciatore	1 breast	(228 gm)	4	6	222
Chicken cacciatore, typical	1 breast	(222 gm)	8	16	298
Carmen's Curry	⅙ recipe	(433 gm)	5	6	293
Curried Chicken Quickie	⅙ recipe	(269 gm)	3	4	415
Chicken rice casserole	⅙ recipe (1 cup)	(242 gm)	10	16	311
Chicken Parmesan	¼ recipe (1 piece)	(100 gm)	6	6	205
Parmesan Yogurt Chicken	⅙ recipe (2 pieces)	(155 gm)	7	10	235
Parmesan chicken	⅙ recipe (2 pieces)	(222 gm)	18	47	606
Cashew Chicken	¼ recipe	(288 gm)	4	10	242
Chicken in Pastry	¼ recipe	(161 gm)	5	10	314
Zesty Stir-Fried Chicken	¼ recipe	(315 gm)	5	9	266
Spicy Chicken with Peppers	⅙ recipe (2 pieces)	(245 gm)	5	8	221
Garlic Chicken with Balsamic Vinegar	¼ recipe (1 piece)	(209 gm)	5	7	220
Chicken with Apricot-Wine Glaze	⅙ recipe (1 piece)	(166 gm)	5	5	270
Chicken Paprika	⅙ recipe (1 piece)	(188 gm)	5	6	214
Chicken Broccoli Roll-Ups	¼ recipe	(221 gm)	6	5	195

The abbreviation *tr.* stands for trace (less than (0.5); the symbol <1 stands for less than one (0.5 to 0.9). Recipes in **bold italics** can be found in Part III.

507

MAIN ENTRÉES: CHICKEN AND TURKEY DISHES (continued)

	SERVING SIZE		CSI	FAT (GM)	CALORIES
Oven-Fried Chicken	2 pieces	(139 gm)	5	6	173
Portland Fried Chicken	2 pieces	(139 gm)	5	5	187
Chicken McNuggets	8 pieces	(146 gm)	11	27	433
Chicken, fried, typical	2 pieces	(177 gm)	11	17	335
Chicken, Kentucky Fried	2 pieces	(232 gm)	11	23	431
Curried Chicken and Peanut Salad	1⅔ cups	(204 gm)	3	8	198
Chicken Salad with Yogurt-Chive Dressing	1 cup	(314 gm)	5	5	252
Chicken salad, with mayonnaise	1 cup	(209 gm)	17	64	705
Thai Barbecued Chicken	2 pieces	(133 gm)	5	5	191
Barbecued chicken (no skin)	2 pieces	(147 gm)	6	7	230
Barbecued chicken (with skin)	2 pieces	(176 gm)	9	16	334
Turkey-Vegetable Chowder	2 cups	(418 gm)	3	7	280
Mulligatawny Stew	1 cup	(244 gm)	3	5	174
Rose Bowl Chili	1 cup	(267 gm)	2	5	213
Sesame Linguini with Chicken	1½ cups	(256 gm)	2	5	311
Turkey Tetrazzini	⅙ recipe	(353 gm)	4	8	422
Poppyseed and Turkey Casserole	¼ recipe	(302 gm)	8	9	344
Chicken Fajitas with Lime	One	(191 gm)	4	9	297
Chicken Fajitas Spicy-Style	One	(253 gm)	4	8	290
Chicken Marbella	⅙ recipe	(218 gm)	5	9	289

MAIN ENTRÉES: FISH AND SHELLFISH DISHES
(SELECT CSIs OF 9 OR LOWER PER SERVING)

Poached	6 ounces	(170 gm)	5	5	2	141
Baked:						
Baked Herbed Fish	7 ounces	(205 gm)	5	5	5	189
Baked Salmon (3 ounces cooked)	3 ounces	(86 gm)		7	11	185
Baked fish with butter	7 ounces	(193 gm)		14	13	246
Fish sticks, commercial	Six	(227 gm)		14	29	405
Broiled or charcoal grilled: no fat added	6 ounces	(170 gm)		5	2	141
Broiled or charcoal grilled: with butter added	6½ ounces	(184 gm)		14	13	241
Skinny Sole	7 ounces	(202 gm)		7	11	303
Panfried	8 ounces	(229 gm)		14	20	420
Deep-fried (batter coated)	11 ounces	(320 gm)		21	52	725
Fish Almondine with Dilly Sauce (6 ounces cooked fish)	9 ounces	(263 gm)		7	8	248
Fish almondine with dilly sauce (6 ounces cooked fish), typical	10½ ounces	(299 gm)		20	44	566
Fancy Baked Scallops	¼ recipe	(280 gm)		5	8	226
Baked Scallops with Feta Cheese	¼ recipe	(320 gm)		15	24	453
Scallops in Creamy Sauce (3 ounces cooked scallops)	6 ounces	(181 gm)		4	6	218
Coquilles St. Jacques (3 ounces cooked scallops)	9 ounces	(252 gm)		34	41	528

The abbreviation tr. stands for trace (less than 0.5); the symbol <1 stands for less than one (0.5 to 0.9). Recipes in **bold italics** can be found in Part III.

MAIN ENTRÉES: FISH AND SHELLFISH DISHES (continued)

	SERVING SIZE		CSI	FAT (GM)	CALORIES
Tuna Noodle Casserole	2 cups	(344 gm)	2	4	292
Tuna noodle casserole, typical	2 cups	(480 gm)	10	30	642
Salmon Loaf	One ¾" slice	(72 gm)	1	4	87
Salmon loaf, typical	One ½" slice	(115 gm)	8	11	212
Salmon Mousse	½ cup	(94 gm)	3	7	140
Salmon mousse, typical	½ cup	(91 gm)	6	19	218
Fish and Leek Chowder	1 cup	(240 gm)	2	2	142
Bouillabaisse	1½ cups	(285 gm)	3	3	123
Northwest Gumbo	2½ cups	(635 gm)	6	5	418
Cioppino	2¼ cups	(529 gm)	8	7	299
Seafood Pilaf	1 cup	(240 gm)	4	3	209
Seafood Strudel	⅙ recipe	(158 gm)	4	6	232
Peppered Salmon Steak	¼ recipe	(135 gm)	5	10	251
Sole with Spring Vegetables	¼ recipe	(241 gm)	5	3	184
Fish à la Mistral	¼ recipe	(324 gm)	6	5	203
Fish Fillets with Walnuts	¼ recipe	(252 gm)	7	11	246
Halibut Mexicana	¼ recipe	(293 gm)	7	6	259
Halibut and Vegetables	¼ recipe	(259 gm)	7	10	289
Lively Lemon Roll-ups	⅙ recipe	(362 gm)	7	6	281
Wonderful Oriental Steamed Fish	¼ recipe	(326 gm)	7	4	268
Oysters Sauté	½ recipe	(229 gm)	7	7	173
Peppers and Prawns	¼ recipe	(200 gm)	9	5	174
Oysters in Crusty French Bread	½ recipe	(318 gm)	9	10	527

MAIN ENTRÉES: INDIAN DISHES
(SELECT CSIs OF 9 OR LOWER PER SERVING)

Curried Chicken Quickie	⅙ recipe	(269 gm)	3	4	415
Chicken rice casserole	⅙ recipe (1 cup)	(242 gm)	10	16	311
Carmen's Curry	⅙ recipe	(433 gm)	5	6	293
Vegetable Pulav	¼ recipe	(349 gm)	1	6	389
Pulihora (tamarind rice)	1 cup	(142 gm)	<1	5	264
Spicy Lentils	1 cup	(201 gm)	<1	4	137

MAIN ENTRÉES: MEXICAN DISHES
(SELECT CSIs OF 9 OR LOWER PER SERVING)

ENCHILADAS

Acapulco Enchilada	One 6"	(177 gm)	3	5	193
Creamy Enchilada	One 6"	(196 gm)	3	4	179
No-Meat enchilada	One 6"	(131 gm)	4	7	202
Chicken enchilada	One 6"	114 (gm)	7	10	197
Beef enchilada	One 6"	(114 gm)	9	15	234
Cheese enchilada	One 6"	(114 gm)	12	17	256

The abbreviation *tr.* stands for trace (less than (0.5); the symbol <1 stands for less than one (0.5 to 0.9). Recipes in **bold italics** can be found in Part III.

MAIN ENTRÉES: MEXICAN DISHES (*continued*)

	SERVING SIZE	CSI	FAT (GM)	CALORIES
BURRITOS (NOT DEEP-FRIED)				
Burritos with Black Beans	One (217 gm)	2	4	242
Your Basic Bean Burrito	One 8" (202 gm)	2	5	269
Baked Burrito Squares	One (149 gm)	4	8	298
Bean burrito	One 8" (161 gm)	7	16	384
Beef burrito	One 8" (125 gm)	9	16	353
CHILE RELLENOS				
Chile Relleno Casserole	One chile (152 gm)	2	4	155
Chile relleno	One chile (110 gm)	19	21	267
SALADS				
Taco Salad	2 cups (261 gm)	4	8	252
Taco salad, typical	2 cups (212 gm)	15	25	336
CASSEROLES				
Tamale Pie	1 cup (276 gm)	3	4	205
Acapulco Bean Casserole	1 cup (201 gm)	5	9	236
Tamale pie, typical	1 cup (286 gm)	16	28	441
SIDE DISHES				
Black Beans with 1,000 Uses	1 cup (212 gm)	tr.	tr.	126
Refried Beans	1 cup (174 gm)	1	6	225
Refried beans (canned)	1 cup (241 gm)	1	4	248
Refried beans, typical	1 cup (243 gm)	12	28	485

FISH

Halibut Mexicana	6 oz. fish	(293 gm)	7	6	259

FAJITAS

Chicken Fajitas with Lime	One	(191 gm)	4	9	297
Chicken Fajitas Spicy-Style	One	(253 gm)	4	8	290

MAIN ENTRÉES: PASTA DISHES
(SPAGHETTI, MACARONI, NOODLES)
(SELECT CSIs OF 9 OR LOWER PER SERVING)

GOULASH TYPE

Garbanzo Goulash	1 cup	(186 gm)	tr.	3	208
Texas Hash	1 cup	(240 gm)	1	3	170
Beef & macaroni casserole	1 cup	(240 gm)	9	19	328

LASAGNA

Bean Lasagna	3" x 3"	(224 gm)	3	5	220
Easy Oven Lasagna	3" x 3"	(321 gm)	3	6	185
Spinach Lasagna	3" x 3"	(245 gm)	3	6	223
Lasagna Primavera	3" x 3"	(221 gm)	4	7	240
Lasagna with meat sauce	3" x 3"	(235 gm)	14	19	390

The abbreviation *tr.* stands for trace (less than (0.5); the symbol <1 stands for less than one (0.5 to 0.9). Recipes in ***bold italics*** can be found in Part III.

MAIN ENTRÉES: PASTA DISHES (*continued*)

	SERVING SIZE		CSI	FAT (GM)	CALORIES
MACARONI & CHEESE					
Macaroni Bake	1 cup	(219 gm)	2	5	246
From packaged mix	1 cup	(209 gm)	6	18	401
Homemade (2% milk)	1 cup	(200 gm)	12	19	336
RAVIOLIS					
Homemade Ravioli (*Chicken*)	6 large, 12 small	(490 gm)	2	10	366
Ravioli, cheese (canned)	1 cup	(223 gm)	4	5	229
Ravioli, meat (canned)	1 cup	(223 gm)	5	7	240
Ravioli, cheese (homemade), with tomato sauce	6 large, 12 small	(131 gm)	10	11	216
Ravioli, meat (homemade), with tomato sauce	6 large, 12 small	(149 gm)	13	20	302
SALADS					
Montana Pasta Salad	1 cup	(196 gm)	<1	4	169
Four-Star Pasta Salad	1 cup	(137 gm)	<1	3	154
Macaroni (with mayonnaise)	1 cup	(184 gm)	7	36	510
STUFFED					
Cheese-Stuffed Manicotti	1 piece	(178 gm)	2	4	135
Manicotti with cheddar cheese	1 piece	(173 gm)	11	10	220
SPAGHETTI					
Spaghetti with *Marinara Sauce*	1½ cups	(302 gm)	tr.	3	251
Spaghetti with *Beef-Mushroom Spaghetti Sauce*	1½ cups	(235 gm)	1	2	267

Spaghetti with **Turkey-Mushroom Spaghetti Sauce**	1½ cups	(250 gm)	1	2	266
Spaghetti with **Light Mushroom Sauce**	1½ cups	(242 gm)	1	3	262
Spaghetti with **Clam Sauce**	1½ cups	(210 gm)	4	6	303
Spaghetti with meat sauce	1½ cups	(259 gm)	6	11	356
TUNA DISHES					
Tuna Noodle Casserole	1 cup	(172 gm)	1	2	146
Tuna noodle casserole, typical	1 cup	(240 gm)	5	15	321
OTHER DISHES					
Fettuccine, at Last!	¼ recipe	(205 gm)	2	5	358
Fettuccine Alfredo	¼ recipe	(234 gm)	31	39	573
Sesame Linguini with Chicken	1½ cups	(256 gm)	2	5	311
Baked Spaghetti Pie	⅙ recipe	(160 gm)	2	3	213
Savory Eggplant Pasta Sauce	1 cup	(250 gm)	1	3	131
Pasta with Fresh Tomato Sauce	⅙ recipe	(362 gm)	2	6	397
Turkey Tetrazzini	⅙ recipe	(353 gm)	4	8	422
Poppyseed and Turkey Casserole	¼ recipe	(302 gm)	8	9	344
Calico Pasta	1 cup	(192 gm)	tr.	3	142

The abbreviation *tr.* stands for trace (less than (0.5); the symbol <1 stands for less than one (0.5 to 0.9). Recipes in **bold italics** can be found in Part III.

MAIN ENTRÉES: PIZZAS
(SELECT CSIs OF 9 OR LOWER PER SERVING)

	SERVING SIZE		CSI	FAT (GM)	CALORIES
THIN CRUST PIZZA					
Spicy Cheese Pizza	¼ of 14" pizza	(357 gm)	5	9	390
Green pepper-mushroom-onion	¼ of 14" pizza	(292 gm)	9	14	419
Canadian bacon	¼ of 14" pizza	(229 gm)	10	16	446
Pepperoni	¼ of 14" pizza	(229 gm)	13	23	509
Cheese	¼ of 14" pizza	(257 gm)	16	24	552
Combination	¼ of 14" pizza	(279 gm)	20	38	676
THICK CRUST PIZZA					
Spicy Cheese Pizza	¼ of 14" pizza	(417 gm)	4	7	565
Green pepper-mushroom-onion	¼ of 14" pizza	(360 gm)	6	9	574
Canadian bacon	¼ of 14" pizza	(334 gm)	7	12	611
Pepperoni	¼ of 14" pizza	(334 gm)	10	19	674
Cheese	¼ of 14" pizza	(343 gm)	11	16	664
Combination	¼ of 14" pizza	(384 gm)	17	33	842
Quick-and-Easy Pan Bread Pizza	⅙ of recipe	(251 gm)	2	11	339
Pita Pizza	1 pizza	(149 gm)	3	5	255
Baguette with Vegetable Filling	½ of recipe	(354 gm)	2	10	500
Vegetable Calzone	¼ of recipe	(301 gm)	5	11	437

MAIN ENTRÉES: QUICHES
(SELECT CSIs OF 9 OR LOWER PER SERVING)

Broccoli Quiche	⅙ of 9" quiche	(229 gm)	2	6	189
Broccoli quiche—no egg yolk, 2% fat milk, typical crust	⅙ of 9" quiche	(209 gm)	9	21	327
Broccoli quiche, typical	⅙ of 9" quiche	(209 gm)	30	38	480
Zucchini Pie	3" x 4½"	(145 gm)	5	7	188
Zucchini casserole	3" x 4½"	(330 gm)	17	14	210

MEAT, FISH, AND POULTRY: BEEF, LAMB, PORK, TOFU, TVP, ETC. (COOKED, BONELESS)
(SELECT CSIs OF 9 OR LOWER FOR 3 OUNCES OR 3 OR LOWER FOR 1 OUNCE)

BEEF

Jerky	1 ounce (13" x ⅝" x ¼")	(28 gm)	2	3	53
Chipped beef	3 ounces	(85 gm)	5	5	173
Oxtails	3 ounces	(85 gm)	11	16	246
Brisket (fresh), corned beef, pastrami	3 ounces	(85 gm)	15	26	316
Shank	3 ounces	(85 gm)	15	27	323
Short ribs	3 ounces	(85 gm)	15	27	323
Ground:					
10% fat	3 ounces	(85 gm)	7	7	170

The abbreviation *tr.* stands for trace (less than (0.5); the symbol <1 stands for less than one (0.5 to 0.9). Recipes in **bold italics** can be found in Part III.

MEAT, FISH, AND POULTRY: BEEF, LAMB, PORK, TOFU, TVP, ETC. (continued)

	SERVING SIZE		CSI	FAT (GM)	CALORIES
15% fat (extra lean)	3 ounces	(85 gm)	9	13	215
20% fat (most "fast-food" restaurants)	3 ounces	(85 gm)	11	16	246
25% fat (lean)	3 ounces	(85 gm)	12	20	278
30% fat (typical)	3 ounces	(85 gm)	15	27	323
Roasts:					
Sirloin tip	3 ounces	(85 gm)	9	13	215
Baron of beef	3 ounces	(85 gm)	9	13	215
Heel of round	3 ounces	(85 gm)	9	13	215
Rump	3 ounces	(85 gm)	12	20	278
Blade, chuck, arm	3 ounces	(85 gm)	15	27	323
Tenderloin	3 ounces	(85 gm)	15	27	323
Standing rib	3 ounces	(85 gm)	15	27	323
Steaks:					
Flank	3 ounces	(85 gm)	5	5	161
Round, cube	3 ounces	(85 gm)	9	13	215
Sirloin	3 ounces	(85 gm)	9	13	215
T-bone, rib, New York	3 ounces	(85 gm)	15	27	323
Porterhouse, filet mignon	3 ounces	(85 gm)	15	27	323
Stew meat, lean	3 ounces	(85 gm)	11	16	246
Stew meat, typical	3 ounces	(85 gm)	15	27	323
GAME					
Venison, rabbit, elk, moose, antelope	3 ounces	(85 gm)	5	5	168
Horsemeat	3 ounces	(85 gm)	5	5	133

LAMB

Stew meat, lean	3 ounces	(85 gm)	7	11	189
Chop, rib	3 ounces	(85 gm)	12	17	238
Chop, shoulder	3 ounces	(85 gm)	17	28	323
Ground	3 ounces	(85 gm)	17	28	323
Leg, roast	3 ounces	(85 gm)	10	15	219
Stew meat, typical	3 ounces	(85 gm)	17	28	323

MEAT SUBSTITUTES

Bacon substitute (Morningstar)	1 ounce	(28 gm)	tr.	3	54
Imitation bacon bits	2 tablespoons	(16 gm)	tr.	3	67
Textured vegetable protein, dehydrated	¼ cup	(24 gm)	tr.	tr.	79
Tofu	2½" x 2½" x 1"	(110 gm)	<1	5	79
Sausage substitute (Morningstar)	1 ounce	(28 gm)	1	5	77

ORGAN MEATS

Tripe, beef	3 ounces	(85 gm)	5	4	85
Tongue, beef	3 ounces	(85 gm)	9	16	230
Heart, beef	3 ounces	(85 gm)	13	5	160
Chitterlings	3 ounces	(85 gm)	15	24	258
Liver, calf	3 ounces	(85 gm)	16	4	153
Giblets	3 ounces	(85 gm)	18	4	135
Liver, beef or pork	3 ounces	(85 gm)	22	8	161
Liver, chicken	3 ounces	(85 gm)	28	5	133

The abbreviation *tr.* stands for trace (less than 0.5); the symbol <1 stands for less than one (0.5 to 0.9). Recipes in **bold italics** can be found in Part III.

519

MEAT, FISH, AND POULTRY: BEEF, LAMB, PORK, TOFU, TVP, ETC. (*continued*)

	SERVING SIZE		CSI	FAT (GM)	CALORIES
Sweetbreads, beef	3 ounces	(85 gm)	28	20	272
Kidney, beef or calf	3 ounces	(85 gm)	39	10	214
Brains, all species	3 ounces	(85 gm)	110	8	117
PORK					
Tenderloin	3 ounces	(85 gm)	5	4	141
Ham, prosciutto	3 ounces	(85 gm)	7	13	192
Chops, center cut	3 ounces	(85 gm)	9	15	227
Ham—center cut, shoulder	3 ounces	(85 gm)	9	18	238
Ham hock	3 ounces	(85 gm)	9	18	238
Pickled pig's feet	3 ounces	(85 gm)	9	14	173
Roast, center cut	3 ounces	(85 gm)	9	15	227
Sausage, link	4 links	(80 gm)	12	25	295
Sausage, patty	3 ounces	(85 gm)	13	26	314
Spareribs, regular and country-style	3 ounces	(85 gm)	13	26	309
Salt pork	3 ounces	(85 gm)	25	60	576
Bacon, Canadian	1 ounce (1½ slices)	(28 gm)	2	2	52
Bacon	1 ounce (4 strips)	(28 gm)	6	14	161
VEAL					
Cutlet	3 ounces	(85 gm)	7	6	176
Roast	3 ounces	(85 gm)	8	8	184
Stew Meat	3 ounces	(85 gm)	8	8	180
Ground	3 ounces	(85 gm)	10	14	229

COLD CUTS, BEEF AND PORK

Thin, pressed	6 slices	(28 gm)	1	1	35
Pastrami, corned beef	2 ounces	(57 gm)	5	5	104
Head cheese	2 ounces	(57 gm)	5	9	120
Salami, beef	2 ounces	(57 gm)	7	11	144
Italian sausage	2 ounces	(57 gm)	7	15	184
Knockwurst	2 ounces	(57 gm)	7	16	174
Bologna	2 ounces	(57 gm)	8	16	180
Polish sausage, kielbasa	2 ounces	(57 gm)	8	16	184
Salami, Genoa (hard)	2 ounces	(57 gm)	9	19	230
Liverwurst	2 ounces	(57 gm)	11	16	184
Braunschweiger	2 ounces	(57 gm)	11	18	204

MEAT, FISH, AND POULTRY: FISH AND SHELLFISH (COOKED)
(SELECT CSIs OF 9 OR LOWER FOR 3 OUNCES, OR 3 OR LOWER FOR 1 OUNCE)

FISH

Anchovies, smoked	6 thin fillets	(24 gm)	1	2	50
Herring, pickled	1" x 1" x ½"	(25 gm)	1	5	65
Tuna, canned (water packed)	½ cup	(80 gm)	2	tr.	105
Fish, smoked	3 ounces	(85 gm)	2	4	99

The abbreviation *tr.* stands for trace (less than 0.5); the symbol <1 stands for less than one (0.5 to 0.9). Recipes in **bold italics** can be found in Part III.

521

MEAT, FISH, AND POULTRY: FISH AND SHELLFISH (*continued*)

	SERVING SIZE		CSI	FAT (GM)	CALORIES
Tuna, canned (drained, oil packed)	½ cup	(80 gm)	2	7	158
Salmon, canned	½ cup	(89 gm)	3	5	124
Sashimi (raw tuna)	3 ounces	(85 gm)	3	4	122
White fish (red snapper, halibut, sole, cod etc.)	3 ounces	(85 gm)	3	1	100
Sardines	½ of 3¾-ounce can	(50 gm)	4	6	104
Trout, rainbow	3 ounces	(85 gm)	4	4	128
Salmon, silver (Coho)	3 ounces	(85 gm)	3	6	157
Salmon, Chinook	3 ounces	(85 gm)	7	10	179
Caviar	2 tablespoons	(32 gm)	11	6	81
Squid, octopus	3 ounces	(85 gm)	13	2	103
SHELLFISH*					
Abalone, canned	3 ounces	(85 gm)	2	tr.	68
Scallops	8 one-inch diameter	(80 gm)	2	1	90
Oysters, raw	6 medium	(85 gm)	3	2	61
Clams, canned	½ of 6½-ounce can	(92 gm)	3	2	136
Clams, steamers	25 medium	(85 gm)	3	2	126
Lobster	1½ tails	(85 gm)	3	<1	83
Crabmeat, canned	½ cup	(85 gm)	4	2	87
Oysters, cooked	8 medium	(85 gm)	4	3	81
Crayfish	3 ounces	(85 gm)	8	1	97
Shrimpmeat	⅔ cup	(85 gm)	9	1	84

* Serving size is with shell removed.

MEAT, FISH, AND POULTRY: POULTRY (COOKED)
(SELECT CSIs OF 9 OR LOWER FOR 3 OUNCES, OR 3 OR LOWER FOR 1 OUNCE)

CHICKEN, CORNISH GAME HEN, OR TURKEY

Light meat (no skin)	3 ounces	(85 gm)	4	3	140
Dark meat (no skin)	3 ounces	(85 gm)	6	7	167
Light meat (with skin)	3 ounces	(85 gm)	6	8	178
Dark meat (with skin)	3 ounces	(85 gm)	7	12	201
Chicken or turkey, ground	3 ounces	(85 gm)	5	5	154
Chicken, canned (boneless)	3 ounces	(85 gm)	5	7	140
Pheasant, wild duck	3 ounces	(85 gm)	8	8	181
Goose, domestic (with skin)	3 ounces	(85 gm)	10	19	259
Duck, domestic (with skin)	3 ounces	(85 gm)	12	24	286
Chicken, giblets	3 ounces	(85 gm)	18	4	135

COLD CUTS, TURKEY & CHICKEN

Ham	2 ounces	(57 gm)	3	3	73
Pastrami	2 ounces	(57 gm)	3	4	80
Bologna	2 ounces	(57 gm)	5	8	113
Salami	2 ounces	(57 gm)	5	8	113

FRANKFURTER

Chicken or turkey	1 wiener	(45 gm)	5	8	102

The abbreviation *tr.* stands for trace (less than 0.5); the symbol <1 stands for less than one (0.5 to 0.9). Recipes in **bold italics** can be found in Part III.

523

MILK, CREAM, AND TOPPINGS

	SERVING SIZE		CSI	FAT (GM)	CALORIES
MILK (SELECT CSIs OF 2 OR LOWER PER CUP)					
Milk, skim or powdered nonfat	1 cup	(245 gm)	<1	tr.	85
Buttermilk, 1% fat	1 cup	(245 gm)	2	2	98
Milk, 1% fat	1 cup	(244 gm)	2	3	102
Milk, 2% fat	1 cup	(244 gm)	4	5	122
Milk, chocolate, 2% fat	1 cup	(250 gm)	5	7	194
Milk, whole	1 cup	(244 gm)	7	8	149
Milk, skim (evaporated)	1 cup	(256 gm)	<1	<1	200
Milk, whole (evaporated)	1 cup	(252 gm)	15	19	338
Milk, condensed	1 cup	(306 gm)	22	27	982
Coconut milk	1 cup	(240 gm)	46	51	473
OTHER DAIRY BEVERAGES (SELECT CSIs OF 2 OR LOWER PER CUP)					
Cocoa, skim milk, sugar-free	1 cup	(260 gm)	2	2	68
Cocoa, skim milk (Swiss Miss, from vending machine)	1 cup	(264 gm)	2	2	154
Cocoa, whole milk	1 cup	(263 gm)	8	10	217
Instant Breakfast, all flavors, made with skim milk	1 cup	(285 gm)	1	1	215
Instant Breakfast, all flavors, made with whole milk	1 cup	(279 gm)	7	9	279
Eggnog	1 cup	(246 gm)	tr.	tr.	200
Eggnog, commercial (no alcohol)	1 cup	(254 gm)	16	19	340

YOGURT (SELECT CSIs OF 3 OR LOWER PER CUP)

Plain:

Nonfat	1 cup	(227 gm)	<1	tr.	127
Low-fat	1 cup	(227 gm)	3	4	143
Whole Milk	1 cup	(227 gm)	7	8	141

All flavors:

Nonfat	1 cup	(227 gm)	<1	tr.	200
Low-fat	1 cup	(227 gm)	3	3	250
Whole milk	1 cup	(227 gm)	7	8	275

COTTAGE CHEESE (SELECT CSIs OF 4 OR LOWER PER CUP)

Dry curd	1 cup	(145 gm)	<1	<1	124
Low-fat (1%)	1 cup	(226 gm)	2	2	163
Low-fat (2%)	1 cup	(226 gm)	4	4	204
Regular	1 cup	(210 gm)	8	9	222

CREAM (SELECT CSIs OF 4 OR LOWER PER CUP)

Evaporated skim milk	1 cup	(256 gm)	<1	<1	200
Liquid non-dairy creamers (soybean oil)	1 cup	(240 gm)	4	24	326
Powdered non-dairy creamer	5⅓ tablespoons*	(32 gm)	11	11	175
Half-and-half	1 cup	(242 gm)	22	28	315
Liquid non-dairy creamers (coconut oil)	1 cup	(240 gm)	23	24	326
Whipping cream	1 cup	(239 gm)	60	74	698

* Equivalent to 1 cup liquid coffee creamer.

The abbreviation tr. stands for trace (less than 0.5); the symbol <1 stands for less than one (0.5 to 0.9). Recipes in *bold italics* can be found in Part III.

MILK, CREAM, AND TOPPINGS (continued)

	SERVING SIZE	CSI	FAT (GM)	CALORIES
TOPPINGS (SELECT CSIs OF 2 OR LOWER PER ¼ CUP)				
Yogurt Dessert Sauce				
Low-fat vanilla yogurt	¼ cup (57 gm)	<1	<1	61
Dream Whip	¼ cup (57 gm)	1	1	50
Whipped cream (aerosol can)	¼ cup (20 gm)	2	3	38
Whipped topping (aerosol can)	¼ cup (15 gm)	3	4	39
Cool Whip	¼ cup (18 gm)	3	4	46
Whipped cream, sweetened	¼ cup (19 gm)	4	5	59
Nonfat plain yogurt	¼ cup (32 gm)	8	9	96
Mock Sour Cream	¼ cup (57 gm)	tr.	tr.	32
Sour cream, light (10% fat)	¼ cup (66 gm)	1	1	55
Sour cream (20% fat)	¼ cup (57 gm)	5	6	90
Imitation sour cream (store brands, IMO)	¼ cup (60 gm)	9	12	117
	¼ cup (58 gm)	10	11	120

NUTS AND SEEDS
(SHELLED)

	SERVING SIZE	CSI	FAT (GM)	CALORIES
Chestnuts	½ cup (72 gm)	1	3	269
Poppyseeds	½ cup (67 gm)	3	30	357
Filberts	½ cup (68 gm)	3	43	430

Pecans	½ cup	(54 gm)	3	37	360
Walnuts	½ cup	(50 gm)	3	31	321
Almonds	½ cup	(71 gm)	4	37	418
Pistachios	½ cup	(64 gm)	4	31	369
Sunflower seeds	½ cup	(72 gm)	4	36	410
Sesame seeds	½ cup	(64 gm)	5	35	376
Peanuts	½ cup	(73 gm)	5	36	423
Cashews	½ cup	(65 gm)	6	31	374
Mixed nuts	½ cup	(72 gm)	6	41	444
Pine nuts	½ cup	(60 gm)	6	37	341
Pumpkin seeds	½ cup	(69 gm)	6	32	373
Macadamia	½ cup	(67 gm)	7	49	470
Brazil	½ cup	(70 gm)	11	46	459

POTATO DISHES
(SELECT CSIs OF 2 OR LOWER PER SERVING)

Baked potato, plain	1 potato/1 cup	(156 gm)	<1	<1	170
Potato Puff	1 potato	(215 gm)	1	2	142
Super Stuffed Potato	½ potato	(131 gm)	1	3	113
Cheese-stuffed baked potato	1 potato	(188 gm)	4	10	236
Plank Potatoes	¼ recipe	(187 gm)	<1	4	231

The abbreviation *tr.* stands for trace (less than (0.5); the symbol <1 stands for less than one (0.5 to 0.9). Recipes in *bold italics* can be found in Part III.

POTATO DISHES (continued)

	SERVING SIZE	CSI	FAT (GM)	CALORIES
Skinny "French Fries"	1 cup (163 gm)	<1	4	134
French fries	1 cup (137 gm)	5	17	392
Skinny Hash Browns	1 cup (155 gm)	<1	5	174
Hash browns	1 cup (155 gm)	5	17	375
Homemade Tatertots	1 cup (93 gm)	2	7	192
Tatertots	1 cup (104 gm)	5	11	222
Mashed Potatoes	1 cup (180 gm)	tr.	tr.	111
Mashed potatoes, typical	1 cup (210 gm)	2	9	241
Potato Salad	1 cup (255 gm)	1	4	206
German potato salad	1 cup (188 gm)	2	5	163
Potato salad, typical	1 cup (240 gm)	10	26	392
Scalloped Potatoes	1 cup (314 gm)	<1	2	219
Scalloped potatoes made with skim milk	1 cup (245 gm)	1	6	232
Scalloped potatoes made with whole milk	1 cup (245 gm)	4	9	259
Au gratin potatoes, homemade	1 cup (245 gm)	15	19	322
Holiday Yams	1 potato (198 gm)	tr.	2	287
Candied sweet potatoes	1 potato (206 gm)	6	8	338
Spuds and Onions	1 cup (146 gm)	tr.	2	185
Italian Potatoes	¼ recipe (161 gm)	<1	4	200

528

GREEN SALADS					
Green salad (1 cup, 55 gm) with: low-calorie blue cheese dressing	2 tablespoons	(31 gm)	1	2	30
Blue cheese dressing	2 tablespoons	(30 gm)	3	16	147
Blue cheese dressing	1/4 cup	(59 gm)	6	32	287
Green salad (1 cup, 55 gm) with: low-calorie French dressing	2 tablespoons	(33 gm)	tr.	2	51
Red French Dressing	2 tablespoons	(31 gm)	<1	5	87
Russian Salad Dressing	2 tablespoons	(30 gm)	<1	4	57
French dressing	2 tablespoons	(32 gm)	3	13	140
French dressing	1/4 cup	(63 gm)	6	25	274
Green salad (1 cup, 55 gm) with: low-calorie Italian dressing	2 tablespoons	(30 gm)	1	3	39
Italian dressing	2 tablespoons	(30 gm)	1	8	97
Italian dressing	1/4 cup	(59 gm)	2	16	187
Green salad (1 cup, 55 gm) with: 3 Tbsp. vinegar + 1 Tbsp. olive oil	1/4 cup	(59 gm)	2	14	129
2 Tbsp. vinegar + 2 Tbsp. olive oil	1/4 cup	(57 gm)	4	27	250
Green salad (1 cup, 55 gm) with: *Western Salad Dressing*	2 tablespoons	(29 gm)	tr.	1	31
Ranch dressing (typical restaurant)	2 tablespoons	(30 gm)	2	11	114
Green salad (1 cup, 55 gm) with: *Thousand Island Salad Dressing*	2 tablespoons	(28 gm)	tr.	1	37
low-calorie Thousand Island dressing	2 tablespoons	(31 gm)	1	3	56

The abbreviation *tr.* stands for trace (less than (0.5); the symbol <1 stands for less than one (0.5 to 0.9). Recipes in **bold italics** can be found in Part III.

SALADS (continued)

	SERVING SIZE	CSI	FAT (GM)	CALORIES
Thousand Island dressing	2 tablespoons (30 gm)	2	10	127
Thousand Island dressing	¼ cup (59 gm)	4	20	247
Sunshine Spinach Salad	1 cup (105 gm)	tr.	2	51
Snowbird Salad	1 cup (120 gm)	<1	5	58
Vinaigrette Salad Dressing with Greens	1 cup (61 gm)	tr.	2	31
Caesar salad	1 cup (87 gm)	6	20	207
CHEF-TYPE SALADS				
Crab Louis without egg, with ¼ cup *Thousand Island Salad Dressing*	1 salad (389 gm)	7	7	232
Crab Louis without egg, with ½ cup low-calorie Thousand Island salad dressing	1 salad (455 gm)	8	18	348
Crab Louis with egg, ½ cup low-calorie Thousand Island salad dressing	1 salad (505 gm)	20	24	427
Crab Louis with egg, ½ cup Thousand Island salad dressing	1 salad (501 gm)	26	51	714
Shrimp Louis without egg, with ¼ cup *Thousand Island Salad Dressing*	1 salad (389 gm)	8	7	232
Shrimp Louis without egg, with ½ cup low-calorie Thousand Island salad dressing	1 salad (455 gm)	10	17	364
Shrimp Louis with egg, ½ cup low-calorie Thousand Island salad dressing	1 salad (505 gm)	22	23	443
Shrimp Louis with egg, ½ cup Thousand Island salad dressing	1 salad (501 gm)	28	50	730

Food	Amount	Weight			
Chef's salad without egg, with Cheddar cheese, ham, turkey, ½ cup low-calorie Thousand Island dressing	1 salad	(466 gm)	19	34	545
Chef's salad with egg, with Cheddar cheese, ham, turkey, ½ cup low-calorie Thousand Island salad dressing	1 salad	(516 gm)	31	40	624
Chef's salad with egg, with Cheddar cheese, ham, turkey, ½ cup Thousand Island salad dressing (typical restaurant)	1 salad	(512 gm)	40	67	910

MISCELLANEOUS SALADS

Food	Amount	Weight			
Confetti Appleslaw	1 cup	(105 gm)	tr.	1	55
Orange Yogurt Fruit Slaw	1 cup	(144 gm)	tr.	2	96
Sesame Slaw	1 cup	(114 gm)	tr.	3	91
Sesame slaw, typical	1 cup	(145 gm)	4	30	331
Cole slaw with salad dressing	1 cup	(120 gm)	4	19	201
Cole slaw with mayonnaise	1 cup	(120 gm)	6	29	282
Potato Salad	1 cup	(255 gm)	1	4	206
German potato salad	1 cup	(188 gm)	2	5	163
Potato salad, typical	1 cup	(240 gm)	10	26	392
California Beans	1 cup	(155 gm)	tr.	2	126
Summer Bean Salad	1 cup	(178 gm)	<1	4	199
Spicy Black Bean Salad	1 cup	(170 gm)	<1	4	228
Chili Bean Salad	1 cup	(221 gm)	<1	5	255
Three-bean salad	1 cup	(167 gm)	4	23	287
Curried Chicken with Peanut Salad	1 cup	(123 gm)	2	5	119

The abbreviation *tr.* stands for trace (less than 0.5); the symbol <1 stands for less than one (0.5 to 0.9). Recipes in **bold italics** can be found in Part III.

SALADS (continued)

	SERVING SIZE		CSI	FAT (GM)	CALORIES
Chicken Salad with Yogurt-Chive Dressing	1 cup	(172 gm)	3	3	169
Simply Wonderful Turkey Salad	1 cup	(171 gm)	1	4	156
Chicken salad with mayonnaise	1 cup	(209 gm)	17	64	705
Orange Bulgur Salad	1 cup	(397 gm)	tr.	1	252
Tabouli	1 cup	(220 gm)	1	8	178
Tabouli, typical	1 cup	(219 gm)	3	19	269
Carrot Raisin Salad	1 cup	(136 gm)	<1	2	166
Carrot raisin salad, typical	1 cup	(108 gm)	6	9	152
Waldorf Salad	1 cup	(147 gm)	2	10	196
Waldorf salad, typical	1 cup	(155 gm)	6	36	382
Greek Salad	1 cup	(114 gm)	<1	3	55
Aspic with mayonnaise, crab, asparagus	1 cup	(209 gm)	3	12	162
Absolutely Delicious Molded Salad	1/15 recipe	(185 gm)	tr.	tr.	150
Holiday Wreath Salad	1 cup	(262 gm)	2	5	274
Fruit salad with marshmallows and whipped cream	1 cup	(152 gm)	7	9	180
Crunchy Vegetable Salad	1 cup	(191 gm)	1	5	136
Crunchy vegetable salad, typical	1 cup	(257 gm)	13	47	561
Cheese and pea salad	1 cup	(187 gm)	15	13	247
Moroccan Salad	1 cup	(163 gm)	<1	4	229
Montana Pasta Salad	1 cup	(196 gm)	<1	4	169
Four-Star Pasta Salad	1 cup	(137 gm)	<1	3	154
Alphabet Seafood Salad	1 cup	(181 gm)	2	3	242

Macaroni (with mayonnaise)	1 cup (184 gm)	7	36	510
Salad Athene	1 cup (69 gm)	1	4	103
Salad Athene, typical	1 cup (137 gm)	3	14	195
Crunchy Confetti Salad	1 cup (186 gm)	<1	6	170
Curried Rice and Artichoke Salad	1 cup (250 gm)	<1	3	206
Fruit and Rice Salad	1 cup (155 gm)	tr.	3	169
Lemony Beets	1/6 recipe (58 gm)	<1	5	66
Green Bean, Mushroom, and Tomato Salad	1/8 recipe (109 gm)	1	4	67

SALAD DRESSINGS AND MAYONNAISE

RANCH-TYPE SALAD DRESSINGS (SELECT CSIs OF 3 OR LOWER PER 4 TABLESPOONS/QUARTER CUP)

Ranch with skim milk or buttermilk and nonfat yogurt	4 tablespoons (59 gm)	tr.	tr.	28
Hearty Ranch Salad Dressing	4 tablespoons (62 gm)	<1	3	51
Western Salad Dressing	4 tablespoons (62 gm)	1	3	51
Ranch-type salad dressing (typical)	4 tablespoons (59 gm)	5	23	213
Russian, low-calorie	4 tablespoons (65 gm)	2	3	92
Russian Salad Dressing	4 tablespoons (60 gm)	1	9	100
Russian salad dressing, typical	4 tablespoons (59 gm)	2	12	180
Fresh Ginger Salad Dressing	4 tablespoons (58 gm)	<1	4	76

The abbreviation *tr.* stands for trace (less than 0.5); the symbol <1 stands for less than one (0.5 to 0.9). Recipes in **bold italics** can be found in Part III.

SALADS DRESSINGS AND MAYONNAISE (continued)

	SERVING SIZE		CSI	FAT (GM)	CALORIES
Vinaigrette Salad Dressing	4 tablespoons	(55 gm)	3	21	196
Oil & vinegar salad dressing	4 tablespoons	(62 gm)	6	32	287
French salad dressing, low-calorie	4 tablespoons	(65 gm)	<1	4	87
Red French Salad Dressing	4 tablespoons	(62 gm)	1	8	148
French salad dressing, typical	4 tablespoons	(63 gm)	6	25	267
Thousand Island Salad Dressing	4 tablespoons	(56 gm)	1	3	68
Thousand Island salad dressing, low-calorie	4 tablespoons	(61 gm)	1	7	97
Thousand Island salad dressing, typical	4 tablespoons	(59 gm)	4	20	240
Blue cheese, low-calorie	4 tablespoons	(61 gm)	2	4	46
Roquefort/blue cheese salad dressing, typical	4 tablespoons	(61 gm)	6	32	280
Italian salad dressing, low-calorie	4 tablespoons	(60 gm)	1	6	63
Italian salad dressing, typical	4 tablespoons	(59 gm)	2	16	180

MAYONNAISE AND MIRACLE WHIP (SELECT CSIs OF 12 OR LOWER PER CUP)

	SERVING SIZE		CSI	FAT (GM)	CALORIES
Tangy Salad Dressing	1 cup	(240 gm)	5	11	224
Mayonnaise, Light (Heart Beat)	1 cup	(224 gm)	7	64	640
Miracle Whip, Light Salad Dressing	1 cup	(224 gm)	10	64	720
Mayonnaise, Light (Best Foods, Kraft)	1 cup	(224 gm)	12	80	800
Miracle Whip Salad Dressing, Cholesterol-free	1 cup	(224 gm)	17	112	1,120
Miracle Whip Salad Dressing, Regular	1 cup	(224 gm)	20	112	1,120
Mayonnaise (Best Foods, Kraft, Saffola), Cholesterol-free	1 cup	(224 gm)	26	175	1,584
Mayonnaise (Best Foods, Kraft, Saffola), Regular	1 cup	(224 gm)	33	175	1,584

SANDWICH FILLINGS
(SELECT CSIs OF 4 OR LOWER PER SERVING)

	SERVING SIZE		CSI	FAT (GM)	CALORIES
Chicken salad (with mayonnaise)	½ cup	(104 gm)	8	32	353
CHEDDAR AND JACK-TYPE CHEESES					
Dorman's Light	1 ounce	(28 gm)	<1	5	70
Scandic Mini Chol or Swedish low-fat	1 ounce	(28 gm)	2	9	113
Olympia's Low Fat	1 ounce	(28 gm)	4	5	72
Green River Part Skim	1 ounce	(28 gm)	4	5	72
Heidi Ann Low-Fat Ched-Style Cheese, Kraft Light Naturals Mild Cheddar	1 ounce	(28 gm)	4	5	80
Swiss	1 ounce	(28 gm)	6	8	107
Cheddar, Monterey Jack, Colby, Havarti, Long Horn	1 ounce	(28 gm)	8	9	114
CHEESE SLICES					
Lite-line	1 ounce	(28 gm)	2	2	51
Lite 'n' Lively	1 ounce	(28 gm)	3	4	74
Kraft Light Naturals (Swiss Reduced Fat)	1 ounce	(28 gm)	4	5	90
American	1 ounce	(28 gm)	7	9	106
COLD CUTS, BEEF & PORK					
Thin, pressed	6 slices	(28 gm)	1	1	35
Pastrami, corned beef	2 ounces	(57 gm)	5	5	104
Head cheese	2 ounces	(57 gm)	5	9	120

The abbreviation *tr.* stands for trace (less than 0.5); the symbol <1 stands for less than one (0.5 to 0.9). Recipes in **bold italics** can be found in Part III.

SANDWICH FILLINGS (continued)

	SERVING SIZE		CSI	FAT (GM)	CALORIES
Ham	2 ounces	(57 gm)	6	12	159
Salami, beef	2 ounces	(57 gm)	7	11	144
Italian sausage	2 ounces	(57 gm)	7	15	184
Knockwurst	2 ounces	(57 gm)	7	16	174
Bologna	2 ounces	(57 gm)	8	16	180
Polish sausage, kielbasa	2 ounces	(57 gm)	8	16	184
Salami, Genoa (hard)	2 ounces	(57 gm)	9	19	230
Liverwurst	2 ounces	(57 gm)	11	16	184
Braunschweiger	2 ounces	(57 gm)	11	18	204
COLD CUTS, TURKEY & CHICKEN					
Ham	2 ounces	(57 gm)	3	3	73
Pastrami	2 ounces	(57 gm)	3	4	80
Bologna	2 ounces	(57 gm)	5	8	113
Salami	2 ounces	(57 gm)	5	8	113
Thin, pressed lunch meats (meat/poultry)	2 slices	(9 gm)	tr.	tr.	12
CHEESE-TYPE SPREADS					
Fruit-Nut Sandwich Spread	¼ cup	(52 gm)	1	4	81
Vegetable-Cottage Cheese Sandwich Spread	¼ cup	(42 gm)	<1	<1	34
Reduced Calories Laughing Cow Cheese	1 ounce	(28 gm)	2	3	113
Denver (egg, ham, green pepper)	1 egg	(84 gm)	15	13	165
"Egg" Salad Sandwich Spread	½ cup	(105 gm)	<1	5	110
Tofu "Egg" Salad Sandwich Spread	½ cup	(75 gm)	<1	5	66

Egg salad (with mayonnaise)	½ cup	(111 gm)	24	23	252
FRANKFURTERS					
Chicken or turkey	1 wiener	(45 gm)	5	8	102
Beef	1 wiener	(45 gm)	7	13	145
Corn Dog or Pronto Pup	One	(111 gm)	13	28	344
Hamburger patty (10% fat)	3 ounces	(85 gm)	7	7	170
Hamburger patty (15% fat)	3 ounces	(85 gm)	9	13	215
Hamburger patty (20% fat)	3 ounces	(85 gm)	11	16	246
Hamburger patty (25% fat)	3 ounces	(85 gm)	12	20	278
Ham, baked	2 ounces	(57 gm)	6	12	159
Ham salad	½ cup	(124 gm)	8	28	338
Peanut butter	2 tablespoons	(32 gm)	3	17	190
Roast beef	2 ounces	(57 gm)	6	9	144
Roast turkey (white meat)	2 ounces	(57 gm)	3	2	94
Spam	2 slices (¼")	(85 gm)	12	26	284
SPREADABLES					
Chicken or turkey	½ cup	(104 gm)	5	14	208
Beef or ham	½ cup	(120 gm)	9	20	271
Ham & cheese	½ cup	(120 gm)	14	22	294
Tuna Salad Sandwich Spread	½ cup	(108 gm)	3	2	111
Tuna salad (with light mayonnaise)	½ cup	(102 gm)	4	15	196
Tuna salad (with mayonnaise)	½ cup	(98 gm)	5	25	272

The abbreviation *tr.* stands for trace (less than 0.5); the symbol <1 stands for less than one (0.5 to 0.9). Recipes in **bold italics** can be found in Part III.

SANDWICH FILLINGS (continued)

	SERVING SIZE		CSI	FAT (GM)	CALORIES
VEGETABLE SANDWICH FILLINGS					
California Beans	½ cup	(78 gm)	tr.	1	63
Spicy Black Bean Salad	½ cup	(85 gm)	tr.	2	114
Falafel	¼ recipe	(79 gm)	tr.	2	124
Chili Bean Salad	½ cup	(111 gm)	<1	3	128
Southern Caviar	½ cup	(104 gm)	<1	3	136
Chowchow	½ cup	(106 gm)	<1	5	94
Refried Beans	½ cup	(87 gm)	<1	3	113
Refried beans (canned)	½ cup	(121 gm)	<1	2	124
Refried beans (typical restaurant)	½ cup	(122 gm)	6	14	243

SPREADS (SELECT CSIs OF 1.0 OR LOWER)

Mustard, prepared	1 tablespoon	(15 gm)	tr.	<1	11
Horseradish	1 tablespoon	(15 gm)	0	tr.	6
Cranberry sauce	1 tablespoon	(17 gm)	0	tr.	30
Ketchup	1 tablespoon	(17 gm)	tr.	tr.	18
Mayonnaise, light	1 tablespoon	(14 gm)	0.8	5	50
Margarine, soft	1 tablespoon	(14 gm)	2.1	11	101
Mayonnaise, typical	1 tablespoon	(14 gm)	2.1	11	101
Butter	1 tablespoon	(14 gm)	9.3	12	102
Jelly, typical	1 tablespoon	(14 gm)	tr.	tr.	55
Jelly, low-sugar	1 tablespoon	(14 gm)	0	0	28

SANDWICHES AND PIZZA
(SELECT CSIs OF 5 OR LOWER PER SERVING)

Baked Bean Special Sandwich	¼ recipe	(280 gm)	<1	3	374
HAMBURGERS					
Very Skinny Burgers	One	(156 gm)	5	10	288
Skinny Burgers	One	(212 gm)	8	15	375
Hamburger, typical	One	(236 gm)	25	50	763
Ham-and-cheese croissant sandwich	One	(196 gm)	35	64	756
BURRITOS (NOT DEEP-FRIED)					
Burritos with Black Beans	One	(217 gm)	2	4	242
Your Basic Bean Burrito	One 8"	(202 gm)	2	5	269
Bean burrito	One 8"	(161 gm)	7	16	384
Beef burrito	One 8"	(125 gm)	9	16	353
THIN CRUST PIZZA					
Spicy Cheese Pizza	¼ of 14" pizza	(357 gm)	5	9	390
Green pepper-mushroom-onion	¼ of 14" pizza	(292 gm)	9	14	419
Canadian bacon	¼ of 14" pizza	(229 gm)	10	16	446
Pepperoni	¼ of 14" pizza	(229 gm)	13	23	509
Cheese	¼ of 14" pizza	(257 gm)	16	24	552
Combination	¼ of 14" pizza	(279 gm)	20	38	676

The abbreviation tr. stands for trace (less than (0.5); the symbol <1 stands for less than one (0.5 to 0.9). Recipes in **bold italics** can be found in Part III.

SANDWICHES AND PIZZA (continued)

	SERVING SIZE		CSI	FAT (GM)	CALORIES
THICK CRUST PIZZA					
Spicy Cheese Pizza	¼ of 14" pizza	(417 gm)	4	7	565
Green pepper-mushroom-onion	¼ of 14" pizza	(360 gm)	6	9	574
Canadian bacon	¼ of 14" pizza	(334 gm)	7	12	611
Pepperoni	¼ of 14" pizza	(334 gm)	10	19	674
Cheese	¼ of 14" pizza	(343 gm)	11	16	664
Combination	¼ of 14" pizza	(384 gm)	17	33	842
Quick-and-Easy Pan Bread Pizza	⅙ of recipe	(251 gm)	2	11	339
Pita Pizza	1 pizza	(149 gm)	3	5	255
Veggie Pockets with Creamy Dressing	2 small pockets or 1 large pocket	(186 gm)	<1	3	234

SAUCES AND GRAVIES
(SELECT CSIs OF 2 OR LOWER PER SERVING)

Basic White Sauce (made with skim milk)	¼ cup	(59 gm)	<1	3	47
White sauce (made with whole milk)	¼ cup	(63 gm)	3	8	101
Cheese sauce, low-fat	¼ cup	(53 gm)	1	3	51
Cheese sauce	¼ cup	(63 gm)	6	11	133
Mock Hollandaise Sauce	¼ cup	(67 gm)	2	7	90
Hollandaise, canned or from a mix	¼ cup	(64 gm)	13	17	176
Hollandaise or Bearnaise, homemade	¼ cup	(65 gm)	16	27	250

Turkey Gravy	¼ cup	(68 gm)	tr.	2	32
Turkey gravy	¼ cup	(65 gm)	1	2	28
Au jus	¼ cup	(63 gm)	tr.	tr.	10
Cream gravy for chicken made with skim milk	¼ cup	(60 gm)	<1	2	39
Cream gravy for chicken made with whole milk	¼ cup	(60 gm)	2	4	55
Tartar Sauce	¼ cup	(47 gm)	<1	<1	40
Tartar sauce, typical	¼ cup	(58 gm)	6	33	305
Cranberry sauce	¼ cup	(68 gm)	0	tr.	103
Baked Cranberry-Nut Relish	¼ cup	(70 gm)	tr.	2	152
Sweet & sour sauce	¼ cup	(78 gm)	0	0	73
Barbecue sauce (bottled)	¼ cup	(63 gm)	tr.	2	70
Marinara Sauce	¼ cup	(86 gm)	tr.	1	29
Italian sauce (meatless)	¼ cup	(60 gm)	tr.	2	42
Italian sauce (with meat)	¼ cup	(64 gm)	3	5	82
Onion Chutney	¼ cup	(53 gm)	tr.	tr.	112
Homemade Enchilada Sauce	¼ cup	(62 gm)	tr.	tr.	14
Cucumber-Dilly Sauce	¼ cup	(60 gm)	tr.	<1	30
Cucumber-dilly sauce, typical	¼ cup	(60 gm)	3	6	64

The abbreviation *tr.* stands for trace (less than 0.5); the symbol <1 stands for less than one (0.5 to 0.9). Recipes in **bold italics** can be found in Part III.

SOUPS
(SELECT CSIs OF 3 OR LOWER PER SERVING)

	SERVING SIZE		CSI	FAT (GM)	CALORIES
BEAN SOUPS					
Greek Lentil	1 cup	(255 gm)	tr.	1	149
Greek-Style Garbanzo	1 cup	(217 gm)	tr.	4	156
Navy Bean	1 cup	(163 gm)	tr.	<1	79
Split Pea	1 cup	(240 gm)	tr.	1	106
Lentil	1 cup	(238 gm)	<1	4	145
Split pea, lentil, etc.	1 cup	(250 gm)	2	6	170
Beer-cheese soup	1 cup	(251 gm)	14	23	308
Broth, beef, diluted	1 cup	(243 gm)	0	0	29
Broth, chicken, diluted	1 cup	(243 gm)	tr.	1	39
Black Bean Chili	1 cup	(244 gm)	<1	4	277
Rick's Chili	1 cup	(215 gm)	<1	3	126
Chicken chili with beans	1 cup	(213 gm)	1	4	190
Rose Bowl Chili	1 cup	(267 gm)	2	5	213
Chili con carne with beans	1 cup	(255 gm)	8	14	282
Chili con carne without beans	1 cup	(255 gm)	11	18	282
Creamy Chicken Noodle Soup	1 cup	(250 gm)	3	3	185
Chicken noodle soup	1 cup	(240 gm)	3	5	170
Clam chowder (tomato base)	1 cup	(251 gm)	1	4	153

Food	Amount				
Clam chowder (New England style) diluted with skim milk	1 cup	(245 gm)	1	3	131
Clam chowder (New England style) diluted with whole milk	1 cup	(244 gm)	4	7	162
Consommé	1 cup	(243 gm)	0	0	29
CREAM SOUPS					
Potato Leek	1 cup	(212 gm)	tr.	1	61
Potato	1 cup	(248 gm)	3	10	169
Mushroom, diluted with skim milk	1 cup	(248 gm)	3	10	173
Mushroom, diluted with whole milk	1 cup	(248 gm)	6	14	204
Broccoli	1 cup	(299 gm)	14	18	230
Egg drop soup	1 cup	(268 gm)	8	4	79
French Onion Soup with bread and low-fat cheese	1 cup	(183 gm)	2	4	109
French onion soup with bread and regular cheese	1 cup	(284 gm)	4	6	212
Gazpacho	1 cup	(267 gm)	1	6	99
Gazpacho, typical	1 cup	(255 gm)	3	17	188
Hearty Fish Soup	1 cup	(228 gm)	2	3	106
Hot and Sour Soup	1 cup	(227 gm)	<1	3	68
Hot and Sour Soup, typical	1 cup	(238 gm)	5	6	124
Minestrone	1 cup	(231 gm)	tr.	2	81
Minestrone, typical	1 cup	(244 gm)	1	3	83
Mock turtle soup	1 cup	(244 gm)	34	16	247

The abbreviation *tr.* stands for trace (less than (0.5); the symbol <1 stands for less than one (0.5 to 0.9). Recipes in **bold italics** can be found in Part III.

SOUPS (continued)

	SERVING SIZE		CSI	FAT (GM)	CALORIES
Oyster stew made with skim milk	1 cup	(245 gm)	3	9	162
Oyster stew made with whole milk	1 cup	(240 gm)	9	16	234
Tomato Soup	1 cup	(117 gm)	tr.	tr.	55
Tomato soup (canned) diluted with skim milk	1 cup	(248 gm)	1	2	128
Tomato soup (canned), diluted with whole milk	1 cup	(248 gm)	4	6	160
Top Raamen	1 cup	(227 gm)	2	8	161
Turkey-Vegetable Chowder	1 cup	(209 gm)	2	3	140
Fish and Leek Chowder	1 cup	(240 gm)	2	2	142
Turtle soup	1 cup	(248 gm)	2	4	92
Moroccan Vegetable Stew	1 cup	(193 gm)	tr.	2	81
Vegetable Beef Soup	1 cup	(257 gm)	1	2	80
Vegetable beef soup (canned)	1 cup	(240 gm)	3	5	170
Mulligatawny Stew	1 cup	(244 gm)	3	5	174
Hungarian Mushroom Soup	1 cup	(255 gm)	<1	3	116
Hungarian mushroom soup, typical	1 cup	(300 gm)	12	16	212

SOUPS FOR CASSEROLES, ETC.

	SERVING SIZE		CSI	FAT (GM)	CALORIES
Homemade Cream Soup Mix	Equivalent of 1 can	(230 gm)	<1	1	131
Cream of celery (condensed, undiluted)	1 can	(305 gm)	5	14	220
Cream of chicken (condensed, undiluted)	1 can	(305 gm)	6	18	284
Cream of mushroom (condensed, undiluted)	1 can	(305 gm)	6	23	314

544

VEGETABLE AND GRAIN DISHES
(SELECT CSIs OF 2 OR LOWER PER SERVING)

Corn Bake	1 cup	(154 gm)	tr.	<1	118
Onion Squares	3" x 3"	(93 gm)	1	5	140
Corn pudding	1 cup	(255 gm)	13	14	280
Calico Pasta	1 cup	(192 gm)	tr.	3	142
Bulgur Pilaf	1 cup	(218 gm)	tr.	3	209
Spicy Peanut Noodles	1 cup	(148 gm)	<1	4	223
Mushroom Barley Pilaf	1 cup	(217 gm)	<1	3	262
Rice pilaf	1 cup	(220 gm)	4	16	365
Barley pilaf	1 cup	(238 gm)	8	13	290
Spanish Rice	1 cup	(219 gm)	tr.	3	149
Spanish rice, typical	1 cup	(245 gm)	<1	3	195
Lemon Rice	1 cup	(167 gm)	tr.	<1	221
Pine Needle Rice	1 cup	(245 gm)	<1	5	318
Gourmet Curried Rice	¼ recipe	(139 gm)	1	4	212
Spinach and Rice Casserole	3" x 4½"	(191 gm)	2	4	174
Broccoli with Rice	1 cup	(182 gm)	2	5	157
Green Rice	1 cup	(130 gm)	3	5	169
Green rice, typical	1 cup	(200 gm)	15	16	299
Eggplant Parmesan	1 cup	(290 gm)	2	6	124
Eggplant Parmesan, typical	1 cup	(209 gm)	10	24	344

The abbreviation *tr.* stands for trace (less than (0.5); the symbol <1 stands for less than one (0.5 to 0.9). Recipes in ***bold italics*** can be found in Part III.

VEGETABLE AND GRAIN DISHES (continued)

	SERVING SIZE		CSI	FAT (GM)	CALORIES
Rancher's Beans	1 cup	(238 gm)	tr.	<1	342
Classic Baked Beans	1 cup	(190 gm)	tr.	2	230
Baked beans with ham	1 cup	(256 gm)	5	12	384
Tomatoes "Provençale"	1 tomato	(197 gm)	tr.	3	73
Ratatouille Provençale	⅛ recipe	(237 gm)	<1	2	72
Stuffed Zucchini Boats	1 boat	(168 gm)	1	4	66
Fettuccine, at Last!	¼ recipe	(205 gm)	2	5	358
Fettuccine Alfredo	¼ recipe	(234 gm)	31	39	573
Vegetable Pulav	2 cups	(349 gm)	1	6	389
Pulihora (Tamarind Rice)	1 cup	(142 gm)	<1	5	264
Spicy Lentils	1 cup	(201 gm)	<1	4	137
Oriental Broccoli	1 cup	(105 gm)	tr.	2	70
Easy Acorn Squash	¼ recipe	(275 gm)	tr.	2	101
Grilled Zucchini	¼ recipe	(200 gm)	tr.	1	32
Lemony Beets	⅙ recipe	(58 gm)	<1	5	66
Acorn Squash with Roasted Onions	⅛ recipe	(315 gm)	<1	3	135
Stir-Fried Mushrooms and Broccoli	⅛ recipe	(101 gm)	<1	3	69
Cheesy Cauliflower	¼ recipe	(167 gm)	2	3	76
Zucchini Puff	¼ recipe	(76 gm)	3	4	93

VEGETABLES
(SELECT CSIs OF 1 OR LOWER PER SERVING)

Vegetables (carrots, celery, green beans, tomatoes, broccoli, cauliflower, etc.) cooked	½ cup	(93 gm)	tr.	tr.	25
raw	1 cup	(123 gm)	tr.	tr.	25
Vegetables (peas, corn, potatoes, winter squash, hominy, etc.)	½ cup	(80 gm)	tr.	tr.	65
Leafy vegetables (lettuce, spinach, etc.), raw	1 cup	(55 gm)	tr.	tr.	10

The abbreviation *tr.* stands for trace (less than (0.5); the symbol <1 stands for less than one (0.5 to 0.9). Recipes in **bold italics** can be found in Part III.

547

GENERAL INDEX

RECIPE INDEX

(Page numbers in **boldface** refer to listings in "CSI Table of Foods.")